Family Therapy Sourcebook

Family Therapy Sourcebook

Second Edition

FRED P. PIERCY
DOUGLAS H. SPRENKLE
JOSEPH L. WETCHLER
and ASSOCIATES

Foreword by William J. Doherty

THE GUILFORD PRESS
New York   London

©1996 The Guilford Press
A Division of Guilford Publications, Inc.
72 Spring Street, New York, NY 10012
Printed in the United States of America

This book is printed on acid-free paper.

Last digit is print number: 9 8 7 6 5 4 3 2 1

Library of Congress Cataloging-in-Publication Data

Piercy, Fred P.
Family therapy sourcebook / Fred P. Piercy, Douglas H. Sprenkle
Joseph L. Wetchler, and associates. — 2nd ed.
p. cm.
Includes bibliographical references and index.
ISBN 1-57230-150-3. — ISBN 1-57230-151-1 (pbk.)
1. Family psychotherapy. I. Sprenkle, Douglas H.   II. Wetchler,
Joseph L. III. Title.
RC488.5.P54 1996   96-34673
616.89′156—dc20
                                                              CIP

Contributors

PRINCIPAL AUTHORS

Fred P. Piercy, Ph.D., Professor and Director, Marriage and Family Therapy Program, Department of Child Development and Family Studies, Purdue University, West Lafayette, Indiana

Douglas H. Sprenkle, Ph.D., Professor, Marriage and Family Therapy Program, Department of Child Development and Family Studies, Purdue University, West Lafayette, Indiana

Joseph L. Wetchler, Ph.D., Associate Professor and Director, Marriage and Family Therapy Program, Department of Behavioral Sciences, Purdue University Calumet, Hammond, Indiana

ASSOCIATES

Judith Myers Avis, Ph.D., Professor, Marriage and Family Therapy Program, Department of Family Studies, University of Guelph, Guelph, Ontario, Canada.

Derek Ball, M.S., Doctoral Student, Marriage and Family Therapy Program, Department of Child Development and Family Studies, Purdue University, West Lafayette, Indiana

Gary Bischof, M.S., Doctoral Student, Marriage and Family Therapy Program, Department of Child Development and Family Studies, Purdue University, West Lafayette, Indiana

James E. Burg, Ph.D., Clinic Coordinator, Marriage and Family Therapy

Program, Department of Child Development and Family Studies, Purdue University, West Lafayette, Indiana

Young Hee Chang, M.S., Doctoral Student, Marriage and Family Therapy Program, Department of Child Development and Family Studies, Purdue University, West Lafayette, Indiana

Pilar Gonzalez-Doupé, M.S., Doctoral Student, Marriage and Family Therapy Program, Department of Child Development and Family Studies, Purdue University, West Lafayette, Indiana

Lisa Aronson Fontes, Ph.D., Visiting Professor, Department of Counseling, University of Massachusetts, Amherst, MA

Jerry E. Gale, Ph.D., Associate Professor and Clinical Director, Marriage and Family Therapy Program, Department of Child and Family Development, University of Georgia, Athens, Georgia

Lorna L. Hecker, Ph.D., Associate Professor and Clinic Director, Marriage and Family Therapy Program, Department of Behavioral Sciences, Purdue University Calumet, Hammond, Indiana

Janie K. Long, Ph.D., Assistant Professor and Director of Clinical Training, Marriage and Family Therapy Program, Department of Child and Family Development, University of Georgia, Athens, Georgia

Volker Thomas, Ph.D., Assistant Professor, Marriage and Family Therapy Program, Department of Child Development and Family Studies, Purdue University, West Lafayette, Indiana

Susan G. Wilkie, M.S., Doctoral Student, Marriage and Family Therapy Program, Department of Child Development and Family Studies, Purdue University, West Lafayette, Indiana

Acknowledgments

No man is an island entire of itself; every man is a piece of the continent, a part of the main . . .

—JOHN DONNE

I get by with a little help from my friends.

—JOHN LENNON & PAUL MCCARTNEY

FROM JOHN DONNE to the Beatles, the message remains the same—no achievement is accomplished in isolation. We exist as parts of an interactional system. As with the first edition of this sourcebook, we again wish to emphasize the collaborative nature of this endeavor. We are indebted not only to the pioneers of family therapy, but to those newer voices who continue to shape the future of our field. We also give thanks to those closest to us who both thrilled and humbled us with their patience and support.

We are particularly indebted to our contributors, Judith Myers Avis, Derek Ball, James Burg, Gary Bischof, Young Hee Chang, Pilar Gonzalez-Doupé, Lisa Aronson Fontes, Jerry Gale, Lorna Hecker, Janie Long, Volker Thomas, and Susan Wilkie for their own contributions to this volume. Their expertise provided a broader perspective consistent with the expansion in our field. Similarly, we thank our students, Tom Carlson and Stacy Hernandez, who conducted massive literature searches to insure that our chapters remained up to date, and Mary Bartram, Maria Bermudez, Mary Dankoski, Julie Hawley, Walter Lowe, Travis Nelson, Gail Ofte-Atha, Tim Ozechowski, David Schmidt, Kate Sori, and Mark Wester who helped write new annotated citations and provided some of the teaching activities for this edition. We also have not forgotten all those that helped with the first edition, the shoulders upon which this second edition was built. We wish to acknowledge the support of Seymour Weingarten of The Guilford Press for knowing when to reign us in and when to let us run. We also thank the School of Liberal Arts and Sciences of Purdue University Calumet for providing partial funding for the completion of this sourcebook. As no endeavor of this kind can be accomplished without excellent clerical support, we thank Pat Geiger and Laura Weiss for their untiring patience with all of our "small requests." Finally, we again wish to offer our sincerest thanks to our parents and immediate family members, Susan, David, Stephen, Char, Mark, Rob, Jay, Chris, Christie, and Jessica for their love, understanding, and so much more.

FRED P. PIERCY, PH.D.
DOUGLAS H. SPRENKLE, PH.D.
JOSEPH L. WETCHLER, PH.D.

Foreword

IN 1986, AFTER YEARS of teaching basic family systems skills to family physicians, I faced the new challenge of teaching family therapy to actual family therapy students. To my good fortune, the first edition of *Family Therapy Sourcebook* was published that same year. The book quickly became my guide and commentary on the family therapy field, a source of lecture notes, a wellspring of teaching ideas, a compendium of up-to-date references. It was the book I wished had been on my desk when I was a family therapy student.

As the years went by and I grew more experienced as a family therapy teacher, and as the field matured beyond where it was in the mid-1980s, I grew less dependent on the *Family Therapy Sourcebook*. But now the second edition arrives to threaten my hard won independence from the irresistible clarity, thoroughness, and educational creativity of Fred Piercy, Doug Sprenkle, Joe Wetchler, and their Purdue associates. They have once again crystallized the field into one highly accessible and practical volume.

How does the second edition of the *Family Therapy Sourcebook* fit into the huge library of books on family therapy? I can describe its unique place with a sports analogy—the "point guard" on a basketball team. The point guard is frequently not the star of the team, not its leading scorer or rebounder. But the point guard stitches together the elements of the team by knowing where to pass the ball, how to balance everyone's contributions, and how to set the pace for the offense. The point guard is almost always the "assist" leader, the player who makes the others look good by passing them the ball when they are in the best position to score.

In the same way, the *Family Therapy Sourcebook* weaves together the elements of family therapy theory and practice in the late 1990s. The authors give us a tour through the history of the field and describe with clarity and brevity the most influential models and areas of emphasis. They update the first edition's highly valuable clinical video recommendations and key books, chapters, and articles. Of particular use for family therapy teachers and trainers are the teaching tools and research examples that accompany every chapter. While other books offer more depth in particular areas, no book in the field matches this eclectic combination of clinical substance, teaching tools and strategies, and research suggestions.

A new edition of a sourcebook marks the emergence of new ideas and practices in a field. The second edition of the *Family Therapy Sourcebook* highlights the advances made by feminist family therapists over the past decade, along with the field's greater sensitivity to cultural issues, medical problems, and sexual abuse. In addition, the advent of postmodern thinking in the field, in particular through narrative therapies, is documented in a number of chapters.

This book is the ideal companion to primary texts in a wide range of family therapy courses, to be read alongside original sources. It will help family therapy students make sense of their studies, it will help practicing therapists keep up with their field, and it will serve as the best single reference book for those studying for the marriage and family therapy licensing examination. As for teachers of family therapy—both experienced teachers and novices (as I was ten years ago)—the second edition of the *Family Therapy Sourcebook* is golden. It updates and expands the best work of a premier teaching group in our field.

WILLIAM J. DOHERTY, PH.D.

Preface

THE FAMILY THERAPY field has grown exponentially since the last edition of the *Sourcebook*. It has also moved toward the center a bit. Who would have thought that family therapy, with its rebel beginnings, would become part of the mainstream? But it has. Virtually all graduate programs in the helping professions offer some family therapy coursework, and graduate family therapy programs are springing up across the nation and around the world.

With this growth has come new theories, techniques, and studies. Social, political, and health-related issues have challenged family therapists to expand their beliefs about clinical practice. As we have become more responsible, some of our cutting-edge ideas have lost their luster. Others sparkle like a diamond.

The second edition of the *Sourcebook* both looks forward to what is new, and backward to our core, foundational ideas. For example, we have added three new chapters to cover social constructionist family therapies, culture and family therapy, and specific problem topics such as AIDS, substance abuse, sexual abuse, and family systems medicine. The "Other Family Therapies" chapter now includes sections on psychoanalytic family therapies, psychoeducation, and internal family systems therapy. We have expanded the feminist family therapy chapter from the first edition to also cover the social construction of gender. Similarly, the original cybernetic foundations chapter now provides a broader view of the historical foundations that influence our field. Finally, we have updated all of the remaining chapters to reflect the growth within each theory or topic.

The *Sourcebook* presents one way of organizing family therapy, but clearly not the only way. While we have attempted to keep our biases in check, we caution readers that none of our categorizations are written in stone.

Similarly, the *Sourcebook* cannot be all things to all people. That is, it is not an exhaustive survey of the field, but remains a useful guidebook for readers wanting to learn more about family therapy. Each chapter contains a brief theoretical overview highlighting key concepts and clinical techniques and an annotated bibliography of the major publications in that area. Family therapy trainers will find a section on teaching exercises for use with their classes while students and researchers can use the "research issues" sections for ideas in developing theses and research projects. While some readers will undoubtedly find us guilty of both sins of omission and commission, our intention is to provide a balanced view of each topic.

We hope that family therapists, students, and teachers will find the *Sourcebook* a useful guide for their continued professional journey. May your ongoing growth be personally rewarding and continue to impact the development of this important field.

Contents

1

Theoretical Foundations of Family Therapy

JERRY E. GALE

JANIE K. LONG

HISTORICAL CONTEXT

Theory development is embedded in and shaped by social and historical contexts. For example, events of culture, economics, politics, gender, race, and family dynamics all influence the evolution of ideas. It is beyond the scope of this chapter to adequately present all the cultural and historical features that have helped to shape the foundations of family therapy. We encourage the reader to read widely on this fascinating subject (cf. Anderson & Goolishian, 1988, 1992; Bateson, 1972, 1991; Broderick & Schrader, 1981; Guerin, 1976; Lipset, 1980; Nichols & Everett, 1986).

Broderick and Schrader (1981), Nichols (1992), and Nichols and Everett (1986), among others, note that marital and family therapy independently emerged in many locations in the 1950s. Therapists began writing about a paradigmatic shift of understanding human interaction in a number of different disciplines and movements. These disciplines included (but are not limited to) social work, child guidance, social psychiatry, sexology, family life education, sociology, and marriage counseling. Up through the 1950s, psychotherapy as a practice was dominated by and limited to physicians practicing the psychoanalytic model. World War II led to a need for assessment and brief but effective clinical approaches, and opened the door to other disciplines. Following World War II, researchers and clinicians of

1

these other disciplines dealt with these problems that helped coalesce the marriage and family therapy movement. These problems related to marital relationships, child behavior problems, and schizophrenia (W. C. Nichols, personal communication, October 27, 1992).

Today, individuals from many disciplines practice family therapy and thus continue to debate theory, the definition of marriage and family therapy, and who represents the field professionally (Anderson, 1994; Hardy, 1994; Shields, Wynne, McDaniel, & Gawinski, 1994). Whereas other chapters of this book present various models of family therapy, this chapter includes the various threads of ideas and people that have contributed to the weave of the family therapy tapestry,[1] key concepts,[2] and a brief summary of key books and articles.

THEORETICAL OVERVIEW (MAJOR IDEAS AND THEORISTS)

The 1950s is the founding decade of family therapy (Guerin, 1976). In this decade, we see the initial contributions of Gregory Bateson, Don Jackson, John Weakland, Jay Haley, and Virginia Satir in Palo Alto; Murray Bowen in Topeka (and later Washington, D.C.); Lyman Wynne and Margaret Singer in Bethesda; Nathan Ackerman in New York; Theodore and Ruth Lidz in Baltimore; Carl Whitaker in Atlanta; R. D. Laing in Great Britain; Ivan Boszormenyi-Nagy, James Framo, and Gerald Zuk in Philadelphia; and Milton Erickson in Phoenix.[3] What follows are some of the major concepts, models, and people that helped lay the theoretical groundwork of the field of family therapy.

CYBERNETICS

In 1942, the Josiah Macy Foundation funded a meeting in New York City that brought together researchers and theorists (including Norbert Wiener, John Von Newmann, Warren Pitts, Arturo Rosenblueth, Julian Bigelow, Warren McCulloch, Gregory Bateson, and Margaret Mead) from many disciplines to discuss the "field of control and communication, whether in

---

[1] In discussing the various schools of therapy, it is important to note that these models are not static and unchanging. Each school has evolved and changed over time. In the descriptions that follow, we are trying to acknowledge only the major assumptions of the various therapeutic schools.

[2] Words in **bold type** are defined in the "Key Concepts" section.

[3] This list is not meant to be exhaustive. Many others have also contributed to the development of the field.

the machine or in the animal" (Wiener, 1948/1961, p. 11). Heims (1977) suggested that this meeting resulted in "a new paradigm of science" one in which "theory would clearly involve the ideas of **information, control and feedback**" (p. 143).

This new paradigm, which Wiener (1948/1961) named cybernetics, had an influential impact on the social sciences. As Keeney (1983) notes, it was Gregory Bateson, an anthropologist, who circulated these ideas back to the marriage and family therapy field. In 1951, Bateson and the psychiatrist Juergen Ruesch wrote the book, *Communication: The Social Matrix of Psychiatry,* which highlighted the importance of feedback and information in communication, and defined all human communication as being simultaneously a **report** and **command.** In 1952, funded by a Rockefeller Foundation grant to study paradox in communication, Bateson invited Jay Haley and John Weakland (and later Don Jackson and William Fry) to work with him in Palo Alto. A subsequent study focused exclusively on schizophrenic communication and produced a landmark article, "Toward a Theory of Schizophrenia" (Bateson, Jackson, Haley, & Weakland, 1956), that introduced the notion of **logical levels** (the **double bind theory**) and led to the assumption of **symptom functionality.** Jackson's (1957) concept of family **homeostasis** further influenced theory development in the field.

GENERAL SYSTEM THEORY

Ludwig von Bertalanffy first wrote of the organism as an open system in the late 1920s. What began as a biological theory later expanded into a general theory with interdisciplinary applications (von Bertalanffy, 1968). General system theory was not an isolated development. Numerous scientists had followed similar lines of thinking in cybernetics, information theory, game theory, decision theory, and factor analysis (von Bertalanffy, 1962). Unlike the conventional categories of physics, von Bertalanffy (1967) developed his theory to offer a comprehensive model that included all living systems and was relevant to all behavioral and social sciences. Von Bertalanffy proposed that the living organism was an open system, characterized by the flow of information in and out of the system. Living systems experience continuous change as they advance toward higher levels of organization and wholeness. He described a system as "a complex of component parts that are in mutual interaction and focus on the relationships between the parts rather than on how the parts contribute to the whole (von Bertalanffy, 1968). Other systems theorists included Walter Buckley (1968), who highlighted the interconnectedness and mutual causality of each part of a system, and Magoroh Maruyama (1968), who introduced the terms **morphogenesis** and **morphostasis.**

COMMUNICATION MODELS

The Mental Research Institute

In late 1958, the Mental Research Institute (MRI) was opened by Don Jackson, Jules Riskin, and Virginia Satir, who were later joined by Jay Haley, Richard Fisch, Paul Watzlawick, and John Weakland. MRI was greatly influenced by Bateson and his ideas about cybernetics and communication. In 1967, Watzlawick, Beavin, and Jackson published *Pragmatics of Human Communications: A Study of Interactional Patterns, Pathologies, and Paradoxes,* which was dedicated to Gregory Bateson. In this book, the authors laid down a framework of cybernetics and communication theory to study interpersonal behavior and build a pragmatic model of therapy, which has been referred to as the MRI model, interactional therapy, and brief therapy. The theoretical principles guiding this school of therapy included a focus on communication and problem solving (Fisch, Weakland, & Segal, 1982; Watzlawick, 1978; Watzlawick & Weakland, 1977; Watzlawick, Weakland, & Fisch, 1974), **logical levels** (Spencer-Brown, 1973; Whitehead & Russell, 1910–1913), and **constructivism** (Watzlawick, 1976, 1984).

It is important to note that a key difference between Bateson's ideological view of cybernetic systems and the MRI pragmatic view was the difference between strategically **intervening** in a system versus respecting the system's own wisdom and thereby avoiding unintended consequences of human interventions (Boscolo, Cecchin, Hoffman, & Penn, 1987; Sluzki & Ransom, 1976). This difference was reflected in different viewpoints between Haley and Bateson regarding the issue of power and control (Allman, 1982; Bateson, 1976; Haley, 1976a). This **epistemological** difference has continued to impact the family therapy field, especially as schools of therapy have developed from the ideas of Bateson, MRI, and others (see Dell, 1989; Goolishian & Anderson, 1992; Keeney, 1983; Keeney & Sprenkle, 1982), and led Rabkin (1978) to conclude that the issues of **power,** control, and intervention were the epistemological core of family therapy. Not all agree. In reaction, at least in part, to the highly instrumental MRI approach, a **second-order family therapy** was developed (Hoffman, 1985), which includes such therapies as the **reflecting team** (Andersen, 1987).

Lyman Wynne

Lyman Wynne was also interested in communication patterns in families with a member with schizophrenia. As head of the Family Studies Section at the National Institute of Mental Health (NIMH) in the mid-1950s, he examined ways that the communicational patterns of these families were different from other families. Wynne introduced the concepts **pseudomutuality, pseudohostility,** and **rubber fence** to the growing area of literature related to the study of schizophrenia and the family. Wynne and associates observed that members who grow up in a pseudomutual family fail to establish a strong sense of personal identity since the predominate family theme is togetherness (Wynne, Ryckoff, Day, & Hirsch, 1958).

Milton Erickson

Another influential person in the family therapy field in the 1950s was the psychiatrist Milton Erickson. Bateson (and Margaret Mead) had previously worked with Erickson, and Bateson arranged a meeting between Haley and Erickson in 1953. As Haley and Weakland continued working with Bateson on their communication project, they also regularly consulted with Erickson regarding **trance** and **paradoxical** communication (Haley, 1967, 1973). Erickson's model emphasized the therapist's active approach to elicit change directly and indirectly, focused on symptoms, and considered problems from a **family life cycle** perspective. Erickson's unorthodox but brilliant clinical interventions had an impact on both Haley and Weakland, and greatly influenced the development of their ideas as well as the MRI, structural, strategic, and solution-focused schools of therapy.

The Milan Team (see also Chapter 3)

In 1972, four psychiatrists (Mara Selvini Palazzoli, Luigi Boscolo, Gianfranco Cecchin, and Giuliana Prata) gathered together in Milan, Italy, and immersed themselves in the writings of Bateson and the MRI group with consultations from Paul Watzlawick (Selvini Palazzoli, Boscolo, Cecchin, & Prata, 1978). Naming their family work a systemic approach, they developed a model that incorporated a male–female team approach with a male–female in the room with the family and a male–female team behind the one-way mirror. The session was divided into five parts: (1) the presession; (2) the session; (3) midsession break and discussion; (4) conclusion of session; and (5) postsession discussion.

Strategic and Structural Therapy (see also Chapter 3)

In the early 1960s, in New York at the Wiltwyck School for delinquent boys, Salvador Minuchin, Braulio Montalvo, E. H. Auerswald, and Richard Rabkin were studying and working with families. This collaboration contributed to the development of both the structural approach and the **ecological approach** of working with families (Hoffman, 1981). In 1967, Jay Haley left MRI to join Salvador Minuchin and Braulio Montalvo at the Philadelphia Child Guidance Clinic. This relationship led to further refinements of structural and strategic therapy.

Structural therapy's main goal is structural change, "which acquires

preeminence over the details of individual change, and the attention paid
to the therapist as an active agent in the process of restructuring the family"
(Colapinto, 1982, p. 112). It is a normative model that is concerned with
organizational features of families and family member roles. This model
tends to work with the entire family, and change is viewed as resulting from
structural changes in the family, often accomplished in-session through such
interventions as enactments, joining, restructuring, and reframing
(Minuchin & Fishman, 1981).

Strategic therapy's focus is on the therapist developing a clear strategy
for changing clients' sequential interactional patterns that revolve around
the presenting problem. These patterns impact the family's organization.
Strategic therapy is primarily concerned with four interrelated elements:
symptoms, **metaphors,** hierarchy, and power (Haley, 1976b). Special issues
of the *Journal of Marital and Family Therapy* (January, 1992) and the *Journal
of Systemic Therapies* (Winter, 1993) have focused on the evolution and
changes in strategic therapy.

Solution-Focused Therapy (see also Chapter 6)

Strongly influenced by both the MRI approach and the work of Erickson,
some of the key figures associated with the development of this model
include Steve de Shazer, Insoo Kim Berg, William O'Hanlon, Michelle
Weiner-Davis, and Eve Lipchick (de Shazer, 1985; O'Hanlon & Weiner-
Davis, 1989; O'Hanlon & Wilk, 1987). The thrust of this model is to help
the client(s) focus on exceptions to the problem, to find times that they are
doing well, and then to do more of this "solution" behavior. This model
tends to be brief and symptom focused. The therapist strives to work from
the client's understanding of the problem and seeks behavioral changes.
Although this model is consistent with strategic approaches of doing
therapy, many solution-focused therapists also describe themselves as post-
modernists and social constructionists, and ground some of their ideas in
the **narrative approach.**

PSYCHODYNAMIC MODELS

Nathan Ackerman

Nathan Ackerman was a child psychiatrist who came to the marriage and
family therapy (MFT) field through his study of children with delinquency
and behavior problems. He began his career in the children's division of
the Menninger Clinic in Topeka, Kansas. As early as 1937, he published
"The Family as a Social and Emotional Unit." Ackerman (1956) noted that
an individual's problem can only be understood in terms of his or her
relationship to others. In 1960, Ackerman founded the Ackerman Family

Institute in New York City in order to organize his work and to teach. His influence can be seen in the early work of Salvador Minuchin. In 1962, he and Don Jackson established *Family Process*, the first and one of the most prestigious journals in the field.

Theodore Lidz

Theodore Lidz began his study of the relationship between schizophrenia and the family in 1940, during his residency at Johns Hopkins University. He contributed several ideas to this burgeoning field of study including the following: (1) He proposed that fathers played at least as important a role as that of mothers in family patterns (Lidz & Lidz, 1949); (2) he rejected the proposals of Fromm-Reichman and Rosen that schizophrenia was caused by maternal rejection; and (3) he proposed that the psychodynamics of the parents, rather than the family system, was predominately culpable for the development of schizophrenic behavior in the child. Lidz and his associates described two patterns of marital interaction as particularly characteristic of these families (Lidz, Cornelison, Fleck, & Terry, 1957). Lidz introduced the concepts of **marital schism** and **marital skew.**

Object Relations (see also Chapter 11)

This theory postulates that the fundamental need of humans is for attachment and relationships. The focus is on parent–infant attachment and the impact of that attachment on the developmental process. Influenced by such people as Melanie Klein, Ronald Fairbairn, Harry Dicks, and Donald Winnicott, object relations considers how people's early experiences and expectations lead to the internalization of these relationships, which, in turn, impacts their adult relationships. Object relations is at variance with Freud's drive-oriented theory and connects the intrapsychic and the interpersonal (Framo, 1981; Scharf & Scharf, 1987). This theory emphasizes that persons relate to others primarily on the basis of their similarity to internalized objects from their past.

INTERGENERATIONAL MODELS

Murray Bowen (see also Chapter 2)

In 1946, Murray Bowen joined the staff of the Menninger Clinic as a psychoanalyst. During this tenure, he developed a groundbreaking treatment plan for schizophrenia in which mothers and their schizophrenic children resided together in cottages on the grounds of the clinic. In 1954, Bowen moved to NIMH, where he instituted and directed a classic study in which the entire family of the schizophrenic was hospitalized for observation and research (Bowen, 1978). In 1956, Bowen joined the faculty of the department of psychiatry at Georgetown University Medical School. While at Georgetown, Bowen developed his theory of family therapy (Bowen, 1978). Bowen believed that theory "was more important than anything else for understanding families, and that a way of thinking, rather than a set of techniques, was the legacy he wanted to leave behind" (Wylie, 1991, p. 26). Theory was also important to Bowen, because it helped to keep the therapist emotionally detached and better able to focus on the problems of the family rather than personal issues (Bowen, 1976).

Ivan Boszormenyi-Nagy (see also Chapter 2)

In 1957, Ivan Boszormenyi-Nagy founded the Family Therapy Department at the Eastern Pennsylvania Psychiatric Institute, a research and training facility with an emphasis on schizophrenia and the family. In 1965, Boszormenyi-Nagy coedited with James Framo *Intensive Family Therapy: Theoretical and Practical Aspects,* one of the earliest volumes in the field. He eventually collaborated with Geraldine Spark to develop a theory of families that featured the impact of intergenerational processes in the family as presented in *Invisible Loyalties: Reciprocity in Intergenerational Family Therapy* (1973). Boszormenyi-Nagy is also known for his emphasis on context and proposes that judging people out of context is unjust. He believes that people operate the best that they can, given their heritage.

James Framo (see also Chapter 2)

James Framo may be described as combining intergenerational and object relations approaches to therapy. Framo believes that understanding both the intrapsychic and the interactional is crucial in understanding the dynamics of relationships. He believes that unresolved intrapsychic conflicts derived from one's family of origin continue to be acted out or replicated with one's current family (Framo, 1976, 1981).

EXPERIENTIAL MODELS

Virginia Satir (see also Chapter 4)

Virginia Satir began her professional life as a schoolteacher who got to know the families of her students, particularly the troubled ones. Later she moved to social work and continued her interest in families. When she joined MRI in the late 1950s, she had been practicing family therapy for several years, had met with Murray Bowen in Washington and the Bateson group in Palo Alto, and had taught family dynamics in Chicago. Satir soon became bored with the research process and opened one of the first training programs in family therapy shortly after the MRI opened (Satir, 1982). *Conjoint Family Therapy,* her introduction to the art of family therapy, was published in 1964 and became one of the first major books in the field. She gained worldwide recognition and was in high demand to demonstrate "her dramatic techniques and deeply empathetic way of working" (Simon, 1989, p. 38).

Carl Whitaker (see also Chapter 4)

Whitaker has been described as "the most dynamic and irreverent" of the colorful founders of family therapy (Nichols, 1984). Whitaker's original training was in obstetrics/gynecology, with early exposure to work with persons who were diagnosed as schizophrenic and child psychiatry. He began seeing families in the mid-1940s, during his tenure as a staff psychiatrist for the army in Oak Ridge, Tennessee. In 1946, he was named the chair of the Department of Psychiatry at Emory University. He recruited a team of colleagues including Thomas Malone and John Warkentin, who practiced a very team-oriented approach to therapy, often allowing Whitaker to work with a cotherapist and develop "his own spontaneity and lay aside the constraining mantle of therapeutic responsibility" (Simon, 1992, p. 105). While at Emory, Whitaker's work focused on the treatment of schizophrenia, and he initiated several conferences on the subject, the last of which was held in 1955 and included Gregory Bateson and Don Jackson.

In 1956, Whitaker left Emory after adverse reaction to his ideas and clinical methods found in *The Roots of Psychotherapy* (Whitaker & Malone, 1953). During this time, Whitaker proposed the idea that both client and therapist were to some degree both client and therapist to the other (Neill & Kniskern, 1982). Whitaker believed that therapists could only be effective if they attended to their own growth. In 1965, after working in private practice in Atlanta for several years as a family therapist, in 1965 he accepted a position in the Department of Psychiatry at the University of Wisconsin School of Medicine, where he stayed until his retirement in 1982. Whitaker described his therapeutic approach as symbolic–experiential family therapy. Whitaker prided himself on being atheoretical. For Whitaker, therapy was an art.

POSTMODERN APPROACHES

In 1985, Lynn Hoffman introduced the term **second-order family therapy.** Her paper emphasized the importance of the "new epistemology" of the MFT paradigm and a concern over issues of power, control, and objectivity. People who influenced the development of second-order family therapy included Humberto Maturana (1978), Francisco Varela (1978), Heinz von Foerster (1981, 1984) and Ernst von Glasersfeld (1984, 1988). Von Foerster presented the issues of **second-order cybernetics.** Maturana and Varela (1987) brought in the concepts of **autopoietic** systems (models of autonomy rather than of control), structurally determined systems, and conversational domains. Von Glasersfeld and von Foerster introduced the tenets of radical **constructivism.** These views and concepts contributed to a view of "the nervous systems as a closed machine," such that "percepts and constructs take shape as the organism bumps against its environment" (Hoffman, 1992, p. 8).

Another postmodern approach also developed from the work of such people as Kenneth Gergen (1982, 1985), John Shotter (1984), Jerome Bruner (1986), and Michel Foucault (1972, 1984). Goolishian and Anderson (1992) state that this approach requires "moving away from the base cybernetic paradigm and machine metaphor of family therapy . . . giving up the focus on 'epistemology' " and moving to "a position informed by hermeneutics, semantics, and narrative" (p. 7). This approach is often referred to as **social constructionism,** which views "ideas, concepts and memories arising from social interchange and mediated through language" and that "all knowledge . . . evolves in the space between people" (Hoffman, 1992, p. 8). The theories organizing these different epistemological perspectives have contributed to various postmodern approaches to family therapy.[4]

Collaborative Language Approach (see also Chapter 6)

The collaborative language approach developed from the work of Harry Goolishian, Harlene Anderson, and associates at the Houston–Galveston Family Institute. The Houston–Galveston Institute traces its origins to the early 1950s (Anderson, Goolishian, Pulliam, & Winderman, 1986). One of the first programs in the country to clinically work with families, their work initially involved multiple-impact therapy (MIT; MacGregor et al., 1964). Bateson was a consultant to this project, and MIT was a "forerunner to . . . systemic family therapy" (Anderson et al., 1986, p. 103). Evolving and developing over time, the Houston–Galveston Institute, led by Harry Goolishian and Harlene Anderson, shifted to a collaborative language approach (Anderson & Goolishian, 1988; Goolishian & Anderson, 1987).

This move developed from what they saw as limitations of the systems paradigm as well as concerns they had over the issues of power, control, and therapist's intervening. Goolishian and Anderson developed a theory and approach that theoretically embraces a **hermeneutic** and linguistic

[4]It can be noted that although radical constructivism and social constructionism have been contrasted as fundamentally different, there are similarities and commonalities between the two epistemologies (see Steffe & Gale, 1995).

paradigm. This epistemological shift moved their work away from a systems perspective to a collaborative language focus (Anderson & Goolishian, 1992; Goolishian & Anderson, 1992).

Narrative Therapy (see also Chapter 6)

Narrative therapy is based on the postmodern **narrative approach** of viewing human interaction from a storied and moral universe. Michael White, David Epston, Jeffery Zimmerman, Victoria Dickerson, Michael Durrant, and Kate Kawalski are some of the people associated with this model. Language and the telling of relational (of self and others) stories are embedded within a cultural and social context. White (1992), following Foucault's ideas, states that "meaning, structures and practices are inseparable" and related to power (p. 122). Therefore, culture's dominant stories can disempower, constrain, and objectify individuals in their actions and meanings. Following Bruner's (1986) ideas that stories are composed in the dual landscape of action and consciousness, White's therapy poses deconstructing types of questions to the clients. Through these practices, clients are able to externalize problems from their self-identity narratives, deobjectify themselves, and reauthor new ways of being.

FEMINIST CONTRIBUTIONS (see also Chapter 9)

In 1978, a new voice emerged in the family therapy arena when Rachel Hare-Mustin's article "A Feminist Approach to Family Therapy" was published in *Family Process*. A common feminist agenda is to examine family therapy in terms of traditional gender-role concepts in order to liberate clients from artificial and unnecessary limitations (Libow, Raskin, & Caust, 1982). Braverman (1988) suggests that "on the level of theory, a feminist approach to family therapy, whatever the school, requires embracing gender as a critical variable in the formulation of the problem definition and problem solution" (p. 9). Feminist family therapists also reject the notion of value-free therapy. Betty Carter (1985) writes, "You cannot not act out of your age, gender, sibling position, experience, belief system, and wisdom, or lack of it. Your only choice is whether to do this consciously or unconsciously" (p. 78).

Feminist family therapists have noted several objections to the heavy reliance on systems theory/cybernetics in the family therapy field, including the following:

1. Comparing the family to a machine divorces it from its historical, social, political, and economic contexts, and ignores the relationship between context and family dysfunction (James & McIntyre, 1983).

2. Ignoring the context dissociates family therapists from the history of the family, including the influence of the Industrial Revolution on family structure and the gendered division of labor (Avis, 1988).
3. Using the systemic concepts of circularity, neutrality, and complementarity ignores differences in power (Bograd, 1984; Goldner, 1985).

KEY CONCEPTS[5]

Analogic communication. The nonverbal aspect of a communication transaction defines the relationship between the participants (Bateson, 1972). The command aspect of the communication is analogic. For example, a boss ordering an employee to "Please open the door!" connotes a much different relationship than a child awakening from a nightmare and begging his father to "Please open the door?" (see also Digital communication).

Autopoiesis. Humberto Maturana, in coining the word autopoiesis, combined auto (meaning self) with poiesis (meaning creation) to describe the "autonomous processes that characterize living systems" (Kenny, 1988, p. i). In autopoiesis, it is the internal structure (nervous system) of a living system that determines its behavior and not the environment. This has also been referred to as structural determinism, in that the structure serves to maintain the organization of the system. Although initially referring to living systems, autopoiesis can also refer to a couple or family (Efran & Lukens, 1985). One implication to therapy of autopoiesis is that a therapist cannot provide instructional interactions to clients, but can only perturb the client system to make changes that the client system structure *itself* will produce.

Biopsychosocial systems approach. Viewing the necessary relationship between a person's health and that person's mental and social conditions (mind–body connection), the physician George Engle (1977) developed the concept of the biopsychosocial model. This model has been adopted by a number of family therapists and medical care practitioners, and has encouraged collaboration between these two disciplines (Griffith & Griffith, 1994; McDaniel, Hepworth, & Doherty, 1992).

Command. See Analogic communication.

Constructivism. Constructivism is an epistemological paradigm that has its roots in the writings of the Greek Skeptics, Kant, Vico, and Piaget, to name a few (von Glasersfeld, 1984). Constructivists view knowledge as actively constructed by the individual, and although not denying an

---

[5]Terms and concepts that are model specific are presented and described in other chapters of this book.

ontological reality, "deny" the human experiencer the possibility of acquiring a "true representation" of reality (von Glasersfeld, 1988, p. 86). Constructivism has been adapted in various ways by different people (e.g., Guba, 1990; Kelly, 1955; Maturana & Varela, 1987). In 1984, in Paul Watzlawick's book *The Invented Reality,* von Glasersfeld introduced the term "radical constructivism" to the family therapy field. The two basic principles of radical constructivism are as follows: (1) Knowledge is actively constructed by the individual and not passively received; and (2) the function of cognition organizes the experiential world rather than seeks to discover ontological reality (von Glasersfeld, 1988). The focus of radical constructivism is on how individuals' cognitions, as active phenomena that are structurally determined by the nervous system, are continuously producing (via assimilation and accommodation) one's adaptation with the environment. Although acknowledging the importance of others (von Foerster, 1984) and the importance of language (von Glasersfeld, 1995), radical constructivists' metaphoric basic unit is the mind as an evolving, adapting organism. The implications to family therapy is radical constructivism's consideration on one's subjective experiential world, for example, in constructing and presenting a therapeutic reframe.

Control. The issue of control has been an important topic in the MFT field. Bateson (1972) argued that no part of a system could have unilateral control of that system, and that the belief of such control was pathological. Bateson wanted to get rid of the concept of control. Haley (1963), on the other hand, viewed the issue of control (and power) as central to understanding family dynamics, and therapy as the struggle for control of the relationship. Issues of control and power are also very important to feminist thinking and narrative therapy, because both models view inequities of control and power as embedded within political, economic, ethnic, sexual, cultural, and gendered contexts.

Cybernetics. Coined by Norbert Weiner (1948/1961), cybernetics is the science of communication and control in man and machine. Cybernetics conceptualizes how patterns of organization (or systems) maintain stability and control through levels of feedback.

Digital communication. This is the verbal content of a communication transaction; for example, the question "Please open the door?" Bateson (1972) viewed messages as having both an analogic and digital component. Although the digital component can remain the same, the message can have a very different meaning when it is the boss ordering an employee to open the door or a small child begging his father to open the door (see also Analogic communication).

Double bind theory. This was initially developed by Bateson and his colleagues in 1954 as a hypothesis about what had happened in the lives of persons who were schizophrenic. The focus was on a pattern of communication that seemed to provoke behavior characteristic of schizophrenia.

The double bind theory was first described in 1956 by the members of Bateson's research project in a paper entitled "Towards a Theory of Schizophrenia." The author described the necessary components of the double bind as follows: (1) The double bind involves two or more persons, one of whom is designated as the "victim"; (2) the double bind is a recurrent theme in the experience of the victim; (3) the "victim" is caught in a situation in which the other person in the relationship is expressing two contradictory or incongruent messages that are both enforced by punishments or signals that threaten survival; (4) the "victim" cannot escape the field and cannot comment on the incongruence of the messages being expressed (Weakland, 1976).

Double description. This is based on Bateson's (1979) idea that no single description accurately describes an event and information is a message of difference. In order to understand relationships, it is necessary to combine two (or more) descriptions (information of differences) of the same event.

Ecological approach. As developed by E. G. Auerswald, this approach takes a holistic view that stresses the importance of working with families within their neighborhood setting and including all members of the community system, from professionals, to extended families, to community figures, to community institutions (Hoffman, 1981). Auerswald developed a model for crisis intervention that had professionals working outside of the office and in the community, in order to be readily available for clients and to better understand the clients' social and economic context.

Epistemology. Epistemology (see Guba, 1990; Steffe & Gale, 1995) is the science (or theory) of methods of knowledge and answers the question "What is knowing?" Different epistemologies provide distinct paradigms (and methods) of discerning knowledge. Positivism is an epistemology that views the world (ontology) as discoverable and knowable. Positivism posits that an inquirer can objectively, and without altering them, uncover facts about the empirical world. Postpositivism adopts a critical realist position, in that this view acknowledges that although one can never discover ultimate truths, there is no question that there is a "reality" out there. Four other epistemologies that are relevant to the theoretical foundations of family therapy include constructivism, radical constructivism, social constructionism, and feminist critical theory. Although constructivism, radical constructivism, and social constructionism have often been used synonymously in the MFT literature, they do have different meanings and implications to the practice of family therapy.

Family life cycle. The progression of the family unit through nodal events or transitional periods (e.g., birth of a child, children leaving home, death of a member) is its life cycle. Nodal events often require the family to rewrite family rules or renegotiate family roles in order to remain functional.

Feedback. A concept from cybernetic theory, feedback is information that produces action in response to change in a system. The change can either increase or decrease a behavior.

First-order cybernetics. The idea that an outside observer can study and make changes in a system while remaining separate and independent of that system is called first-order cybernetics.

Hermeneutics. Hermeneutics (or exegesis) is the activity of understanding achieved through the interpretation of texts (Frank, 1987). It is a phenomenological and contextual approach that offers no transcendental ground from which to attain absolute meaning. Analytical (and clinical) insight is developed through a continuous process of interpreting levels of contexts of meaning. The hermeneutic circle is the recursive loop of interpretations.

Homeostasis. A term introduced by Don Jackson (1965), homeostasis is the notion that families develop recurring interactional patterns to maintain stability and balance, especially in times of stress. Jackson viewed families as rule-governed systems that seek to maintain a normal range of behavior.

Information. As defined by Bateson (1972), information is "a difference which makes a difference" (p. 459).

Logical levels. Logical types are based on the philosophical writings of Whitehead and Russell (1910–1913) and were used by Bateson to account for levels of communication and paradoxes. For example, the statement "Did you do your homework?" presents both a content question ("Did you do it?") and also (in context) provides a metastatement about the relationship between the speaker and respondent ("I am in charge of seeing that you do it."). The metamessage is of a different logical type than the content aspect of the message. The study of the confusion, or paradox, of messages that give conflicting injunctions led to the development of the double bind theory (Bateson, 1972).

Marital schism. Marital schism refers to spouses who are unable to achieve role reciprocity due to preoccupation with their own problems. Each spouse then may try to undermine the other, especially with the children, and compete for their support.

Marital skew. Marital skew refers to a marital relationship in which one spouse is viewed as strong and the other as weak. The strong spouse dominates the home, while the weak spouse accepts the domination and proposes to the children that this situation is normal. This denial by the parent may lead to further denial and distortion by the children.

Metaphors. Kenneth Burke (1945/1969) states that "metaphor is a device for seeing something in terms of something else. It brings out the thisness of a that, or the thatness of a this" (p. 503). From a postmodern perspective, human experience can only be expressed (and understood) metaphorically.

Morphogenesis. Morphogenesis is the process by which a system changes its structure to adapt to new contexts. From a second-order cybernetic perspective, morphostasis (stability) and morphogenesis (change) function together to help a system maintain a well-functioning balance (Keeney, 1983).

Morphostasis. Morphostasis is a system's tendency toward stability and dynamic equilibrium, and the ability of a system to maintain stability in the context of change.

Negative restraints. Bateson (1972) describes cybernetic explanation as a shift from causal explanation of the type *A* causes *B* (which offers a positive account) to the notion of restraints (which provide negative accounts). Positive and negative do not refer to being good or bad, but rather point to how logical choices are made. Cybernetic explanations offer negative restraints and provide logical proofs through eliminating all choices but one (*reductio ad absurdum*). For example, a person placing a jigsaw puzzle piece is restrained by the shape of the other pieces to select only one piece. In a family system, the various relationships cybernetically contribute to constrain the perceptions and actions of each member.

Power. See Control.

Pseudohostility. Pseudohostility refers to the use of superficial anger to mask family members needs for intimacy and affection or deeper issues of chronic conflict and alienation.

Pseudomutuality. Pseudomutual families fail to establish a strong sense of personal identity since the predominate family theme is togetherness. Efforts to establish an individual identity are viewed as a threat to the family and discouraged.

Recursiveness. Describing the repeating connectedness of a process, Bateson (1979) notes that logical levels present a "hierarchy of orders of recursiveness" (p. 201). Keeney and Thomas (1986) provide the example of a recursive view as "the client directs the therapist how to direct the client, who in turn redirects the therapist how to subsequently direct the client" (p. 282).

Report. The report aspect of a message conveys information or data and is synonymous with the content of the message (see also Digital Communication).

Rubber fence. As coined by Lyman Wynne, rubber fence describes how psychotic and schizophrenic families resist outside influences.

Rules. Rules are repeated communication patterns that serve to stabilize family relationships. Rules can be both overt (acknowledged, e.g., father makes all the decisions in the family) or covert (unspoken, e.g., scapegoating the oldest son for all family problems). Jackson (1965) views rules (rather than roles) as organizing family identities and interactions.

Second-order cybernetics. Heinz von Foerster (Howe & von Foerster, 1974) conceived of second-order cybernetics as the cybernetics of observing systems. From this perspective, there can be no independent observer of a system because any observer is a participant who both influences and is influenced by that system. Also referred to as cybernetics of cybernetics (Mead, 1968).

Second-order family therapy. A distinction first suggested by Hoffman (1985) to deal with the issue of power and control as applied to family therapy, Hoffman (1988) states that second-order family therapy is an approach "that truly respects second-order cybernetics" (p. 65), such that the therapist is always reflexively and collaboratively involved with that system. Second-order family therapy strives to adopt a noninterventionist approach to conducting therapy.

Social constructionism. Introduced by Ken Gergen (1982, 1985), the emphasis of social constructionism is that knowing and knowledge are socially constructed through language and discourse and are context dependent. Social constructionism, like constructivism, challenges that there is an objective basis for achieving knowledge. But unlike radical constructivism's emphasis on the mind and cognitive processes, social constructionism attends to the world of intersubjectively shared meaning making. The implications for family therapy include (1) social constructionism's emphasis of context; (2) self-identity (viewed as multiple selves) as being socially and reflexively created; and (3) the understanding of the world as seen through studying the construction of stories and narratives, from both a micro- and macrolevel.

Structural determinism. The structure of the system (e.g., human body, family, etc.) acts to self-maintain the organization of the system. Living systems are informationally closed and can only understand the world in terms of their own structure.

System. A system is a complex of interacting components (von Bertalanffy, 1962). It is an invention used to describe regularities or redundant patterns we observe between people and other phenomena.

Trance. Trance was viewed by Erickson as both an ordinary and clinical phenomenon in which a person's attention is focused and he or she is able "to utilize the competencies that exist within him[her] at both a psychological level and physiological level" (1983, p. 76). A key element of trance is that communication within a person occurs at multiple levels (e.g., conscious–unconscious), such that there may be different logical levels of information. Erickson viewed the unconscious as a positive resource.

KEY BOOKS, CHAPTERS, AND ARTICLES

Bateson, G. (1972). *Steps to an ecology of mind.* New York: Ballantine.

    A collection of Bateson's writings that highlight his contribution to family therapy as well as to other fields.

Bateson, G. (1979). *Mind and nature: A necessary unity.* New York: Dutton.

Bateson's final book before his death, which strives to integrate his ideas.

Bruner, J. (1986). *Actual minds, possible worlds.* Cambridge, MA: Harvard University Press.

One of Bruner's key works that highlights his contributions to narrative and cognitive psychology.

Erickson, M. H. (1980). *The collected papers of Milton H. Erickson* (Vols. I, II, & III) (E. L. Rossi, Ed.). New York: Irvington.

This three-volume classic contains many of Erickson's foundational articles describing his clinical innovations. These volumes provide excellent descriptions of utilization, deep-trance phenomenon, and Erickson's approach to brief therapy. Many clinical examples are provided.

Foucault, M. (1984). *Foucault reader* (P. Rabinow, Ed.). New York: Pantheon.

This reader contains selections of Foucault's writings as well as an interview with Foucault. This is a good book to orient the reader to Foucault's influential and complex ideas.

Gergen, K. J. (1985). The social constructionist movement in modern psychology. *American Psychologist, 40,* 266–275.

This article helped bring Gergen to the forefront of psychology. Gergen's ideas on social constructionism are summarized in this concise article.

Hoffman, L. (1981). *Foundations of family therapy.* New York: Basic Books.

Although written in 1981, and not representing Hoffman's current thinking, this book captures the theory, practice, and history of the marriage and family therapy field at that time.

Keeney, B. P. (1983). *Aesthetics of change.* New York: Guilford Press.

Keeney clearly applies Bateson's ideas and cybernetics to the marriage and family therapy field. A clear understanding of Bateson's dialectic ladder of process and form is included.

Maturana, H. R., & Varela, F. J. (1987). *The tree of knowledge.* Boston: New Science Library.

This well-written book clearly presents Maturana's and Varela's ideas about autopoiesis, structural determinism, constructionism, emotions, and more.

Sluzki, C., & Ransom, D. (Eds.). (1976). *Double bind: The foundation of the communicational approach to the family.* New York: Grune & Stratton.

A collection of chapters that provide a fundamental understanding of Bateson and his colleagues' ideas about the influence of cybernetics, logical levels, and communication theory on family therapy. Authors provide various perspectives on the development of the double bind theory.

von Bertalanffy, L. (1962). General system theory—A critical review. *General Systems, 7,* 1–20.

A reassessment of general system theory, its foundations, achievements, criticisms, and prospects.

Watzlawick, P., Beavin, J., & Jackson, D. (1967). *Pragmatics of human communication.* New York: Norton.

A basic introduction to the pragmatics of human communication, with special attention to behavior disorders.

Weiner, N. (1961). *Cybernetics or control and communication in the animal and the machine.* Cambridge, MA: MIT Press. (Original work published 1948)

Originally published in 1948, this book was considered "one of the most influential books of the 20th century." This book impacted many different disciplines and fields.

REFERENCES

Ackerman, N. W. (1937). The family as a social and emotional unit. *Bulletin of the Kansas Mental Hygiene Society, 12.*

Ackerman, N. W. (1956). Interlocking pathology in family relationships. In S. Rado & G. Daniels (Eds.), *Changing conceptions of psychoanalytic medicine.* New York: Grune & Stratton.

Allman, L. R. (1982). The aesthetic preference: Overcoming the pragmatic error. *Family Process, 21,* 43–56.

Andersen, T. (1987). The reflecting team: Dialogue and meta-dialogue in clinical work. *Family Process, 26*(4), 415–428.

Anderson, H. (1994). Rethinking family therapy: A delicate balance. *Journal of Marital and Family Therapy, 20*(2), 145–149.

Anderson, H., & Goolishian, H. (1988). Human systems as linguistic systems: Evolving ideas about the implications for theory and practice. *Family Process, 27,* 371–393.

Anderson, H., & Goolishian, H. (1992). The client is the expert: A not-knowing approach to therapy. In S. McNamee & K. J. Gergen (Eds.), *Therapy as social construction.* London: Sage.

Anderson, H., Goolishian, H., Pulliam, G., & Winderman, L. (1986). The Galveston Family Institute: A personal and historical perspective. In D. Efron (Ed.), *Journeys: Expansions of the strategic–systemic therapies.* New York: Brunner/Mazel.

Avis, J. M. (1988). Deepening awareness: A private study guide to feminism and family therapy. In L. Braverman (Ed.), *A guide to feminist family therapy.* New York: Harrington Park Press.

Bateson, G. (1972). *Steps to an ecology of mind.* New York: Ballantine.

Bateson, G. (1976). Comments on Haley's history. In C. Sluzki & D. Ransom (Eds.), *Double bind: The foundation of the communicational approach to the family.* New York: Grune & Stratton.

Bateson, G. (1979). *Mind and nature: A necessary unity.* New York: Dutton.

20 FAMILY THERAPY SOURCEBOOK

Bateson, G. (1991). *A sacred unity* (R. E. Donaldson, Ed.). New York: HarperCollins.

Bateson, G., Jackson, D. D., Haley, J., & Weakland, J. (1956). Toward a theory of schizophrenia. *Behavioral Science, 1,* 251–264.

Bateson, G., & Ruesch, J. (1951). *Communication: The social matrix of psychiatry.* New York: Norton.

Bograd, M. (1984). Family systems approaches to wife battering: A feminist critique. *American Journal of Orthopsychiatry, 54,* 558–563.

Boscolo, L., Cecchin, G., Hoffman, L., & Penn, P. (1987). *Milan systemic family therapy: Conversations in theory and practice.* New York: Basic Books.

Boszormenyi-Nagy, I., & Framo, J. (Eds.). (1965). *Intensive family therapy: Theoretical and practical aspects.* New York: Harper & Row.

Boszormenyi-Nagy, I., & Spark, G. (1973). *Invisible loyalties: Reciprocity in intergenerational family therapy.* New York: Harper & Row.

Bowen, M. (1976). Theory in the practice of psychotherapy. In P. J. Guerin (Ed.), *Family therapy: Theory and practice.* New York: Gardner.

Bowen, M. (1978). *Family therapy in clinical practice.* New York: Jason Aronson.

Braverman, L. (Ed.). (1988). *A guide to feminist family therapy.* New York: Harrington Park Press.

Broderick, C. B., & Schrader, S. S. (1981). The history of professional marriage and family therapy. In A. S. Gurman & D. P. Kniskern (Eds.), *Handbook of family therapy.* New York: Brunner/Mazel.

Brunner, J. (1986). *Actual minds, possible worlds.* Cambridge, MA: Harvard University Press.

Buckley, W. (1968). Society as a complex adaptive system. In W. Buckley (Ed.), *Modern systems research for the behavioral scientist.* Chicago: Aldine.

Burke, K. (1969). *A grammar of motives.* Berkeley: University of California Press. (Original work published 1945)

Carter, B. (1985). Ms. intervention's guide to "correct" feminist family therapy. *Family Therapy Networker, 9,* 78–79.

Colapinto, J. (1982). Structural family therapy. In A. M. Horne & M. M. Ohlsen (Eds.), *Family counseling and therapy.* Itasca, IL: Peacock.

Dell, P. (1989). Violence and the systemic view: The problem of power. *Family Process, 28,* 1–14.

de Shazer, S. (1985). *Keys to solutions in brief therapy.* New York: Norton.

Efran, J., & Luken, M. D. (1985, May–June). The world according to Humberto Maturana. *Family Therapy Networker,* pp. 23–28, 72–75.

Engle, G. L. (1977). The need for a new medical model: A challenge for biomedicine. *Science, 196,* 129–136.

Erickson, M. H. (1983). *Healing in hypnosis.* New York: Irvington.

Fisch, R., Weakland, J., & Segal, L. (1982). *The tactics of change: Doing therapy briefly.* San Francisco: Jossey-Bass.

Foucault, M. (1972). *The archaeology of knowledge and the discourse on language* (A. M. Sheridan Smith, Ed. & Trans.). New York: Pantheon Books.

Foucault, M. (1984). *Foucault reader* (P. Rabinow, Ed.). New York: Pantheon Books.

Framo, J. L. (1976). Family of origin as a therapeutic resource for adults in marital and family therapy: You can and should go home again. *Family Process, 15,* 193–210.

Framo, J. L. (1981). The integration of marital therapy with sessions with family of origin. In A. S. Gurman & D. P. Kniskern (Eds.), *Handbook of family therapy.* New York: Brunner/Mazel.

Frank, J. D. (1987). Psychotherapy, rhetoric, and hermeneutics: Implications for practice and research. *Psychotherapy, 24*(3), 293–302.

Gergen, K. J. (1982). *Towards transformation in social knowledge.* New York: Springer.

Gergen, K. J. (1985). The social constructionist movement in modern psychology. *American Psychologist, 40,* 266–275.

Goldner, V. (1985). Feminism and family therapy. *Family Process, 24,* 31–47.

Goolishian, H., & Anderson, H. (1987). Language systems and therapy: An evolving idea. *Psychotherapy, 24,* 529–538.

Goolishian, H., & Anderson, H. (1992). Strategy and intervention versus nonintervention: A matter of theory. *Journal of Marital and Family Therapy, 18*(1), 5–15.

Griffith, J. L., & Griffith, M. E. (1994). *The body speaks: Therapeutic dialogues for mind–body problems.* New York: Basic Books.

Guba, E. G. (Ed.). (1990). *The paradigm dialogues.* Newbury Park, CA: Sage.

Guerin, P. J., Jr. (1976). Family therapy: The first twenty-five years. In P. J. Guerin, Jr. (Ed.), *Family therapy: Theory and practice.* New York: Gardner.

Haley, J. (1963). *Strategies of psychotherapy.* New York: Grune & Stratton.

Haley, J. (1967). (Ed.). *Advanced techniques of hypnosis and therapy: Selected papers of Milton H. Erickson, MD.* New York: Grune & Stratton.

Haley, J. (1973). *Uncommon therapy.* New York: Norton.

Haley, J. (1976a). Development of a theory: A historical review of a research project. In C. Sluzki & D. Ramson, (Eds.), *Double bind: The foundation of the communicational approach to the family.* New York: Grune & Stratton.

Haley, J. (1976b). *Problem-solving therapy.* New York: Harper Colophon.

Hardy, K. (1994). Marginalization or development: A response to Shields, Wynne, McDaniel, and Gawinski. *Journal of Marital and Family Therapy, 20*(2), 139–144.

Heims, S. (1977). Gregory Bateson and the mathematicians: From interdisciplinary interaction to societal functions. *Journal of the History of the Behavioral Sciences, 13,* 141–159.

Hoffman, L. (1981). *Foundations of family therapy.* New York: Basic Books.

Hoffman, L. (1985). Beyond power and control: Toward a second-order family systems therapy. *Family Systems, 3,* 381–396.

Hoffman, L. (1988). Reply to Stuart Golann. *Family Process, 27,* 65–68.

Hoffman, L. (1992). A reflexive stance for family therapy. In S. McNamee & K. J. Gergen (Eds.), *Therapy as social construction.* London: Sage.

Howe, R., & von Foerster, H. (1974). Cybernetics at Illinois. *Forum, 6,* 15–17.

Jackson, D. D. (1957). The question of family homeostasis: *Psychiatric Quarterly Supplement, 31,* 79–90.

Jackson, D. D. (1965). The study of the family. *Family Process, 4,* 1–20.

James, K., & McIntyre, D. (1983). The reproduction of families: The social role of family therapy? *Journal of Marital and Family Therapy, 9,* 119–129.

Kelly, G. A. (1955). *The psychology of personal constructs.* New York: Norton.

Keeney, B. P. (1983). *Aesthetics of change.* New York: Guilford Press.

Keeney, B. P., & Sprenkle, D. (1982). Ecosystemic epistemology: Critical implications for the aesthetics and pragmatics of family therapy. *Family Process, 21,* 1–19.

Keeney, B. P., & Thomas, F. N. (1986). Cybernetic foundations of family therapy. In F. P. Piercy, D. H. Sprenkle, & associates. *Family therapy sourcebook.* New York: Guilford Press.

Kenny, V. (1988). Guest editor's foreword. Radical constructivism and autopoiesis and psychotherapy [Special issue]. *Irish Journal of Psychology, 9,* i–iii.

Keim, J. (1995). Strategic therapy. In M. Elkaim (Ed.), *Panorama des thérapies familiales.* Paris: Editions du Seuil.

Libow, J. A., Raskin, P. A., & Caust, B. L. (1982). Feminist and family systems therapy: Are they irreconcilable? *American Journal of Family Therapy, 10,* 3–12.

Lidz, R. W., & Lidz, T. (1949). The family environment of schizophrenic patients. *Journal of Psychiatry, 106,* 332–345.

Lidz, T., Cornelison, A., Fleck, S., & Terry, D. (1957). The intrafamilial environment of schizophrenic patients: II. Marital schism and marital skew. *American Journal of Psychiatry, 106,* 241–248.

Lipset, D. (1980). *Gregory Bateson: The legacy of a scientist.* Englewood Cliffs, NJ: Prentice-Hall.

MacGregor, R., Ritchie, S., Serrano, A., Schuster, F., McDanald, E., & Goolishian, H. (1964). *Multiple impact therapy with families.* New York: McGraw-Hill.

Maruyama, M. (1968). The second cybernetics: Deviation–amplifying mutual cause process. In W. Buckley (Ed.), *Modern systems research for the behavioral scientist.* Chicago: Aldine.

Maturana, H. R. (1978). Biology of language: The epistemology of reality. In G. A. Miller & E. Lennenberg (Eds.), *Psychology and biology of language and thought.* New York: Academic Press.

Maturana, H. R., & Varela, F. J. (1987). *The tree of knowledge.* Boston: New Science Library.

McDaniel, S. H., Hepworth, J., & Doherty, W. J. (1992). *Medical family therapy: A biopsychosocial approach to families with health problems.* New York: Basic Books.

Mead, M. (1968). Cybernetics of cybernetics. In H. von Foerster, J. D. White, L. J. Peterson, & J. K. Russell (Eds.), *Purposive systems: The first annual symposium of the American Society of Cybernetics.* New York: Spartan.

Minuchin, S., & Fishman, C. H. (1981). *Family therapy techniques.* Cambridge, MA: Harvard University Press.

Neill, J. R., & Kniskern, D. P. (Eds.). (1982). *From psyche to system: The evolving therapy of Carl Whitaker.* New York: Guilford Press.

Nichols, M. P. (1984). *Family therapy—Concepts and methods.* New York: Gardner.

Nichols, W. C. (1992). *Fifty years of marital and family therapy.* Washington, DC: AAMFT.

Nichols, W. C., & Everett, C. A. (1986). The field of family therapy. In W. C. Nichols & C. A. Everett (Eds.), *Systemic family therapy: An integrative approach.* New York: Guilford Press.

O'Hanlon, W. H., & Weiner-Davis, M. (1989). *In search of solutions: A new direction in psychotherapy.* New York: Norton.

O'Hanlon, W. H., & Wilk, J. (1987). *Shifting contexts: The generation of effective psychotherapy.* New York: Guilford Press.

Rabkin, R. (1978). *Strategic psychotherapy.* New York: Basic Books.

Satir, V. (1964). *Conjoint family therapy.* Palo Alto, CA: Science and Behavior Books.

Satir, V. (1982). The therapist and family therapy: Process model. In A. M. Horne & M. M. Ohlsen (Eds.), *Family counseling and therapy.* Itasca, IL: Peacock.

Scharf, D. E., & Scharf, J. S. (1987). *Object relations family therapy.* Northvale, NJ: Jason Aronson.

Selvini Palazzoli, M. (Ed.). (1988). *The work of Mara Selvini Palazzoli.* Northvale, NJ: Jason Aronson.

Selvini Palazzoli, M., Boscolo, L., Cecchin, G., & Prata, G. (1978). *Paradox and counter-paradox.* New York: Jason Aronson.

Selvini Palazzoli, M., Boscolo, L., Cecchin, G., & Prata, G. (1980). Hypothesizing–circularity–neutrality: Three guidelines for the conductor of the session. *Family Process, 19,* 3–12.

Shields, G. C., Wynne, L. C., McDaniel, S. H., & Gawinski, B. A. (1994). The marginalization of family therapy: A historical and continuing problem. *Journal of Marital and Family Therapy, 20*(1), 117–138.

Shotter, J. (1984). *Social accountability and selfhood.* Oxford: Blackwell.

Simon, R. (1989). Reaching out to life: An interview with Virginia Satir. *Family Therapy Networker, 13,* 37–43.

Simon, R. (1992). Take it or leave it: An interview with Carl Whitaker. In R. Simon (Ed.), *One on one: Conversations with the shapers of family therapy.* New York: Guilford Press.

Sluzki, C., & Ransom, D. (Eds.). (1976). *Double bind: The foundation of the communicational approach to the family.* New York: Grune & Stratton.

Spencer-Brown, G. (1973). *Laws of form.* New York: Bantam.

Steffe, L., & Gale, J. (1995). *Constructivism in education.* Hillsdale, NJ: Erlbaum.

Varela, F. J. (1979). *Principles of biological autonomy.* New York: Elsevier North Holland.

von Bertalanffy, L. (1962). General system theory: A critical review. *General Systems, 7,* 1–20.

von Bertalanffy, L. (1967). *Robots, men, and minds: Psychology in the modern world.* New York: George Braziller.

von Bertalanffy, L. (1968). *General system theory.* New York: George Braziller.

von Foerster, H. (1981). *Observing systems.* Seaside, CA: Intersystems.

von Foerster, H. (1984). On constructing a reality. In P. Watzlawick (Ed.), *The invented reality*. New York: W. W. Norton.

von Glasersfeld, E. (1984). An introduction to radical constructivism. In P. Watzlawick (Ed.), *The invented reality*. New York: Norton.

von Glasersfeld, E. (1988). The reluctance to change a way of thinking. Radical constructivism and autopoiesis and psychotherapy [Special issue]. *Irish Journal of Psychology, 9,* 83–90

von Glasersfeld, E. (1995). Sensory experience, abstraction and teaching. In L. Steffe & J. Gale (Eds.), *Constructivism in education*. Hillsdale, NJ: Erlbaum.

Watzlawick, P. (1976). *How real is real?* New York: Random House.

Watzlawick, P. (1978). *The language of change*. New York: Basic Books.

Watzlawick, P. (1984). *The invented reality*. New York: Norton.

Watzlawick, P., Beavin, J., & Jackson, D. (1967). *Pragmatics of human communication: A study of interactional patterns, pathologies, and paradoxes*. New York: Norton.

Watzlawick, P., & Weakland, J. (Eds.). (1977). *The interactional view: Studies at the Mental Research Institute, Palo Alto, 1965–1974*. New York: Norton.

Watzlawick, P., Weakland, J., & Fisch, R. (1974). *Change: Principles of problem formation and problem resolution*. New York: Norton.

Weakland, J. (1976). The "double bind" hypothesis of schizophrenia and three-party interaction (1960). In C. E. Sluzki & D. C. Ransom (Eds.), *Double bind: The foundation of the communicational approach to the family*. New York: Grune & Stratton.

Weiner, N. (1961). *Cybernetics or control and communication in the animal and the machine*. Cambridge, MA: MIT Press. (Original work published 1948)

Whitaker, C. A., & Malone, T. P. (1953). *The roots of psychotherapy*. New York: Blakiston.

White, M. (1992). Deconstruction and therapy. In D. Epston & M. White (Eds.), *Experience, contradiction, narrative and imagination*. South Australia: Dulwich Centre Publications.

Whitehead, A. N., & Russell, B. (1910–1913). *Principa mathematica* (3 vols., 2nd ed.). Cambridge: Cambridge University Press.

Wylie, M. S. (1991). Family therapy's neglected prophet. *Family Therapy Networker, 15,* 24–37.

Wynne, L. C., Ryckoff, I. M., Day, J., & Hirsch, S. I. (1958). Pseudomutuality in the family relationships of schizophrenics. *Psychiatry, 21,* 205–220.

2

Transgenerational Family Therapies

JOSEPH L. WETCHLER
FRED P. PIERCY

TRANSGENERATIONAL approaches to family therapy have grown out of the work of such pioneers as Murray Bowen, Ivan Boszormenyi-Nagy, James Framo, Norman Paul, and Donald Williamson. These theorists share the belief that present-day problems are related to issues in a person's family of origin. Although their theories and practice may differ, all agree that the royal road to problem resolution involves working with more than one generation in therapy. A common misconception is that these models espouse a linear approach, in which people's problems are "caused by their families of origin." In fact, all of these are larger systems models that view problems as being maintained in ongoing patterns that span generations. Each of these key theorists and their basic theoretical tenets are introduced briefly here.

MURRAY BOWEN

Murray Bowen's (1960) ideas about the interactional nature of pathology began during the 1950s when he conducted clinical studies at the National Institute of Mental Health (NIMH) in which entire families lived on a psychiatric ward with their schizophrenic family members. During this project, Bowen noticed the patients and their parents acted in predictable interactional patterns. Anxiety could often be transmitted from one family member to another, and even to other staff members working on the unit. In fact, a family's anxiety often subsided as various members of the unit staff began to take on the anxiety for them. These observations led Bowen to develop a systems concept for schizophrenia and other disorders.

Bowen's ideas evolved through his attempt to bridge the dichotomy between the social and the biological sciences (Bowen, 1978; Friedman, 1991; Kerr & Bowen, 1988). In doing this, he developed a model that moves beyond explaining how families resolve problems to a broadscale theory that attempts to explain humanity's relationship to other natural systems (Friedman, 1991).

A core assumption of Bowen Systems Theory is that families and other natural systems respond in organized, patterned behaviors. This patterned interdependency exists in biological groupings from cells, to individuals, to families, to society in general. This instinctual organizing into repetitive patterns is called the emotional system. Bowen therapists contend that all natural systems are emotional systems, in that they respond in repetitive, predictable ways (Kerr & Bowen, 1988).

Within all living systems is the pull between togetherness and separateness, between being an individual and being part of a group. Bowen coined the term "differentiation" (Bowen, 1978) to address the lifelong process individuals go through to define the self within the family emotional system. Individuals with low levels of differentiation respond in patterned behaviors learned within their families of origin. Those more differentiated individuals are capable of more independent thought and feelings. They know where they end and others begin. Those individuals with lower levels of differentiation respond more reactively, whereas those with higher levels of differentiation respond more proactively. A differentiated individual can respond with either emotions or intellect, as the situation appropriately demands. Therefore, a person who tends to intellectualize in most situations may not necessarily be differentiated. To alleviate this confusion, Friedman (1991) uses the terms "reactive" and "clearheaded."

Differentiation is both an individual and a family phenomenon. Low levels of family differentiation are often maintained in families through the process of emotional cutoff; that is, although individuals may appear to behave more functionally by staying away from certain family members, the anxiety around the cutoff still exists, and other family members may become involved in the process.

Triangles are the basic building blocks of an emotional system and serve to connect individuals to each other. As anxiety builds between two members of a family, a third individual is involved (i.e., triangled) to stabilize the relationship or bind the anxiety (Kerr & Bowen, 1988). Continued repetitions of this pattern over time eventually stabilize it. Triangles and emotionality may be passed down from generation to generation. This is called the multigenerational transmission process. Those children most triangled into parental anxiety have lower levels of differentiation than their siblings. Bowen (1978) believes that individuals marry others of the same level of differentiation. Therefore, over several generations of lower differentiated family members marrying lower differentiated individuals, according to Bowen, a schizophrenic offspring will be the result. Of course, a similar evolution of highly differentiated families is also developing as higher differentiated family members are simultaneously marrying other highly differentiated individuals.

A critical goal of Bowen therapy is to help individuals differentiate from their family's emotional "togetherness." This means that an individual, while staying in contact with key family members, is able to remain an autonomous, clearheaded individual and not fall back into old family patterns. This is accomplished through teaching individuals about family triangles and coaching them to stay outside of them. In doing this, the person disrupts the family pattern and creates a ripple effect that raises the level of differentiation of close family members. This is done, in part, by staying in contact with key family members, and not through emotional cutoffs. As Michael Kerr (1981) states: "The best measure of change in self is the long-term effect it has on others that are important to you. If you 'change' and your family does not, then either you have not changed as much as you think you have or you are using a lot of distance to deal with others" (p. 257).

In March 1967, at a national conference, Bowen described how he had employed his theoretical concepts with his own family of origin (Anonymous, 1972). His provocative presentation helped focus attention on his theory and emphasized the importance of family-of-origin therapy as a viable therapeutic tool. Subsequently, Bowen began using family-of-origin strategies to teach young family therapy residents. Several of these therapists began using detriangling procedures with their own parental families. Bowen noticed that it was these therapists who seemed to be more effective with patient families. Consequently, family-of-origin work with trainees themselves has become one of the most important aspects of training in the Bowen model.

Similarly, Bowen found that helping adult family members differentiate from their own families of origin often has surprisingly positive effects on the patients' relationships with their spouses and children. His findings have led to the use of family-of-origin procedures as the treatment of choice for most family problems. Bowen (1978) states:

Families in which the focus is on the differentiation of self in the families of origin automatically make as much or more progress in working out the relationship system

with spouses and children as families seen in formal family therapy in which there is
a principal focus on the interdependence in the marriage. My experience is going
in the direction of saying that the most productive route to change, for
families who are motivated, is to work at defining self in the family of origin,
and to specifically avoid focus on the emotional issues in the nuclear family.
(p. 545, italics in original)

Bowen coaches his patients to differentiate from their families of origin
by such methods as developing person-to-person relationships with significant family members, becoming better observers, controlling emotional
reactiveness, and learning how to detriangle from emotional family situations (Bowen, 1974).

IVAN BOSZORMENYI-NAGY

Ivan Boszormenyi-Nagy and his colleagues have developed an integrated
systems model, contextual therapy, that focuses on four interacting dimensions of relationships (Boszormenyi-Nagy, Grunebaum, & Ulrich, 1991;
Boszormenyi-Nagy & Krasner, 1986; Boszormenyi-Nagy & Ulrich, 1981).
The first dimension, facts, deals with what is provided by destiny. This has
to do with things that are actually a part of one's life, such as ethnic identity,
gender, physical handicaps, parental divorce, abuse, illness, and so forth.
Psychology, the second dimension, focuses on the meanings individuals
attribute to relationships and facts. Psychological phenomena include cognitions, emotions, fantasies, and other symbolic processes (Boszormenyi-
Nagy et al., 1991).

Transactions, the third dimension, are concerned with the patterns of
organization within the family, such as hierarchy, triangles, and interactional
sequence. The majority of family therapy models have focused on this
dimension.

Dimension four, relational ethics, supersedes the others and serves as
the theoretical cornerstone of contextual therapy. Boszormenyi-Nagy and
colleagues (Boszormenyi-Nagy et al., 1991) state:

> We consider relational ethics to be a fundamental dynamic force, holding
> family and societal relationships together through reliability and trustworthi-
> ness. According to multilateral logic, the balance of fairness among people is
> the most profound and inclusive "cluster" of relationship phenomena. This
> is the context to which the term "contextual therapy" applies. (p. 204)

Innately tied to the focus on relational ethics is the clinical technique
of multidirected partiality. Contextual therapists make sure that the needs
and concerns of all family members are attended to, both as a source of

relational resources for resolving problems and to make sure that family solutions are fair and just for all members. Inherent in this concern are the needs of children and future generations (Boszormenyi-Nagy & Krasner, 1986). Keeping with the ecological imperative of this approach, a solution that negatively affects the needs of future generations is neither ethical nor just.

Key to the relational context of this model is the emphasis on transgenerational entitlements and indebtedness in the formation of symptoms within the family (e.g., Boszormenyi-Nagy, 1965, 1972; Boszormenyi-Nagy et al., 1991; Boszormenyi-Nagy & Krasner, 1986; Boszormenyi-Nagy & Spark, 1973). According to Boszormenyi-Nagy, invisible, often unconscious loyalties or bonds across generations greatly influence present behavior. For example, a scapegoated child's misbehavior may be his or her means of loyally acting out his or her parents' need for a focus of anger (a cycle that may have connections to behavioral sequences begun generations before). Such loyalties arise from the basic human concern for fairness and result in unconscious "ledgers" of what has been given and what is owed. One accumulates merit by the extent to which he or she "balances the ledger." Individuals receive entitlement not only through receiving positive attributions from others, but also through providing to others their fair due.

Boszormenyi-Nagy's concept of the family ledger provides an interesting rationale for a variety of maladaptive behaviors. For example, an abused child may grow up to balance his or her ledger in the only way he or she may know how: by becoming an abusive parent. This is a complicated situation, in that the adult child of abuse has been destructively entitled and has the right to bear a grudge; however, this person lessens his or her own entitlement by destructively entitling his or her own child. This is the continuation of an invisible loyalty with the parent that initially abused the adult as a child. This pattern is altered when the adult chooses to deal with the issues related to the abusive parent and not take them out on the child. The adult can further earn entitlement in this situation by viewing his or her own childhood abuse as a situation that can be overcome through the positive parenting of one's own offspring.

The process of exoneration is a means by which adults earn entitlement by dealing with issues with their own parents. In doing this, adults first recognize how they were victimized by their parents, and then how those parents were also victimized by preceding generations. In this manner, adults come to view their parents less as monsters and more as struggling humans, themselves acting out invisible loyalties. This blocks the transgenerational pattern of destructive entitlement and allows the positive transmission of relational resources.

Ledgers carry a statement of entitlement and indebtedness for each individual in the family. However, the parent–child relationship is asymmetrical, in that the child's entitlement naturally exceeds his or her indebtedness. This is the child's birthright as a member of the future generation (Boszormenyi-Nagy & Krasner, 1986). Although no child can ever fully compensate his or her parents for all they have done, payback occurs through the positive parenting of ones own offspring and/or through dealing with society at large in a just manner. This is a source of entitlement for the individual and his or her parents.

Boszormenyi-Nagy and Ulrich (1981) discuss contextual therapy as a means of dealing directly with the web of invisible loyalties influencing family members' behavior. In contextual therapy, the therapist explores legacies, invisible loyalties, and ledger balances, and thus guides family members toward those tasks necessary to restore some balance in the ledger. The therapist's aim is to "loosen the chains of invisible loyalty and legacy, so each person can give up symptomatic behaviors and explore new options" (Boszormenyi-Nagy & Ulrich, 1981, p. 174). Through contextual therapy, the family's resources for trustworthiness are unlocked, and these allow them to meet the relational needs of all members, exonerate previous generations, and provide a more healthy world for children of future generations to grow and prosper.

JAMES FRAMO

For James Framo, the relationship between intrapsychic and transactional influences is primary. Framo (1980) states:

> It is just as important to know what goes on inside people as to know what goes on between them. . . . I think it is the relationship between the intrapsychic and interpersonal that will provide the greatest understanding and therapeutic leverage, that is, how internalized conflicts from past family relationships are being lived through the spouse and the children in the present. (p. 58)

Framo's (1981, 1982, 1992) theory of symptoms is based largely on the object relations concepts of Fairbairn (1952) and Dicks (1967), described later in this book (see Chapter 11). Framo emphasizes transgenerational projective identification, in which children subtly collude in identifying and acting out the projected "introjects" (i.e., bad objects) of their parents on their spouses and children.

Framo's therapeutic approach employs varied intervention formats, such as couples groups and family-of-origin therapy sessions. Framo (1981) believes that couples group therapy (with groups of three couples) is the treatment of choice in premarital, living-together, marital, and separation or divorce relationship problems. His couples groups place a lesser emphasis on group process than on each couple working for a specified period of time in front of the others and receiving feedback from them. From an object relations perspective, this format enables Framo to avoid some of the projected introjects of the couple as feedback is diffused throughout the group. This enables him to use group leverage to encourage couples to engage in family-of-origin sessions (Framo, 1982).

In virtually all of his couple therapy, Framo suggests that it is extremely helpful to bring in the partners' families of origin at some point during the course of treatment, typically toward the end. This intervention has become the hallmark of his approach. In doing this, each member of the couple is able to decrease the amount of parental introjects projected onto his or her spouse. In effect, they are able to see their spouses without the ghosts of their family of origin occluding their vision (Framo, 1992). The primary goals of these sessions is to "put the burden of responsibility on the individuals to think about and take up with their family the issues about the family relationships that have concerned them throughout the years" (Framo, 1982, p. 174).

Family-of-origin sessions typically include two sessions, each approximately 2 hours long, over the course of a weekend. All family members are expected to attend, with the knowledge that the session can be cancelled if an important member chooses not to come. The therapist coaches the individual on how to approach family members and set an agenda for the session. Framo prefers to conduct these sessions with a cotherapist, as they often can be unpredictable. The cotherapist serves as a life net in case of projective identification on the part of the family to the therapist or vice versa. The individual's spouse is not invited to these sessions to avoid cross-generational triangulation but is allowed to listen to audiotaped recordings (Framo, 1991).

Framo's (1982, 1992) family-of-origin sessions provide important diagnostic information regarding how past family problems are being lived in the present. More important, however, are the corrective experiences of (1) discovering previously unknown information about the family; (2) clarifying old misunderstandings rooted in childhood misperceptions; (3) demystifying magical meanings that family members have for one another; (4) getting to know one's parents as real people; and (5) opening up the possibility of establishing adult-to-adult relationships with one's aging parents. Moreover, Framo (1976, 1992) contends that dealing with the real, external figures (i.e., the adult clients' parents) within the therapy session loosens the grip of the internalized representatives of these figures, with the result that both the adult clients and their parents are freer to be themselves in the future. Having "returned" to their families of origin, the adult clients are subsequently more able to respond to their spouses and children as real people and not as the targets of disowned parts of themselves.

NORMAN PAUL

Norman Paul believes that the feelings family members most tenaciously withhold are those associated with grief. His major contribution involves treatment procedures derived from his contention that a direct relationship exists between family members' maladaptive responses to the death of a loved one and the subsequent rigidity of family patterns. Paul believes that the family tends to return to a "pathological stable equilibrium" when they do not express grief appropriately. A family scapegoat generally maintains this steady state by averting the family's attention away from their recognition of grief (Paul, 1974; Paul & Grosser, 1965).

Paul (1986; Paul & Paul, 1990) believes that a person who does not deal with transgenerational issues is also not able to be empathic to others. By connecting with past issues, the person dissolves the projections they placed previously on others.

The goal of therapy is "operational mourning," in which the family dislodges pathologically fixed patterns, and the grief feelings that they have distorted to maintain the rigid family equilibrium are exposed, released, neutralized, and resolved within therapy (Paul & Grosser, 1965).

In operational mourning, Paul deliberately introduces a belated grief experience through "cross-confrontation" (Paul, 1977). For example, he may directly ask about past losses or may play audio- or videotapes of family members' discussions of such losses.

Paul also has used labels such as "sympathy" and "loyalty" rather than "grief" or "depression" to positively connote what appear to be depressive patterns and incompetent behaviors of family members. His hope is that all family members, scapegoat included, can unite as partners in the same project—mourning a mutual loss rather than being locked into a rigid system of family equilibrium. In all of his work, Paul enables clients to consider unpleasant feelings as normal consequences of living, thus making them easier to be shared.

DONALD WILLIAMSON

Donald Williamson (1981, 1991) hypothesizes that a family life-cycle stage occurs at about the fourth decade of life, the goal of which is to terminate the hierarchical power structures governing the relationships between adults and their older parents. This process involves the redistribution of power between the two generations. Williamson contends that the termination of hierarchical boundaries between adult clients and their "former parents" facilitates the clients' own "personal authority" and encourages a more intimate peer relationship across generations. Williamson believes that the goal of developing "personal authority in the family system" is to promote differentiation between the adults of the second generation and their parents. It is through this process that they begin to see their parents as humans in their own right and not parent figures. This enables the development of true intimacy between the generations. Williamson (1991) states:

> Distinguishing of self from all others and all else begins with the discovery of the self as existing apart from that older man and woman who used to be "Daddy" and "Mummy." One may then move on to be able both to identify with and to find oneself in the face of every other human being (beginning with parents), regardless of all those many things that make us different, sometimes for a brief time even "special." (p. 266)

Williamson (1991) describes his work as being theoretically consistent with transgenerational therapy, stylistically consistent with experiential therapy (see Chapter 4), and technically consistent with strategic therapy (see Chapter 3). Running through all of his work is a strong thread of social constructionism. Personal authority work is a way for individuals to rewrite their perception of their family's story by creating a new narrative of equalitarianism and intimacy with their parents (Williamson, 1991).

Williamson (1982a, 1991), perhaps more than any other intergenerational family therapist, has clearly described the procedures he uses to effect change in the power structure across generations. He suggests the assignment of a series of tasks (e.g., the writing of an autobiography, the making of audiotaped letters to each parent, the audiotaping of telephone conversations with each parent), much of which is presented and practiced in a group with other clients over several months. This serves as preparation for a 3-day, in-office consultation with the adult client and his or her parents.

In this consultation, the therapist allows the client freedom and authority to renegotiate the politics of his or her relationship with the parents. The adult client, first talking with each parent separately and then together, deals with a variety of issues and at some point simply and poignantly declares, "I am no longer your little girl (or little boy)" (Williamson, 1982a, p. 34). After an appropriate period of debriefing, a supportive peer relationship develops in which grief, anxiety, happiness, guilt, and other strong emotions are shared freely among all members of the family.

Although Williamson's goal of intergenerational "peerhood" may seem solemn and forbidding, he addresses therapy with playfulness and humor that both support the family members and remind them of the absurdity of the human condition (Williamson, 1982b, 1991). Williamson's humor also helps diffuse the intensity of emotional issues and often takes the form of relabeling and paradoxical statements, which are more typically associated with structural and strategic therapies.

Williamson's work is unique among the transgenerational theorists, in that he has tested his ideas through an organized research program. From this, Williamson and colleagues developed the Personal Authority in the Family System Questionnaire (Bray, Williamson, & Malone, 1984) and have generated initial support for the theory (Bray, Harvey, & Williamson, 1987; Harvey & Bray, 1991; Harvey, Curry, & Bray, 1991) and the clinical model (Bray, Williamson, & Malone, 1986).

KEY CONCEPTS

Differentiation of self. This is the extent to which one's emotional and intellectual systems are distinguishable. According to Bowen's (1978) theory, the more autonomous one's intellect is from automatic emotional forces, the more differentiated one is.

Differentiation of Self Scale. This theoretical scale was postulated by Bowen (1978) for evaluating the lowest possible level of "undifferentiation," which is 0 on the scale, to the highest level of "differentiation," which is 100 on the scale. One's degree of undifferentiation (no self) is directly correlated with one's degree of emotional fusion into a common self with others. The scale, then, is a means of conceptualizing one's basic level of self.

Emotional cutoff. In the process of separation, isolation, withdrawal, running away, or denying the importance of one's parental family, dealing with unresolved attachment may be problematic. According to Bowen (1978), "the more intense the cutoff with the past, the more likely the individual is to have an exaggerated version of his parental family problem in his own marriage" (p. 382).

Emotional system. Kerr and Bowen (1988) believe that all natural systems respond in a patterned, reactive manner. Due to the development of the cerebral cortex, humans have the ability to operate as individuals rather than fuse into old family patterns. However, the greater the amount of anxiety in a system, the greater the likelihood that its members will behave in a reactive manner rather than as clearheaded individuals.

Entitlement. This is the amount of merit a person accrues for behaving in an ethical manner with others. Boszormenyi-Nagy and Krasner (1986) believe that the amount of entitlement individuals earn is related to the freedom they have in relating to others.

Family projection process. According to Bowen (1978), this is a process in which parents may project part of their immaturity onto one or more of their children. The child who is the object of the projection develops the lowest level of differentiation of self and is more likely to be symptomatic in the future.

Ledger. According to Boszormenyi-Nagy and Ulrich (1981), this is an accumulation of the accounts of what has been given and what is owed. Merit may be accumulated through contribution to the welfare of another, whereas debts and entitlements relate to the relative balance of the ledger. For example, a kind, alcoholic father may accrue entitlements from his daughter that she then unconsciously "pays back" by becoming a nun.

Legacy. According to Boszormenyi-Nagy (1976), legacy is a specific configuration of expectations that originate, not from the merit of the parents, but simply from the universal implication of being born of parents. In other words, there is a chain of destiny anchored in every parent–child relationship. Certain debts and entitlements are dictated by one's legacy, and payment of debts typically occurs in the way one has been taught to pay. For example, an abused child may become a child-abusing parent.

Loyalty. Loyalty is a central concept of Boszormenyi-Nagy and Spark (1973) in understanding family behavior. Internalized expectations, injunctions, and obligations in relation to one's family of origin have powerful interpersonal influences. What to an outsider may seem like irrational or pathological behavior may, in fact, conform to a basic family loyalty. For example, a scapegoated, irresponsible child may be unconsciously acting out this loyalty message: "I will be the bad one to help you look good, since you have done so much for me."

Multigenerational transmission process. This is a pattern that develops over several generations, in which children grow up and marry partners with similar levels of differentiation to themselves. Bowen (1978) believes that schizophrenia is the result of several generations of individuals with low levels of differentiating ("weak links") marrying other low-level individuals and producing one or more children with low levels of differentiation. Bowen believes it may take several generations for such a process to develop a schizophrenic offspring.

Nuclear family emotional system. Bowen (1978) uses the term "emotional system" to describe the triangular emotional patterns typical of all close relationships. In the nuclear family emotional system, parental undifferentiation may produce (1) marital conflict, (2) dysfunction in a spouse, and/or (3) projection to one or more children.

Personal authority in the family system. This is described by Williamson (1982b) as a synthesizing construct arising from the Hegelian dialectic of autonomy and intimacy. When an individual has personal authority, he or she is in charge of his or her own thoughts and opinions, acts freely and responsibly, and maintains appropriate social connection with others.

Relational ethics. Boszormenyi-Nagy and Krasner (1986) state that life is a chain of interlocking consequences between the generations. The behavior of an individual is both rooted in the past and has the ability to affect future generations. Because of this, individuals are ethically responsible for the consequences of their behaviors.

Sibling position. Birth order is emphasized by both Toman (1961) and

Bowen (1978) as an important factor in the development of personality characteristics. Bowen also suggests that sibling position is useful in understanding how a particular child is chosen as the object of the family projection process.

Societal regression. This is a concept applying Bowen's (Kerr & Bowen, 1988) theory to society in general; that is, during periods of societal anxiety, society responds emotionally with problematic "Band-Aid" legislation that simply increases problems. What is needed is better differentiation between emotion and intellect, allowing more constructive societal decisions to be made.

Triangle. A triangle is a three-person system, according to Bowen (1978), the smallest stable relationship system. Bowen contends that a two-person system is an unstable system that forms a triangle under stress. More than three people in a system form themselves into a series of interlocking triangles.

KEY CLINICAL SKILLS

Transgenerational family therapy skills are not as easily isolated, identified, or operationalized as are those in present-centered, problem-focused therapies, such as behavioral and strategic family therapy. Perhaps this is because such goals as differentiation, insight, and renegotiation of interpersonal power are emphasized more in transgenerational family therapies than are explicit problem-centered techniques. This is not to say that transgenerational family therapies are void of systematic procedures to meet these goals (cf. Framo, 1992; Williamson, 1991), but simply that these procedures can more typically be considered clinical processes than skills. The following are several representative clinical processes/skills.

Coaching. A term used by Bowen (1978), "coaching" describes his role in supervising patients and trainees in the process of differentiation of self. Bowen believes that his relationship is similar to that of a coach's relationship to an athlete, in that his initial goal is to get the patient (and trainee) started. However, the actual work is done by the patient, and the learning comes as the patient works toward his or her goal outside the therapy session.

Cross-confrontation and self-confrontation. Norman Paul uses with his clients emotionally charged "stressor stimuli" in the form of audio- and videotapes (often of former clients), letters, pieces of literature, and poems in order to normalize unpleasant feeling states. His clients' reactions to these stressor stimuli are also audio- or videotaped and are later played back to them as a type of self-confrontation (Paul, 1977).

Detriangling. This is the process whereby an individual keeps him- or herself (or someone else) outside the emotional field of two others. For example, because spouses will automatically attempt to involve a third person when anxiety increases, if the therapist can stay rational and not respond as others do to their emotional attempts at triangulation, then the spouses can begin to deal more directly with each other, and patterns can change.

Exoneration. In contextual family therapy (Boszormenyi-Nagy & Krasner, 1986), exoneration is a process by which the therapist attempts to help the client see the positive intent and intergenerational loyalty issues behind the behavior of members of previous generations. Regardless of how destructive their behavior may have been to the client, if their behavior can be seen in a human context, exoneration occurs, loosening the hold of the past behavior on the client.

Genogram. A written symbolic diagram of the family system, the genogram is not unlike a "family tree." Many transgenerational therapists use the genogram both diagnostically and therapeutically (e.g., McGoldrick & Gersen, 1985).

Multidirected partiality. At the core of the practice of contextual therapy (Boszormenyi-Nagy & Krasner, 1986) is the clinical stance that therapists are accountable to everyone whose well being is potentially affected by their interventions. This stance requires that therapists keep channels open among all family members and that all solutions serve the best interests of everyone.

Operational mourning. Norman Paul (1974) states that "there is a direct relationship between the maladaptive response to the death of a loved one and the fixity of symbolic relationships within the family." Operational mourning, according to Paul, involves dislodging those fixed and distorted feelings through introducing a belated grief experience. In therapy, these feelings, which are often associated with grief, can be neutralized and resolved through empathic intervention and procedures such as cross-confrontation.

Person-to-person relationships. This is a relationship in which two family members relate personally to each other about each other; that is, they do not talk about others (triangling) and do not talk about impersonal issues. Person-to-person relationships among family members may be facilitated, for example, by having an adult patient write separate letters to "Mother" and "Father," and by having him or her spend portions of visits home in personal discussions with each alone.

TEACHING TOOLS AND TECHNIQUES

Training Videotapes

A list and description of videotapes that discuss and/or demonstrate transgenerational family therapies may be secured from the following:

- *AAMFT Master Series*, AAMFT, 1133 15th Street, N.W., Suite 300, Washington, DC 20005-2710.

- Georgetown Family Center, 4400 MacArthur Boulevard, N.W., Washington, DC 20007.
- Menninger Video Productions, exclusively distributed by Altschul Group Corporation, 1560 Sherman Avenue, Suite 100, Evanston, IL 60201.

Family Autobiography

Students may be asked to write a 15- to 20-page family autobiography in which they discuss the dynamics of their own families of origin, utilizing the terminology and theoretical rational of such writers as Bowen (1978), Framo (1992), Williamson (1991), and Boszormenyi-Nagy and Krasner (1986). Although such a retrospective analysis is obviously biased, it does provide students the opportunity to apply ideas from family-of-origin readings to personally meaningful family relationships.

Nicknames from the Past

As an introductory exercise, students/trainees can each be asked to think of two labels (nicknames, adjectives, or phrases) that were often applied to them as children—one that felt positive and one that felt negative. Then have them mill around the room and introduce themselves to each person in the room by these traits. For example, one student might say, "Hi, I'm Joe. I'm irresponsible and can really catch a football." After the milling, ask each person to find a partner and discuss the derivation of the descriptions or labels he or she used, where they came from, and what they mean. Each dyad should also discuss whether the labels are true today. If not, what happened to them? (This exercise is adapted from Duhl, 1983.)

Family-of-Origin Audiotape

One of the sequential steps that Williamson (1982a) suggests adult clients engage in to begin negotiating "peership" with their parents is an audiotape exercise. Williamson's clients are asked to make an audiotape to each of their parents in which they tell each parent reactions to growing up in their family, as well as any "unfinished business" related to their past and/or present relationships with their parents. Students may be asked to do the same thing in order to make Williamson's process more immediate and meaningful. Students are then asked to write reaction papers describing how they felt while making the audiotapes to their parents and what they may have learned. In order to make this assignment less anxiety provoking, students are not required to turn in the audiotapes or give them to their parent.

Simulation Activities

Simulation activities may include written papers that allow students to apply the concepts they are learning from their readings. For example, the following is a simulation assignment intended to strengthen students' understanding of transgenerational concepts:

> Choose a character from literature, stage, screen, radio, or TV who has some problematic characteristic or personality trait. Using concepts from transgenerational theory, discuss possible etiology and present purpose of this characteristic. Also discuss how a psychotherapy based on transgenerational theory might be employed to deal with your character's problematic trait.

Birth-Order Exercise

The students/trainees may be asked to divide into the following four groups based upon their sibling positions in their own families of origin: (1) oldest child, (2) youngest child, (3) middle child, and (4) only child. The members of these groups then discuss their early growing-up years and what roles and ways of "fitting in" they developed within their families. Each person should note any trends within his or her group. These trends are later presented by a group spokesperson to the rest of the class. After each group spokesperson's report, the instructor summarizes what Toman (1961) has written about the particular sibling position of that group.

Open-Ended Sentences

In groups of three or four, students are asked to briefly discuss their answers to the following open-ended sentences related to their own families of origin:

- The family I come from could best be described as . . .
- In my family, my mother was always the one who . . .
- In my family, my father was always the one who . . .
- In my family, I was always the one who . . .
- If there was a topic that couldn't be discussed in my family, it was . . .
- The greatest strength about my family was . . .
- Disagreement in my family was handled by . . .
- I learned from my mother that . . .
- I learned from my father that . . .
- My siblings taught me . . .
- To me, family "events" (birthdays, holidays, etc.) were . . .

- An emotion rarely expressed in my family was . . .
- In my family, I usually felt closest to . . .
- In my family, I usually felt most distant from . . .
- When I was out in public with my family, I usually felt . . .
- A myth my family perpetuated was . . .
- If I were to supply a title for a book about living with my family, it would be entitled . . .
- What I like best about my family is . . .
- If I could change anything about my family, it would be . . .

(This exercise is adapted from Janine Roberts, personal communication, 1984.)

Family Myths

1. Students/trainees may be asked to write down stories about their families of origin for each of these categories:
   a. Interactional scenarios of events that were repetitive.
   b. Legends that have been passed down from generation to generation.
   c. A story commonly told to outsiders about the family.

2. Then students/trainees are asked to write down and/or discuss rules of communication within their family, highlighting the following:
   a. What could be discussed within the family?
   b. What could be discussed outside the family?
   c. What could not be discussed directly?

3. Students/trainees then identify family-of-origin themes emerging from the preceding information:
   a. Themes that can be discussed and challenged.
   b. Themes, or family myths, that are not discussed or challenged openly (i.e., people tend to share the same "party line").

(This exercise is also adapted from Janine Roberts, personal communication, 1984.)

RESEARCH ISSUES

Charismatic figures such as Murray Bowen and James Framo have identified some important concepts that have considerable clinical utility.

Unfortunately, they defend their therapies with more vigor than rigor. Although family-of-origin issues are beginning to be examined empirically (e.g., Bray et al., 1984; Hovestadt, Anderson, Piercy, Cochran, & Fine, 1985), virtually no experimental research has been conducted on the effectiveness of transgenerational family therapies; however, these therapies are researchable at both the micro- and macrolevels, as are their underpinning theoretical assumptions. The first necessary step is to operationalize such fuzzy concepts as "triangling," "detriangling," and "personal authority." For example, degree of differentiation could be measured by an appropriately developed self-report scale or operationally defined as the peripheral skin temperature and/or heart rate of a family member at the time he or she is criticized by two other family members. Given appropriate concretization of terms, research questions such as the following could begin to be addressed:

- Is triangling likely to occur at times of high anxiety?
- Which of the differentiation procedures mentioned by Bowen (1978), Williamson (1982a, 1991), and Framo (1976, 1992) are most likely to result in differentiation of self?
- Do people marry partners with the same general level of differentiation?
- What effects do family-of-origin therapies have on present family functioning?
- Is complete separation and isolation from one's family of origin (i.e., "emotional cutoff") detrimental to one's present marriage?
- To what extent is one's degree of differentiation of self related to measures of individual, marital, and family health?
- Is level of therapist differentiation positively related to the degree of change in differentiation achieved by clients?
- Is therapy training that incorporates family-of-origin activities more effective than similar therapy training that does not incorporate such activities? (Many outcome measures could be used for such a study. An important one, however, would be the extent to which the clients of the therapists in each group achieve their goals in therapy.)
- Which of the therapist skills associated with a particular family-of-origin therapy (e.g., the contextual family therapy of Boszormenyi-Nagy) are most positively related to symptom reduction?
- What is the degree of the relationship between unresolved grief and the severity of particular presenting problems? When unresolved grief is dealt with in therapy, do presenting problems decrease in severity? Are changes maintained over time?
- What is the relationship between level of differentiation in a therapist's family of origin and his or her effectiveness in therapy?

KEY BOOKS, CHAPTERS, AND ARTICLES

Anonymous. (1972). On the differentiation of self. In J. Framo (Ed.), *Family interaction: A dialogue between family researchers and family therapists.* New York: Springer.

This classic chapter, written anonymously by Murray Bowen, describes his long-term efforts to differentiate from his own family of origin. His account is often moving and provides an excellent example of Bowen Systems Theory in practice.

Boszormenyi-Nagy, I. (1987). *Foundations of contextual therapy: Collected papers of Ivan Boszormenyi-Nagy, M.D.* New York: Brunner/Mazel.

This book is a collection of the important papers of Ivan Boszormenyi-Nagy, presenting a historic account of the theoretical development of contextual therapy. Each chapter is preceded by a brief discussion placing it in historical and theoretical context. Issues related to loyalty, trust, and ethics are discussed.

Boszormenyi-Nagy, I., Grunebaum, J., & Ulrich, D. (1991). Contextual therapy. In A. S. Gurman & D. P. Kniskern (Eds.), *Handbook of family therapy* (Vol. 2). New York: Brunner/Mazel.

This chapter presents a concise, up-to-date overview of contextual therapy. The authors discuss relational ethics in both the family and therapy contexts. Perhaps this chapter's greatest strength is as a good introduction to contextual therapy.

Boszormenyi-Nagy, I, & Krasner, B. R. (1986). *Between give and take: A clinical guide to contextual therapy.* New York: Brunner/Mazel.

This excellent text provides an in-depth look at the theory and practice of contextual therapy. It provides a detailed discussion of the interrelationship of the dimensions of relational reality and is especially noteworthy for its solid presentation on the issues of relational ethics. The authors illustrate concepts through numerous clinical studies and vignettes. This is perhaps the best single source on contextual therapy to date.

Boszormenyi-Nagy, I., & Spark, G. M. (1973). *Invisible loyalties: Reciprocity in intergenerational family therapy.* New York: Harper & Row.

In this classic, Boszormenyi-Nagy and Spark describe the powerful influences of loyalty commitments across generations. Presenting problems are explained in terms of "balancing the ledger" within the family. Although the obfuscatory style of this book makes for difficult reading, its influence on the field renders it an important text for those interested in transgenerational family therapy.

Bowen, M. (1978). *Family therapy in clinical practice.* Northvale, NJ: Jason Aronson.

This book is a collection of Murray Bowen's most important papers from 1957 to 1977, including reports on his clinical research at NIMH with schizophrenics and their families between 1954 and 1959, important papers on the development of his theory, and the much-discussed "Anonymous" piece in which Bowen chronicles his attempts at differentiation from his own family of origin.

Bray, J. H., Williamson, D. S., & Malone, P. E. (1984). Personal authority in the family system: Development of a questionnaire to measure personal authority in intergenerational family processes. *Journal of Marital and Family Therapy, 10,* 167–178.

This article presents the development of the Personal Authority in the Family System Questionnaire. The reliability and validity of this scale, derived from Williamson's theory, is discussed.

Framo, J. L. (1976). Family of origin as a therapeutic resource for adults in marital and family therapy: You can and should go home again. *Family Process, 15,* 193–210.

This is a pioneering article on Framo's brand of family-of-origin therapy. Framo clearly describes both the theory and practice of his approach. His theory, based on the object relations concepts of Fairbairn and Dicks, emphasizes the importance of clients confronting their parents face-to-face in order to "loosen the grip of the internal representatives of these figures" (p. 194). This article is must reading for any student of family-of-origin therapy.

Framo, J. L. (1982). *Explorations in marital and family therapy: Selected papers of James L. Framo, Ph.D.* New York: Springer.

This book includes some of the most important papers of James Framo, whose approach to therapy includes both intrapsychic and interpersonal dimensions. In this collection he writes about his theoretical orientation and his methods of working with families, couples, couples groups, divorcing couples, and family of origin. He also discusses personal aspects of being a family therapist. His article on conducting family-of-origin work is destined to become a classic.

Framo, J. L. (1992). *Family-of-origin therapy: An intergenerational approach.* New York: Brunner/Mazel.

This is the most comprehensive text on Framo's model of family therapy. While focusing primarily on the family-of-origin sessions, he combines a solid theoretical rationale with excellent case examples. This book is a first-rate treatment manual for understanding and replicating this model. Framo concludes this book with a moving autobiography.

Freeman, D. S. (1992). *Family therapy with couples: The family-of-origin approach.* Northvale, NJ: Jason Aronson.

This book proposes that by resolving family-of-origin issues, clients are better able to form intimate relationships with their spouses. The middle phase of marital therapy is exemplified in a three-step process that includes (1) rethinking one's family story, (2) returning home to interview family members, and (3) engaging with one's parents and siblings in a family-of-origin session.

Freeman, D. S. (1992). *Multigenerational family therapy.* Binghamton, NY: Haworth.

This well-written book provides a harmonious interplay between verbatim therapy segments and explanations of theory and technique. It presents a step-by-step guide to conducting family therapy that substantively fleshes out the framework of Bowen's family systems theory. Specific characteristics of change are identified as contextualized in the beginning, middle, and ending stages of therapy. The book provides innovative methods of transgenerational family therapy with couples, individuals, siblings, and parents.

Friedman, E. H. (1985). *Generation to generation: Family process in church and synagogue.* New York: Guilford Press.

This book provides a thorough discussion of Bowen Systems Theory as it applies to emotional process in religious institutions. Although geared toward the clergy, it is an excellent source for clinicians wishing to deepen their understanding of Bowen's ideas.

Friedman, E. H. (1991). Bowen theory and therapy. In A. S. Gurman & D. S. Kniskern (Eds.), *Handbook of family therapy* (Vol. 2). New York: Brunner/Mazel.

This is perhaps the single best chapter for those wishing to understand the premises of Bowen Systems Theory. Rather than briefly describing the whole theory, Friedman focuses on the constructs of chronic anxiety, differentiation, emotional system, and multigenerational transmission. Especially important is Friedman's discussion on continuity versus dichotomies in understanding natural systems.

Hovestadt, A., Anderson, W., Piercy, F., Fine, M., & Cochran, S. (1985). A family-of-origin scale. *Journal of Marital and Family Therapy, 11*(3), 287–298.

This article presents the development and psychometric properties of a scale for measuring the perceived health of one's family of origin. The scale is easy to administer and has acceptable reliability and validity data. It provides a useful measure for those interested in conducting family-of-origin research.

Kerr, M. E., & Bowen, M. (1988). *Family evaluation.* New York: Norton.

This excellent text is the most comprehensive source on Bowen Systems Theory to date. The authors thoroughly discuss concepts such as the emotional system, individuality versus togetherness, anxiety, triangles, and the multigenerational transmission process. Furthermore, the book provides a fine explanation of the biological relationship between families and other natural systems. The book concludes with a chapter by Bowen on the evolution of his approach.

Kramer, J. R. (1985). *Family interfaces: Transgenerational patterns.* New York: Brunner/Mazel.

This book does an excellent job of presenting the multiple levels of family interactions that exist in therapy. The author examines how transgenerational patterns affect families in therapy, as well as how therapists' families of origin affect their behavior. The final section of the book presents the use of family-of-origin groups as a training format for family therapists.

McGoldrick, M., & Gerson, R. (1985). *Genograms in family assessment.* New York: Norton.

This readable little book provides a rationale and specific procedures for constructing, interpreting, and using genograms. The usefulness of genograms in family assessment is clearly illustrated in the many examples provided. The authors creatively maintain the reader's interest by providing fascinating, illustrative genograms of the families of such notables as Sigmund Freud, Gregory Bateson, John Quincy Adams, Alfred Adler, Jane Fonda, the Brontë sisters, F. Scott Fitzgerald, Virginia Woolf, and John F. Kennedy.

Papero, D. V. (1990). *Bowen family systems theory.* Needham Heights, MA: Allyn & Bacon.

This excellent book provides a concise yet extensive overview of Bowen theory and practice. The family unit is placed in the context of other biological systems and evolution. The authors explain the core tenets of the theory, provide clinical examples, and describe the process and elements that go into training in family systems theory.

Paul, N. L. (1967). The role of mourning and empathy in conjoint marital therapy. In G. H. Zuk & I. Boszormenyi-Nagy (Eds.), *Family therapy and disturbed families.* Palo Alto, CA: Science and Behavior Books.

This key chapter discusses how incompletely mourned losses are often hidden in marital difficulties. With his classic "Lewis couple" case study, Paul demonstrates the use of operational mourning combined with therapist empathy in neutralizing the long-term effects of hidden grief.

Paul, N. L., & Grosser, G. (1965). Operational mourning and its role in conjoint family therapy. *Community Mental Health Journal, 1*(4), 339–345.

This cornerstone work of Norman Paul is well written and is still not outdated. Paul and Grosser maintain that incompleted mourning is a defense against further losses and is often transmitted unwittingly to other family members, especially offspring. The resulting interaction patterns promote a fixated family equilibrium. The authors describe their technique of operational mourning, which is designed to involve the family in a belated grief reaction. The shared affective experience can create empathy and understanding of the origins of current relational difficulties, and can weaken the maladaptive family equilibrium. The authors furnish a case illustration.

Paul, N. L., & Paul, B. B. (1975). *The marital puzzle.* New York: Norton.

This book demonstrates the importance of transgenerational themes in affecting present marital interactions. The Pauls' ideas are presented through the use of a full-length transcription of a marital case study and added comments on diagnosis and treatment procedures. The authors present the use of operational mourning and cross-confrontation within the flow of the therapy process.

Paul, N. L., & Paul, B. B. (1990). Enhancing empathy in couples: A transgenerational approach. In R. Chasin, H. Grunebaum, & M. Herzig (Eds.), *One couple, four realities: Multiple perspectives on couple therapy.* New York: Guilford Press.

This chapter presents concise discussions on the interplay of transgenerational themes, empathy, and videotape playback in marital therapy. The highlight of the chapter is an interesting case study exemplifying the Pauls' ideas.

Roberto, L. G. (1992). *Transgenerational family therapies.* New York: Guilford Press.

This book provides an extensive overview of transgenerational family therapies. The first section summarizes the transgenerational theories and contributions made by Bowen, Whitaker, Boszormenyi-Nagy, and psychoanalytic theorists. The second section expands the theory of transgenerational work to therapy and demonstrates how the therapist may best select goals, make effective use of genograms, assess transgenerational systems, create a frame for therapy, and conduct therapy. The concluding section offers suggestions for training transgenerational family therapists.

Sager, C. J. (1976). *Marriage contracts and couple therapy.* New York: Brunner/Mazel.

The central concept of this book is that each partner in a marriage brings to it an individual, unwritten contract, a set of conscious and unconscious expectations and promises based in part on transgenerational influences. Sager presents procedures for helping couples uncover and explore the various written and unspoken terms of their individual contracts. The goal of Sager's approach to therapy is to help partners make quid pro quo concessions, working toward a single joint contract that is agreed upon at all levels of awareness.

Titleman, P. (Ed.). (1987). *The therapist's own family: Toward differentiation of self.* Northvale, NJ: Jason Aronson.

This book is a collection of many therapists' work within their own families of origin. It provides a unique perspective into this process, due to the fact that each chapter is written by a different therapist. The chapters were chosen carefully so that no two focus on the same principles. The reader is left with a variety of examples on how to deal with their own family issues.

van Heusden, A., & van den Eerenbeemt, E. (1987). *Balance in motion: Ivan Boszormenyi-Nagy and his vision of individual and family therapy.* New York: Brunner/Mazel.

This book is an excellent primer on contextual therapy. It is especially noteworthy for its clear, concise discussion of theoretical ideas. Furthermore, it presents an interview with Boszormenyi-Nagy on the development of contextual therapy and one of his clinical consultations with a couple.

Williamson, D. S. (1981). Termination of the intergenerational hierarchical boundary between the first and second generation: A "new" stage in the family life cycle. *Journal of Marital and Family Therapy, 7,* 441–452.

This is the first of Williamson's excellent trilogy on renegotiating the power structures between adults and their older parents. This well-written article presents a compelling rationale for the need to redistribute intergenerational power in the direction of equality.

Williamson, D. S. (1982a). Personal authority via termination of the intergenerational hierarchical boundary: Part II. The consultation process and the therapeutic method. *Journal of Marital and Family Therapy, 8,* 23–37.

The author describes his family-of-origin approach by outlining the successive steps used in helping adult clients renegotiate a more emotionally equal peer relationship with their older parents. These steps culminate in a 3-day in-office consultation between the client and his or her parents. This is one of the most specific, pragmatic, and well-written papers on conducting family-of-origin therapy.

Williamson, D. S. (1982b). Personal authority in family experience via termination of the intergenerational hierarchical boundary: Part III. Personal authority defined, and the power of play in the change process. *Journal of Marital and Family Therapy, 8,* 309–323.

Williamson suggests personal authority as a synthesizing construct arising from the Hegelian dialectic of autonomy and intimacy; however, the real contribution of the article is in Williamson's enchanting and clever uses of paradox and play in the application of his transgenerational approach.

Williamson, D. S. (1991). *The intimacy paradox: Personal authority in the family system.* New York: Guilford Press.

This book provides a thorough presentation of the theoretical and clinical aspects of Williamson's "personal authority in the family system" model. This book serves as a comprehensive treatment manual for utilizing Williamson's approach. Furthermore, personal authority is discussed as it relates to gender issues and family health. Also of note is a chapter discussing the current research on the theory and practice of this approach.

REFERENCES

Anonymous. (1972). On the differentiation of self. In J. Framo (Ed.), *Family interaction: A dialogue between family researchers and family therapists.* New York: Springer.

Boszormenyi-Nagy, I. (1965). A theory of relationships: Experience and transaction. In I. Boszormenyi-Nagy & J. Framo (Eds.), *Intensive family therapy: Theoretical and practical aspects.* New York: Harper & Row.

Boszormenyi-Nagy, I. (1972). Loyalty implications of the transference model in psychotherapy. *Archives of General Psychiatry, 27,* 374–380.

Boszormenyi-Nagy, I. (1976). Behavior change through family change. In A. Burton (Ed.), *What makes behavior change possible?* New York: Brunner/Mazel.

Boszormenyi-Nagy, I., Grunebaum, J., & Ulrich, D. (1991). Contextual therapy. In

A. S. Gurman & D. S. Kniskern (Eds.), *Handbook of family therapy* (Vol. II). New York: Brunner/Mazel.

Boszormenyi-Nagy, I., & Krasner, B. R. (1986). *Between give and take: A clinical guide to contextual therapy.* New York: Guilford Press.

Boszormenyi-Nagy, I., & Spark, G. M. (1973). *Invisible loyalties: Reciprocity in intergenerational family therapy.* New York: Harper & Row.

Boszormenyi-Nagy, I., & Ulrich, D. N. (1981). Contextual family therapy. In A. S. Gurman & D. P. Kniskern (Eds.), *Handbook of family therapy.* New York: Brunner/Mazel.

Bowen, M. (1960). A family concept of schizophrenia. In D. D. Jackson (Ed.), *The etiology of schizophrenia.* New York: Basic Books.

Bowen, M. (1974). Toward the differentiation of self in one's family of origin. In F. Andres & J. Loris (Eds.), *Georgetown Family Symposium papers.* Washington,DC: Georgetown University Press.

Bowen, M. (1978). *Family therapy in clinical practice.* Northvale, NJ: Jason Aronson.

Bray, J. H., Harvey, D. M., & Williamson, D. S. (1987). Intergenerational family relationships: An evaluation of theory and measurement. *Psychotherapy, 24,* 516–528.

Bray, J. H., Williamson, D. S., & Malone, P. E. (1984). Personal authority in the family system: Development of a questionnaire to measure personal authority in intergenerational family processes. *Journal of Marital and Family Therapy, 10,* 167–178.

Bray, J. H., Williamson, D. S., & Malone, P. E. (1986). An evaluation of the effects of intergenerational consultation process to increase personal authority in the family system. *Family Process, 25,* 423–436.

Dicks, H. (1967). *Marital tensions.* New York: Basic Books.

Duhl, B. S. (1983). *From the inside out and other metaphors: Creative and integrative approaches to training in systems thinking.* New York: Brunner/Mazel.

Fairbairn, W. R. D. (1952). *An object-relations theory of the personality.* New York: Basic Books.

Framo, J. L. (1976). Family of origin as a therapeutic resource for adults in marital and family therapy: You can and should go home again. *Family Process, 15,* 193–210.

Framo, J. L. (1980). Marriage and marital therapy: Issues and initial interview techniques. In M. Andolfi & I. Zwerling (Eds.), *Dimensions of family therapy.* New York: Guilford Press.

Framo, J. L. (1981). The integration of marital therapy with sessions with family of origin. In A. S. Gurman & D. P. Kniskern (Eds.), *Handbook of family therapy.* New York: Brunner/Mazel.

Framo, J. L. (1982). *Explorations in marital and family therapy: Selected papers of James L. Framo.* New York: Springer.

Framo, J. L. (1992). *Family-of-origin therapy: An intergenerational approach.* New York: Brunner/Mazel.

Friedman, E. H. (1991). Bowen theory and therapy. In A. S. Gurman & D. P. Kniskern (Eds.), *Handbook of family therapy*. New York: Brunner/Mazel.

Harvey, D. M., & Bray, J. H. (1991). An evaluation of an intergenerational theory of personal development: Family process determinants of psychological and health distress. *Journal of Family Psychology, 4*, 42–69.

Harvey, D. M., Curry, C. J., & Bray, J. H. (1991). Individuation/intimacy in intergenerational relationships and health: Patterns across two generations. *Journal of Family Psychology, 4*, 204–236.

Hovestadt, A., Anderson, W., Piercy, F., Cochran, S., & Fine, M. (1985). A family of origin scale. *Journal of Marital and Family Therapy, 11*(3), 287–297.

Kerr, M. E. (1981). Family systems theory and therapy. In A. S. Gurman & D. P. Kniskern (Eds.), *Handbook of family therapy*. New York: Brunner/Mazel.

Kerr, M. E., & Bowen, M. (1988). *Family evaluation*. New York: Norton.

McGoldrick, M., & Gerson, R. (1985). *Genograms in family assessment*. New York: Norton.

Paul, N. (1974). The use of empathy in the resolution of grief. In J. Ellard et al., (Eds.), *Normal and pathological responses to bereavement*. New York: MSS Information Corporation.

Paul, N. (1977). Cross-confrontation. In P. Guerin (Ed.), *Family therapy: Theory and practice*. New York: Gardner.

Paul, N. (1986). The paradoxical nature of the grief experience. *Contemporary Family Therapy, 8*, 5–19.

Paul, N., & Grosser, G. (1965). Operational mourning and its role in conjoint family therapy. *Community Mental Health Journal, 1*(4), 339–345.

Paul, N., & Paul, B. B. (1990). Enhancing empathy in couples: A transgenerational approach. In R. Chasin, H. Grunebaum, & M. Herzig (Eds.), *One couple, four realities: Multiple perspectives on couple therapy*. New York: Guilford Press.

Toman, W. (1961). *Family constellation*. New York: Springer.

Williamson, D. S. (1981). Personal authority via termination of the intergenerational hierarchical boundary: A "new" stage in the family life cycle. *Journal of Marital and Family Therapy, 7*, 441–452.

Williamson, D. S. (1982a). Personal authority in family experience via termination of the intergenerational hierarchical boundary: Part II. The consultation process and the therapeutic method. *Journal of Marital and Family Therapy, 8*, 23–37.

Williamson, D. S. (1982b). Personal authority in family experience via termination of the intergenerational hierarchical boundary: Part III. Personal authority defined, and the power of play in the change process. *Journal of Marital and Family Therapy, 8*(3), 309–323.

Williamson, D. S. (1991). *The intimacy paradox: Personal authority in the family system*. New York: Guilford Press.

3

Structural, Strategic, and Systemic Family Therapies

FRED P. PIERCY
JOSEPH L. WETCHLER

STRATEGIC FAMILY THERAPY

Strategic family therapy and structural family therapy were born on different coasts of the United States. Strategic family therapy has its roots in the Palo Alto research group led by Gregory Bateson in the early 1950s. As part of his research on family communication, Bateson began to look at schizophrenia as a discrepancy between levels of communication. Jay Haley, John Weakland, and Don D. Jackson joined the Bateson project, and in 1956 their paper "Toward a Theory of Schizophrenia" influenced therapists throughout the country to examine the double-binding communications of family members.

During the 1960s, many articles were written by Jackson and his associates at the Mental Research Institute (MRI) in Palo Alto, describing communicational strategies as devices for escaping or establishing definitions of intrafamilial relationships (see Hoffman, 1981, p. 23). Strategic family therapy evolved largely from this work at the MRI. It was also influenced by the work of Milton Erickson, with his emphasis on hypnosis and paradoxical therapeutic strategies. Haley, who also worked at the MRI and was a biographer of Erickson, continues to influence the growth and direction of strategic family therapy today.

Strategic family therapy generally is characterized by the use of specific strategies for addressing family problems (Haley, 1987; Madanes & Haley, 1977). Therapy is directly geared toward changing the presenting complaint and is typically accomplished by the therapist's first assessing the cycle of family interaction, then breaking that cycle through straightforward or paradoxical directives. Therapy is not growth- but change-oriented, and the therapist is responsible for successful therapeutic outcomes (Haley, 1987; Watzlawick, Weakland, & Fisch, 1974). The therapist focuses on present interaction; he or she does not interpret family members' behavior or explore the past. Therapy is terminated when the presenting problems have ceased.

Although these characteristics are common to all strategic family therapies, the ways in which strategic therapy is practiced vary considerably. For example, the two approaches most associated with strategic family therapy, collectively described as the Haley–Madanes approach (e.g., Haley, 1980, 1987; Madanes, 1981, 1990), and the Brief Therapy Model, developed at the MRI (e.g., Fisch, Weakland, & Segal, 1983; Weakland & Ray, 1995; Watzlawick et al., 1974), have some clear differences in emphasis.

Haley–Madanes

Both Haley and Madanes believe that problems are maintained by a faulty hierarchy within the family. The goal of therapy is to alter the family's interactions, thereby changing the family's structure (Haley, 1987). Also, they contend that the presenting problem is often a metaphor for the actual problem (Haley, 1987; Madanes, 1981). Regarding a patient with a fear of dying of a heart attack, Haley (1987) states the following:

> A family-oriented directive therapist . . . will assume that the patient's statement about his heart is analogic to his current situation. He will inquire about how the client relates to his wife, about his job, about his children, and so on. The therapist will also want the wife present in a session so that he can examine how they deal with each other and how the complaints about the heart are used in the ongoing interchange between husband and wife. When he interviews husband and wife together, the therapist will take an interest in the wife's response when the husband is feeling better and when he is feeling worse. . . . The family-oriented therapist will construct a theory that the husband's communication about his heart is a way of stabilizing the marriage. (p. 98)

Haley will often align himself with the parental generation when dealing with child-focused problems (Haley, 1980). When he brings parents together to work on their child's problem, he also realigns problematic hierarchies and strengthens the couple's relationship. Haley and Madanes alter malfunctioning triangles (Haley, 1980, 1987) and incongruous hierarchies (Madanes, 1980, 1981) through such diverse interventions as paradox, reframing, ordeals, "pretending," and unbalancing through creating alternative coalitions.

Recently, Madanes (1990, 1991) has come to view all problems as stemming from the dilemma between love and violence and categorizes them into one of four types. The first, *to dominate and to control*, contains symptoms such as delinquency, drug abuse, and assorted behavior problems. Second is *the desire to be loved*, which is associated with eating disorders, phobias, anxiety, depression, and psychosomatic symptoms. The third type, *to love and protect*, is related to problems such as abuse, neglect, obsessions, and suicide. Finally, *to repent and to forgive* is associated with incest, sexual abuse, murder, and sadistic acts. Her ultimate goal with all of these problems is to utilize a 16-step model to steer the family from violence back to love (Madanes, 1990).

Mental Research Institute

The MRI group operates from a process rather than an organizational model. Issues of hierarchy and power are not as important as those of interactional sequence. It is the family's sequence of behavior around their attempted solution that is assumed to maintain, and perhaps exacerbate, the presenting problem (Watzlawick et al., 1974; Weakland, Fisch, Watzlawick, & Bodin, 1974). Segal (1991) states: "The original difficulty becomes a problem when mishandling leads clients to use more of the same 'solution.' A vicious circle is set in motion, producing a problem whose severity and nature may have little similarity to the original difficulty" (p. 175). The MRI therapist tracks this cycle of behavior within the family by asking questions in the session and then prescribing a homework assignment (either direct or paradoxical) designed to break up the existing sequence of behavior.

Consistent with Bateson's (1972) concern about overintervention, the MRI approach is a minimalist one. Treatment goals may not involve changing the family at all. MRI therapists may look at a problem maintaining sequence within an individual. For example, Watzlawick et al. (1974) describe a case in which a college student had problems procrastinating when writing papers due to his fear of doing a poor job. He was told to write one paper his usual way and complete a second paper for a different class, writing only a quick first draft. The quick first draft received a better grade and the problem-maintaining sequence was broken.

Because MRI therapists do not place as much importance on hierarchy as Haley or Madanes, they often exhibit a less direct, more one-down position in dealing with a family in order to gain greater maneuverability (Fisch et al., 1983). Furthermore, MRI therapists usually limit treatment to within 10 sessions (Weakland et al., 1974).

STRUCTURAL FAMILY THERAPY

The structural school of family therapy has its roots in a residential institution for ghetto boys in New York. In the 1960s, Salvador Minuchin and his colleagues worked at the Wiltwyck School for boys and served a population primarily from New York's inner-city ghettos. They found psychoanalytic, long-term, passive, growth-oriented therapy to be extremely ineffective with these children, whose issues were immediate and survival-based. Minuchin and his associates experimented with a more active approach to therapy in which they worked with the boys and their families together (Aponte & VanDeusen, 1981; Colapinto, 1991; Minuchin & Nichols, 1993). *Families of the Slums* (Minuchin, Montalvo, Guerney, Rosman, & Schumer, 1967) was written about the Wiltwyck School experiences and is the first book to present the structural approach to family therapy.

Born out of this work with low-socioeconomic-status families, structural family therapy is an active, problem-solving approach to a dysfunctional family context. Although Minuchin's work with psychosomatic families is well known (e.g., Minuchin, Rosman, & Baker, 1978), Minuchin has applied his approach to patients of varying socioeconomic classes with a variety of presenting problems (Minuchin & Fishman, 1981; Minuchin & Nichols, 1993). Furthermore, structural family therapists increasingly examine isomorphic patterns between larger systems and families that may maintain individual problems (Fishman, 1993).

Structural family therapy generally is characterized by its emphasis on organizational issues (Colapinto, 1991; Minuchin, 1974). Typical goals of therapy include correcting dysfunctional hierarchies by putting parents in charge of their children and differentiating between subsystems within families. Therapy usually involves changing the family structure by modifying the way people relate to one another. This is done with a focus on the present, using direct, indirect, and paradoxical directives (Minuchin & Fishman, 1981). The structural therapist terminates therapy when the family structure is altered in a way that it can maintain itself without the use of the presenting problem (Minuchin, 1974).

SIMILARITIES

Although we have presented structural and strategic therapy as theoretically distinct schools, certain similarities exist. Some of these similarities may be due to previous interaction among prominent structural and strategic family therapists. For example, Haley, one of the founders of strategic family therapy, greatly influenced Minuchin's structural approach during his tenure at the Philadelphia Child Guidance Clinic. Haley was also influenced by Minuchin, as reflected in Haley's (1980, 1987) emphasis on hierarchy and boundaries.

The theoretical similarities between structural and strategic family therapies include their view of families as rule-governing systems that can best be understood in context. For Haley and Minuchin, the presenting problem often serves a function within the family and can best be understood by examining present family interactions. Both consider the family life cycle, and both employ general systems concepts (e.g., homeostasis, positive feedback) in their conceptualizations of family functioning.

Strategic and structural therapies also are similar in practice. For example, both employ assessment in the form of observing the results of therapeutic interventions in order to plan future interventions. Although adherents of both therapies maintain that they use whatever "works," techniques obviously common to both include joining, reframing, and therapeutic paradox (e.g., Fisch et al., 1983; Haley, 1987; Madanes, 1981; Minuchin & Fishman, 1981). Both emphasize process over content and present behavior over past behavior. Both utilize therapeutic contracts and behavioral tasks to change family interactions, believing that if the family context changes, so will individual behaviors. In both, the therapist takes a directive role to relieve the presenting problem. Finally, both approaches tend to be brief, usually between 10 and 20 sessions.

DIFFERENCES

Theoretically, structural and strategic therapies differ regarding the negative- or positive-feedback view of symptom dysfunction. In structural family therapy and Haley–Madanes strategic therapy, dysfunction is seen in terms of rigid, homeostatic transactions that must be broken. In terms of general system theory, a family's response to change is negative feedback, an attempt to maintain the family's status quo (e.g., a daughter's asthma keeps the mother and father together). In contrast, MRI strategic family therapy conceptualizes family dysfunction in terms of positive feedback or the vicious cycle created when an attempt to solve a problem (e.g., a wife's nagging) inadvertently worsens the symptomatic behavior (e.g., her husband's drinking). Thus, the MRI strategic therapist's view of family problems arising from positive feedback (deviation amplification) necessitates a therapeutic focus on behavioral sequence as the locus of analysis and the target for change. On the other hand, Haley–Madanes strategic therapy, with its assumption of a rigid, negative-loop, attempts to alter those sequences that maintain the homeostatic family structure. Structural family therapy attempts to alter the family's organization. Haley–Madanes, MRI, and structural therapists assess and alter interactional sequences, but for different reasons. Structural family therapists are more concerned than the others with the subsequent organizational structure of the family system.

Perhaps Colapinto (1991) best describes the theoretical difference between structural and strategic therapies through his discussion of the differences between "complementarity" (a structural term) and "circular causality" (a strategic concept):

> Circular causality designates a *sequential* two-way interaction (A's *behavior* causes B's *behavior,* and vice versa), represented by arrowed lines connecting A and B. . . . Complementarity, on the other hand, designates a spatial configuration (A's and B's *shapes* fit), represented by the interlocking pieces of the puzzle. This semantic difference is not trivial, but is consistent with the structural therapist's preference for tackling spatial arrangements (literal and metaphorical) among family members rather than sequences of behavior. (p. 423, italics in original)

A final difference exists between MRI strategic and Haley–Madanes strategic therapies. Similar to structural family therapy, Haley (1987) and Madanes (1981) assume that symptoms serve a function in the family. To bring about lasting change, interventions must be geared to altering the family organization. Proponents of the MRI approach espouse a strict interactional view of problem maintenance. The MRI makes no mention of the need of a family for a symptom.

The differences in therapeutic interventions between the two approaches are not always clear-cut but are more a matter of emphasis. For example, structural family therapy is typically more confrontive than strategic, perhaps owing to Minuchin's own personal style. Although both are present-oriented, structural family therapy focuses more on in-session behaviors and is more likely to employ in-session enactments. Strategic therapy, on the other hand, generally explores current out-of-session behavioral sequences and employs directives to be completed outside the session to disrupt these sequences. Strategic therapy (particularly at the Brief Family Therapy Project of the MRI) is also more likely than structural therapy to work with only one or two members of a family system to bring about change in the entire system (Stone Fish & Piercy, 1987).

SYSTEMIC FAMILY THERAPY

Systemic family therapy as practiced by the original Milan team, Mara Selvini Palazzoli, Luigi Boscolo, Gianfranco Cecchin, and Giuliana Prata, shares similar roots with both the MRI and Haley–Madanes versions of strategic family therapy in that they were all influenced by the work of Gregory Bateson. This has led all three groups to view problems as being maintained by interactional sequences; however, MRI and Haley became further influenced by the work of Milton Erickson, whereas the Milan group held true to Bateson's original works. With their book, *Paradox and*

Counterparadox (Selvini Palazzoli, Boscolo, Cecchin, & Prata, 1978), the Milan team presented a model in which individual symptoms were maintained by family homeostasis. To counteract this tendency to resist change, the Milan team relied heavily on paradoxical interventions in hopes of ending therapeutic impasses.

Prior to their split in 1979, the Milan team wrote a major paper, "Hypothesizing–Circularity–Neutrality: Three Guidelines for the Conductor of the Session" (Selvini Palazzoli, Boscolo, Cecchin, & Prata, 1980), in which they presented some important departures from their original model in *Paradox and Counterparadox*. Most notable was their growing disenchantment with paradoxical interventions (Campbell, Draper, & Crutchley, 1991; Selvini Palazzoli, Cirillo, Selvini, & Sorrentino, 1989) and their evolving belief in the importance of the process of the therapy session. Boscolo and Cecchin's ideas have remained consistent with those initially presented in "Hypothesizing–Circularity–Neutrality," whereas Selvini Palazzoli and Prata began experimenting with the concept of an invariant prescription for treating severe psychopathology (Prata, 1990; Selvini Palazzoli et al., 1989).

Boscolo and Cecchin

Systemic therapy as practiced by Boscolo and Cecchin views the family as a constantly evolving system. Problems exist when the family's old epistemology does not fit its current pattern of behaviors (Tomm, 1984a). The therapist does not develop specific goals for the family or overtly attempt to alter behavior. Instead, the team helps the family develop an alternative epistemology by introducing new information into the family system, information that invites spontaneous change (Boscolo, Cecchin, Hoffman, & Penn, 1987). Their in-session behavior is guided by three themes: hypothesizing, circularity, and neutrality (Selvini Palazzoli et al., 1980). The therapist is constantly generating hypotheses regarding why the family behaves as it does. These hypotheses create a map that guides them as they question the family. Boscolo and Cecchin consider all hypotheses, including those developed by the family, as equally valid.

Circularity exists in the way the therapist conducts the session. Through the use of triadic or circular questions, in which one family member is asked to comment on the interactional behaviors of the others, the therapist develops a systemic picture of the family's behavior (Penn, 1982). By conducting the session in this way, new information is introduced, in which family members experience themselves in a new context. Furthermore, therapist hypotheses also evolve as the therapist receives feedback from the family as the family responds to the questions. The original Milan team contended that simply conducting a session in this way may introduce enough new information to produce change (Selvini Palazzoli et al., 1980). Although this, as yet, is an untested hypothesis, it has led to several theoretical papers on the importance of therapist questions in the therapy process (Penn, 1985; Tomm, 1987a, 1987b, 1988).

Therapist neutrality is the glue that holds this process together. By avoiding issues of hierarchy, power, and side taking, the therapist is free to experience the system in its entirety (Boscolo et al., 1987). He or she is free to generate new hypotheses. Also, the family develops at its own pace in its own way. Within this sense of neutrality, the family is free to decide whether it wishes to change (Tomm, 1984b). Because some therapists associate the term neutrality with noninvolvement, Cecchin (1987) now prefers the term curiosity. Cecchin states: "Curiosity leads to exploration and invention of alternative views and moves, and views breed curiosity. In this recursive fashion, neutrality and curiosity contextualize one another in a commitment to evolving differences, with a concomitant nonattachment to any particular position" (p. 406).

Milan therapists typically intervene by asking circular questions, positively connoting the entire family system and providing end-of-session tasks designed to provide more information about the family. Milan interventions differ from those used in strategic therapies in that their aim is simply to infuse new information into the system, not necessarily to alter patterns of interaction (Boscolo et al., 1987). Interventions connect family members' behaviors through the development of a systemic hypothesis. Whether the family does the task or accepts the hypothesis is irrelevant. The important thing is that they are exposed to a different way of viewing their problems.

In systemic therapy, sessions often occur 1 month apart. This period, according to the Milan group, allows time for the intervention to take effect. As each family member reacts to the intervention, his or her behavior sets off a chain reaction that alters other members' perceptions and actions, creating a vortex of feedbacks (Tomm, 1984a).

Selvini Palazzoli and Prata

Since the split of the Milan team, Selvini Palazzoli and Prata have focused their work on researching the effectiveness of the "invariant prescription" in the treatment of severe psychopathology, (Prata, 1990; Selvini Palazzoli et al., 1989). The invariant prescription is based on a six-stage model of psychotic family games (Selvini Palazzoli, 1986). The first stage is based on a marital stalemate between the parents. The second stage consists of the child allying with the perceived loser of the marital stalemate against the perceived winner. In the third stage, the child displays symptomatology to challenge the perceived winner and to show the loser how to cope with the winner. In stage four, the "loser" fails to understand the purpose of the child's symptomatology and sides with the "winner" to disapprove of this behavior. In the fifth stage, the child feels misunderstood by the parents yet is determined to continue his or her game at all costs to eventually prove his or her point. The sixth stage happens when the family arrives at the belief that the child is "crazy" and develops strategies based on the assumption that the child will always be this way. This stabilizes the family game and maintains the pathological behavior.

The invariant prescription involves having the parents join in a secret coalition against the other family members. Initially they have confidential therapy sessions without the rest of the family. They then progress through secret outings and eventually make extended trips of several days without the others' knowledge. The couple is asked to make extensive notes on the reactions of the family and report them to the therapists. The goal of the invariant prescription is to alter the numerous patterns of family interaction by developing a stable alliance that is resistant to the pull of other family members (Prata, 1990; Selvini Palazzoli et al., 1989).

KEY CONCEPTS

Structural Family Therapy

Boundaries. Invisible lines of demarcation in a family, which may be defined, strengthened, loosened, or changed as a result of structural family therapy. Boundaries range from "disengaged" (extreme separateness) to "enmeshed" (extreme togetherness). Ideally, boundaries are "clear."

Coalition. A (usually) covert alliance between two family members against a third. When one parent joins a child in a rigidly bounded, cross-generational coalition against the other parent, this is called a "stable coalition" (Minuchin, 1974; cf. "detouring" and "triangulation").

Detouring. A process whereby stresses between spouses get redirected through a child so that the spouse subsystem gives the impression of harmony (cf. "stable coalition" and "triangulation").

Disengaged family. An extreme pattern of family organization in which members are so separate they seem oblivious to the effects of their actions on each other. Boundaries among family members are typically impermeable (the opposite of an "enmeshed family").

Enmeshed family. An extreme pattern of family organization in which family members are so tightly locked that autonomy is impossible. Boundaries among family members are typically diffuse (the opposite of a disengaged family).

Family mapping. The diagramming of a family's organizational structure, boundaries, and patterns of interaction. Family mapping is useful in hypothesizing family functioning and forming goals for structural change (see Minuchin, 1974, Chap. 3).

Generational boundaries. Invisible lines of demarcation between generations. Healthy generational boundaries allow parents to maintain parental roles and children to maintain child roles.

Hierarchy. A boundary that differentiates the leader of an organization from the other members. In a family, the parents are often higher in the hierarchy, meaning they have a greater say when it comes to making decisions on how the children are expected to behave.

Isomorphism. Situations in which the structure of a larger system is similar to a family's structure. When this happens, the larger system also serves to maintain the family's problematic behavior. In these situations, the therapist needs to alter the structure of the larger system as well as the family (Fishman, 1993).

Parental child. An overly responsible child who has power and authority that more appropriately belongs to the parents. This typically reflects an inappropriate generational boundary within the family.

Subsystems. Units within a family, based on characteristics such as sex, age, or interest (e.g., mother and daughter may represent the female subsystem in a family).

Triangulation. A process in which two family members demand that a third family member (often the child) side with each against the other. Siding with one is defined as attacking by the other, and the triangulated family member may feel paralyzed (cf. "stable coalition" and "detouring").

Strategic Family Therapy

Analogical message. A metaphorical or symbolic message. For example, certain behaviors (fighting over who cleans the bathroom) may have a metaphoric meaning for a couple (who is in charge?).

Circular causality. A contextual, cyclic view of behavior, as opposed to linear, cause-and-effect explanations of behavior. For example, a father's withdrawal from arguments is not because of anything the mother has done, but is seen in terms of circularity; that is, it is one point in a repetitive, predictable, circular pattern of behaviors in which the family is engaged.

Digital message. The content of a message. In the preceding example of an analogical message, the digital message is the fight over who cleans the bathroom. Analogical messages reflect the metaphoric meaning of digital messages.

Double bind. Originally noted by Bateson and his colleagues; a communication that leaves the responder "damned if you do and damned if you don't." A double bind includes (1) a double message (e.g., saying "I'm glad to see you" while looking away) (2) within an emotionally important relationship (3) in which the receiver of the message is unable to comment on the message. Bateson proposed that double-bind messages are important ingredients in the etiology of schizophrenia. Therapeutic paradox may be seen as a therapeutic application of double-bind messages.

First-order change. Change in which the fundamental rules of the system remain the same. For example, a disengaged alcoholic may quit drinking alcohol but stay disengaged from his wife by working long hours. Although change has occurred (he's quit drinking), the basic rules of the system have not (his disengagement from his wife). Another way to think of it is that first-order change is more of the same behavior (e.g., going faster in first gear as opposed to a more discrete fundamental change in rules (e.g., switching gears).

Homeostasis. The tendency within a system to seek equilibrium or balance through maintaining the status quo and resisting change. Theorists differ as to whether family pathology is maintained by resisting change (homeostasis or negative feedback) or by engaging in vicious cycles of change-attempting behavior (positive feedback or error amplification).

Metacommunication. Communication about communication. This term usually refers to the covert, nonverbal message (tone of voice, inflection, body language) that gives additional meaning to an overt, verbal message.

Negative feedback. A process to correct system deviations by reestablishing the previous state of equilibrium. For example, this process is at work in families in which a child acts out in order to bring quarreling parents back together again.

Positive feedback. The morphogenic, change-activating process within systems. Any tactic from a therapist or a family that challenges family homeostasis and changes a family's way of behaving is an example of positive feedback. In strategic family therapy, a dysfunctional family's solution to its problem is assumed to involve positive feedback (i.e., deviation amplification) that exacerbates the problem rather than solves it. For example, increasingly chiding a nonresponsive spouse (the "solution") often makes the spouse less responsive rather than more responsive (the "problem").

Punctuation. Human interaction is typically complex and cyclical, in which people often attribute different meanings to events because they arbitrarily bracket or focus on different parts of the cycle. For example, if a son's misbehavior and his parents' restrictiveness have produced a vicious cycle, the parents might say, "We are strict because you misbehave," whereas the son would retort, "If I misbehave, it's because you are so strict."

Second-order change. Strategies involving alteration of the fundamental rules or context in which a problem is embedded to solve the problem. This often involves changing the meaning of a problem-maintaining interactional sequence (MRI) or a family's interactional pattern (Haley–Madanes) in a way that discourages the previous more-of-the-same behavior.

Systemic Family Therapy

Circularity. As discussed by the Milan team (Selvini Palazzoli et al., 1980), circularity actually has two definitions. The first definition refers to the interactional nature of families. An individual's behavior is part of a sequence of behaviors or cognitions in a family. The second definition refers to the interactional relationship between the therapist and the treatment family. Therapist hypotheses develop through an interactional relationship with the family. Therapists' hypotheses change due to families' responses to their questions. New hypotheses lead to new questions, which, in turn, lead to new changes.

Curiosity. Cecchin (1987) uses the term curiosity to deal with misconceptions about the concept of neutrality. Curiosity refers to the therapist stance of being open to multiple hypotheses about client behavior. By limiting one's hypotheses, one constrains the number of options that can lead to a treatment family's change.

Hypothesizing. Hypothesizing refers to the therapist developing systemic theories about a family's behavior. These hypotheses guide the use of circular questions and lead to new ideas in the family system. If a therapist is without hypotheses, his or her questions will lack a coherent meaning and bring no new information to the family.

Neutrality. See Curiosity.

Psychotic family games. Selvini Palazzoli (1986) describes a 6-stage sequence for the development of a psychotic child. In this process, the child aligns with the perceived loser of a marital difficulty against the perceived winner. Failing to see the child's behavior as a tactic for beating the "winner," the "loser" aligns with the "winner" against this symptom. The child persists in this behavior, and the system eventually stabilizes around the psychotic behavior.

Time. Boscolo and Bertrando (1993) add the dimension of time to systemic therapy. A family's view of the history of a problem affects their current view, which in turn affects both their view of the past and the future. If they view Billy as bad, based on his misbehavior in the past, they will rewrite their view of the past to remember predominantly bad events and continue their actions based on viewing him as bad in the future. By altering a family's view of its future, and possibly its past, the therapist can help them to alter their behaviors in the present.

KEY CLINICAL SKILLS

Structural Family Therapy

Accommodation. A general term referring to the adjustments a therapist may make to a family (e.g., joining, maintenance, mimesis) in order to achieve a therapeutic alliance with them.

Boundary marking. A strategy in which the therapist reinforces appropriate boundaries and diffuses inappropriate boundaries by modifying transactional patterns (e.g., a therapist may sit between an intrusive mother and her child so that the mother will have difficulty speaking for the child).

Enactment. The acting out of dysfunctional transactional patterns within the family therapy session, encouraged by the therapist. Through setting up these transactions in the present, the therapist learns much about the family's structure and interactional patterns. The therapist is then able to intervene in the process by increasing its intensity, indicating alternative transactions, marking boundaries, and so forth. The therapist may also have the family enact more positive transactional patterns within the therapy session, which will serve as a template for more positive interactions outside therapy.

Intensity. The degree of impact of a therapeutic message, selectively regulated by the therapist. The therapist can achieve intensity by increasing the affective component of a family transaction, by increasing the length of a transaction, or by frequently repeating the same message in different transactions.

Joining. An accommodating maneuver in which the therapist establishes rapport with family members and temporarily becomes part of the family system. The family accepts the therapist more openly, making it easier for the therapist to bring about change.

Mimesis. The paralleling of a family's mood or behavior, which solidifies a therapeutic alliance. For example, a therapist may talk slowly with a slow-talking family or be animated with an animated family.

Restructuring. Any therapeutic intervention that confronts and challenges a family and facilitates structural changes. Examples of restructuring maneuvers include assigning tasks, shifting power systems, escalating stress, and marking boundaries.

Unbalancing. Any therapeutic intervention that supports one member of the family, thus interfering with the homeostasis of the family system.

Strategic Family Therapy

Directives. Therapeutic tasks aimed at breaking inappropriate sequences of behavior.

Ordeals. Interventions in which clients are directed to engage in a mildly noxious activity (that is also good for them) each time they engage in the targeted symptomatic behavior. For example, a man having trouble sleeping might be told to clean the entire house each night he is unable to sleep.

Pretending. A therapist's prescribing that a symptomatic person "pretend" to exhibit his or her symptom, which reclassifies that symptom as voluntary and not really "real." This may alter the family's reaction to that symptom. For example, when a depressed husband is told to pretend to be depressed a certain number of times during the week, his wife may assume he is pretending and thus begin to respond to him differently. Similarly, the husband is now in charge of "acting" depressed, which reflects his ability to be in charge of his depression. In essence, he is more volitional and powerful than if he were simply "being" depressed (see Madanes, 1981).

Reframing. Use of language to give new meaning to a situation. The alteration of meaning invites the possibility of change. For example, relabeling a youth's depression as stubbornness or laziness suggests personal responsibility for that behavior and may change the family's response to that behavior.

Therapeutic paradox. A strategic intervention that has been defined and implemented in many ways (see Weeks & L'Abate, 1979). Generally, it involves a seemingly illogical intervention to bring about change. This entails maneuvers that are in apparent contradiction to the goals of therapy, yet are actually designed to achieve them (Haley, 1987). Major classes of therapeutic paradox are (1) prescribing the symptom, (2) restraining change, and (3) positioning, in which the therapist accepts and exaggerates the client's position on an issue.

Systemic Family Therapy

Circular questions. Introduced by Selvini Palazzoli and her associates (1978), circular questions are interview questions used to learn more about changes and differences in family relationships. These differences, in turn, may provide clues to recursive family patterns. Circular questions are useful in generating systemic hypotheses and interventions, and in allowing family members to begin viewing themselves systemically. For more on the theory and practice of circular questioning, see Fleuridas, Nelson, and Rosenthal (1986) and Penn (1982).

Extending time between sessions. A central concern of Milan-style therapists is allowing an adequate amount of time between sessions to assess whether an intervention works. By extending the length of time between sessions to 1 month (and in some cases even longer), interventions have enough time to affect all aspects of the family system. With an extended time frame, therapists won't be thrown off track by a family's initial reaction to an intervention on their way toward change.

Invariant prescription. This is a specific intervention designed and studied by Selvini Palazzoli and Prata to treat psychotic families. It involves having the parents form a secret alliance without the rest of the family. The parents engage in a series of cloistered meetings that range from a few hours to several days. The purpose of this alliance is to disrupt the multiple interactional sequences existing in the family, allowing new patterns to develop.

Positive connotation. Positive connotation expands on the notion of a reframe in that rather than relabeling a behavior, the therapist positively describes the entire family interaction. This ties the symptomatic behavior to its context (the family) and enables the family to view both the symptom and itself in a new light.

Rituals. Used extensively by Selvini Palazzoli and her associates (1978), a ritual is an individualized prescription of an action or series of actions that are designed to alter the family's roles. For example, the parents of a family with an intrusive, live-in grandmother might be given the following message to read to the grandmother each night: "Thank you for your many suggestions regarding how we should discipline our son. If it weren't for your loving help we would surely fail." The grandmother is told to read this message in response: "I love you and am willing to completely sacrifice my own life and happiness to make sure you don't fail to discipline your child the right way." Any rejection of the positively connoted messages should shift the family members toward more functional interactions.

Triadic questions. See Circular questioning.

TEACHING TOOLS AND TECHNIQUES

Training Videotapes

Several excellent videotapes are available that demonstrate structural and strategic approaches to family therapy. Lists and descriptions of available tapes can be secured from the following sources:

- *AAMFT Master Series*, AAMFT, 1133 15th Street, N.W., Suite 300, Washington, DC 20005-2710
- Family Therapy Institute, 5850 Hubbard Drive, Rockville, MD 20852
- The Minuchin Center for the Family, 114 East 32nd Street, New York, NY 10016
- Nathan W. Ackerman Institute for Family Therapy, 149 East 78th Street, New York, NY 10021
- Philadelphia Child Guidance Clinic, Two Children's Center, 34th Street & Civic Center Boulevard, Philadelphia, PA 19104

Journal Days

In order to expose students to as many key journal articles as possible, every month each student chooses two articles form an extensive bibliography to read and summarize to the class. Many of these 5-minute summaries generate provocative discussions regarding the theory, research, and practice of strategic, structural, and systemic family therapies.

Debates and Panels

A debate on "how change occurs" may be set up between students identifying themselves as structural and those identifying themselves as strategic. Also, students may take the role of central figures such as Haley, Minuchin, Bateson, Selvini Palazzoli, Watzlawick, Erickson, Stanton, and Madanes for a panel discussion or debate. Needless to say, a student must know the writings of a central figure quite well to be able to step into his or her shoes.

Choreographic History of Strategic, Structural, and Systemic Family Therapies

The instructor writes the names of key individuals in the history of strategic, structural and systemic family therapies on separate 5" × 8" cards. On the back of each card, the instructor writes a saying that captures an essential point of each respective key individual's theory. Names and sayings we have used include the following:

Name	Saying
Norbert Wiener	"Cybernetics explains information flow in systems."
Gregory Bateson	"Don't chop up the ecology."
Don D. Jackson	"Families resist change."
Jay Haley	"But how can I bring about change?"
Paul Watzlawick	"You're absolutely right."
John Weakland	"Go slow."
Richard Fisch	"Change can be dangerous."
Milton Erickson	"My voice will go with you."
Salvador Minuchin	"Sit over here."
Braulio Montalvo	"I'm a clinician."
Cloé Madanes	"Let's pretend."
Mara Selvini Palazzoli	"The observers have an important message for each of you."
Luigi Boscolo	"I focus on training."
Gianfranco Cecchin	"The context is everything."
Giuliana Prata	"The prescription is invariant."

The instructor tells the history of strategic, structural, and systemic family therapies: He or she begins with the work of Norbert Wiener, explains how Wiener's work affected the thinking of Gregory Bateson, describes how Bateson subsequently moved to California and worked on a research grant on levels of communication with Jay Haley and John Weakland, and so on (for a short history of strategic and structural family therapies, see Stanton, 1981, or Bodin, 1981). As different names are mentioned, the instructor gives a member of the class a card with that person's name on it, and has him or her read the saying on the back of the card. Also, as people move in and out of the historical overview, the instructor has them physically move around the room. For example, such a historical choreography will trace Haley's travels from Palo Alto to his consultations with Milton Erickson, to his work with Minuchin in Philadelphia, and finally to his present position in Washington. Similarly, students learn that Watzlawick consulted frequently with Selvini Palazzoli in the development of the systemic approach and how the Milan team divided so Boscolo and Cecchin could focus on training and Selvini Palazzoli and Prata could research the invariant prescription. This kind of choreographic history brings the key figures alive and underlines the influences these leaders had on one another.

Responding to Ethical Concerns

Haley (1987, Chapter 8) addresses quite well a variety of ethical concerns related to strategic therapy. After students have read Haley's ethical justification of strategic therapy, they are given classroom practice in thinking through and responding to similar ethical concerns. Specifically, they are divided into seven small groups, with each group given a provocative ethical concern for discussion and formulation of a response. After about 20 minutes, the instructor dramatically questions each group about the particular concern that the group has been discussing. A predetermined spokesperson from the group then responds to the concern the instructor raised. The entire class is given the opportunity to discuss each issue after the group response is given.

The ethical concerns discussed in the groups include the following:

1. Strategic therapy seems manipulative and underhanded. Don't you agree?
2. Do the ends justify the means?
3. What place does honesty play in this kind of therapy? How acceptable is lying?
4. Isn't it unethical to change someone outside his or her awareness? Why keep therapeutic techniques secret?
5. If a therapist is "in charge" of change, how is the client supposed to become self-sufficient?
6. Who is the therapist to say what is best for a client to do? Isn't nondirective therapy much more respectful and ethical?
7. What right do you have to consider yourself an expert on how people should live their lives?

Read–Summarize–React Exercise

A read–summarize–react exercise may be used to help students learn the various explanations and rationales of therapeutic paradox (cf. Hoffman, 1981; Raskin & Klein, 1976; Weeks & L'Abate, 1979). Each explanation is typed on a 5″ × 7″ card. Students form groups of five, with 10 cards in the middle of each group. The teacher instructs them, in turn, to (1) take a card and silently read the explanation; (2) paraphrase the explanation; (3) give their own reactions to it; and (4) allow any other member of the group to respond. After this exercise, the class comes together, and the instructor answers any questions regarding the various explanations of paradox. (This exercise is drawn from Piercy & Sprenkle, 1984.)

Reframing Exercise

Reframing invokes giving a new meaning to a presenting problem in a way that facilitates change. To practice this skill, students are asked to write down situations or characteristics in the left-hand column and attempt to give them new meaning in the right hand column. This may be done individually or in small groups. The instructor shares alternative realities in the right-hand column if students have difficulty reframing the symptom or problem behavior. An alternative exercise is to have each small group responsible for role-playing the reframing of one or more of the symptoms. Of course there is no such thing as a "correct reframe." Reframes must be tailored to the belief systems of a specific family.

Symptom or problem behavior	*An alternative reality*
Depression	"You are just a little lazy."
Overinvolved mother	"You really care about your child."
Distant husband	"You care enough to take the back seat and give the spotlight to others."
Jealousy	"You really care about your wife and don't want to lose the relationship you have."
Adolescent running away	"I compliment you. This is a very creative way to achieve autonomy."
Nagging	"You want to matter to your family—to be closer—and this is the way you are asking for this closeness."
Disrespectful teenager	"You are telling your folks you want to grow up and be more responsible for yourself."

Alcoholic husband   "Your family needed help, and you
                                  were selfless enough to sacrifice your-
                                  self so they could get that help."

Strategic Directives

The instructor presents problems from Haley's (1987) *Problem-Solving Therapy* (pp. 60–63). The instructor then asks students to brainstorm possible
directives for interrupting behavioral sequences. After the brainstorming, he
or she shares and discusses the directives Haley uses.

Family Mapping

Family mapping (see Minuchin, 1974, Chapter 3) is a helpful way of visually
depicting the structure of a dysfunctional family. The class is given para-
graphs depicting certain dysfunctional family hierarchies and asked to (1)
draw a map of the family's present structure; (2) draw a map of the ideal
family structure at the termination of therapy; and (3) give the rationale
and therapeutic strategy to be used to reach this structuring goal. The
following is an example:

> *Question:* The husband criticizes the wife, who then seeks a coalition
> with the child against the father. Map this structure and map your goal.
> Also, briefly discuss how you would achieve your goal.
> *Possible answer:*

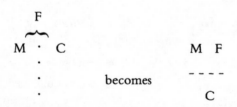

To achieve this, I would see the mother and father alone for therapy and
give a directive that the mother could only speak with the child through
the father. I would also provide opportunities in therapy for the mother
and father to deal directly with each other without the child.

Milan-Style Rituals

The instructor presents cases to the class, who in groups of five act as therapy
teams in developing Milan-style rituals (see Boscolo et al., 1987). The
following is an illustrative situation and one possible Milan-style team
message:

Situation: Bill, a conduct-disordered 9-year-old, is the identified patient. The father, usually mild-mannered and withdrawn, has taken major responsibility in trying to discipline and lecture Bill. The overworked mother is a borderline alcoholic, but this fact is not discussed by the family. Mary, an 11-year-old, is the model child in her parents' eyes, although she is only doing average work in school.

Milan-style ritual: "Each night at dinner, the family is to thank Bill for his helpfulness. The mother is to thank him for engaging father so she can rest. The father is to thank him for keeping him so busy that he does not have to notice mother's problem. Mary is to thank him for allowing her to look so good in her parents' eyes and keeping the pressure off her."

RESEARCH ISSUES

Most of the articles and books written about structural, strategic, and systemic therapies are nonempirical and anecdotal in nature. The few data-based research studies that have been conducted (e.g., Minuchin et al., 1978; Stanton, Todd, & Associates, 1982) have used relatively specific presenting problems (e.g., psychosomatic illness, drug addiction) and have not employed alternative family therapy control groups. Future research should probe the relative effectiveness of each approach, as well as various components of each approach, with certain presenting problems and/or family types. Researchers should also consider single-case studies using multiple baselines. Examples of research questions that warrant investigation include the following:

- Which structural family therapy interventions account for the greatest change in family therapy outcome?
- Are paradoxical directives more effective than straightforward directives for specific symptoms (with certain types of families)?
- How do effective and ineffective strategic interventions differ?
- Which family types respond best to structural, strategic, or systemic therapies?
- Madanes (1990, 1991) divides symptomatic families into four types: (1) to dominate and control; (2) to be loved; (3) to love and protect; (4) to repent and to forgive. Can these four quadrants be empirically validated? Are the treatment strategies she suggests for these problems effective (Gurman & Kniskern, 1991)?
- How does Haley's (1980) "leaving home" strategy compare to psychoeducational approaches (see Chapter 11) in the treatment of schizophrenia?

- Are tasks given within the session more effective than those given outside the session?
- Do families with a psychotic member actually engage in a 6-stage family game as described by Selvini Palazzoli (1986)?
- How effective is the invariant prescription (Selvini Palazzoli et al., 1989) in clinical outcome trials?
- Is it necessary to provide a task at the end of Milan-style treatment, or are circular questions enough to bring about change (Selvini Palazzoli et al., 1980).
- What treatment schedule (e.g., once a week, once a month) is most effective for Milan-style systemic therapy?

KEY BOOKS, CHAPTERS, AND ARTICLES

Bateson, G., Jackson, D. D., Haley, J., & Weakland, J. (1956). Toward a theory of schizophrenia. *Behavioral Science, 1,* 251–264.

In this classic article, the authors hypothesize the origin of schizophrenia to be rooted in dysfunctional, double-binding communication between family members. The impact of this article on family therapy has been tremendous. This is must reading!

Boscolo, L., & Bertrando, P. (1993). *The times of time: A new perspective in systemic therapy and consultation.* New York: Norton.

The authors discuss how a family's construction of time can serve to maintain symptomatic behavior. Through detailed theoretical and clinical presentation, they show how therapists can include the construct of time in diagnosis and treatment. This book adds an important dimension to the practice of systemic therapy.

Boscolo, L., Cecchin, G., Hoffman, L., & Penn, P. (1987). *Milan systemic family therapy: Conversations in theory and practice.* New York: Basic Books.

This is the single, best source for understanding the work of Boscolo and Cecchin. The format of the book focuses on transcribed sessions interspersed with questions by Hoffman and Penn to Boscolo and Cecchin as they view the sessions. This is a circular model for understanding a circular theory.

Campbell, D., Draper, R., & Crutchley, E. (1991). The Milan systemic approach to family therapy. In A. S. Gurman & D. P. Kniskern (Eds.), *Handbook of family therapy* (Vol. 2). New York: Brunner/Mazel.

This is a useful chapter for those wishing to understand the various stages of development of the Milan teams. The authors also illustrate the effects of the Milan teams on the development of the field and highlight the various theoretical concepts and techniques.

Cecchin, G. (1987). Hypothesizing, circularity, and neutrality revisited: An invitation to curiosity. *Family Process, 26,* 405–413.

Cecchin challenges the misconception that "neutrality" means noninvolvement on the part of the therapist. He utilizes the term "curiosity" to argue that therapists need to be open to many views on problem maintenance and not be seduced by a tantalizing few. Curiosity is an active process and not a cool, detached position.

Colapinto, J. (1991). Structural family therapy. In A. S. Gurman & D. P. Kniskern (Eds.), *Handbook of family therapy* (Vol. 2). New York: Brunner/Mazel.

This chapter presents a comprehensive overview of structural family therapy. It provides a historical context for the theory as well as discussing several current issues. This is a good source for those wanting a brief update on how structural family therapy has evolved since *Families and Family Therapy*.

Coyne, J. C. (1985). Toward a theory of frames and reframing: The social nature of frames. *Journal of Marital and Family Therapy, 11,* 337–344.

This largely conceptual article describes certain critical elements of effective reframes. Coyne discusses the contributions and limitations of "radical constructivism" to the understanding of reframes, and emphasizes their social and intersubjective nature. Coyne's use of clear examples makes this largely theoretical article surprisingly readable.

Fisch, R., Weakland, J. H., & Segal, L. (1983). *The tactics of change.* San Francisco: Jossey-Bass.

This is perhaps the most pragmatic, usable, compelling book on the MRI approach to "doing therapy briefly." It is clearly written and provides excellent case illustrations. Particularly helpful are the chapters on therapist maneuverability, patient position, and interventions.

Fishman, H. C., (1988). *Treating troubled adolescents: A family therapy approach.* New York: Basic Books.

Fishman makes the case that structural family therapy is the treatment of choice for troubled adolescents. Focusing on the role of homeostasis, Fishman presents a wide variety of clinical examples.

Fishman, H. C. (1993). *Intensive structural family therapy: Treating families in their social context.* New York: Basic Books.

Structural family therapy comes of age with this excellent book. Fishman updates structural concepts in a way that answers earlier critiques (e.g., not focusing on a traditional family model). Focusing on the issues of homeostasis and isomorphism, he discusses the importance of clinicians using the larger system in which families are embedded.

Fleuridas, C., Nelson, T., & Rosenthal, D. (1986). The evolution of circular questions: Training family therapists. *Journal of Marital and Family Therapy, 12,* 113–127.

This article provides a helpful taxonomy for understanding circular questioning, as well as a variety of useful examples of circular questions. The table of circular questions make particularly good instructional handouts.

Fraser, J. S. (1984). Paradox and orthodox: Folie à deux? *Journal of Marital and Family Therapy, 10,* 361–372.

Fraser critiques the contraindications of the use of paradox identified by others on the grounds that what is paradoxical is dependent on what does or does not make "sense" to the therapist (i.e., what he or she sees as "orthodox"). Fraser contends that what some see as paradoxical may often be elected by therapists with a "systemic orthodox" as a logical and effective first choice in therapy. This is a thought-provoking article.

Haley, J. (1980). *Leaving home.* New York: McGraw-Hill.

Haley emphasizes hierarchical issues in this succinct, step-by-step guide to disengaging the disturbed young person from his or her parents. His use of verbatim family therapy transcripts makes this an interesting as well as useful volume. Haley's inclusion of both structural and strategic concepts underlines the overlap of these two family therapy approaches.

Haley, J. (1984). *Ordeal therapy.* San Francisco: Jossey-Bass.

Haley builds upon the work of Milton Erickson by providing a strong and detailed theoretical rationale for the use of ordeals in therapy. He uses excellent case histories to illustrate the application of ordeal therapy with a variety of clients and presenting problems.

Haley, J. (1987). *Problem-solving therapy* (2nd ed.). San Francisco: Jossey-Bass.

This book remains one of the clearest expositions of the basic tenets underlying Haley's approach to family therapy. The book is updated to incorporate many of the changes that have taken place in family therapy since the first edition. Especially informative is the expanded chapter on conducting the first session.

Held, B. S. (1992). The problem of strategy within the systemic therapies. *Journal of Marital and Family Therapy, 18,* 25–34.

Held addresses the debate over the role of therapist power and influence in strategic therapy that exists within the systemic therapy movement. By considering a distinction between therapeutic process and content and a distinction between realist and antirealist epistemologies, she makes a convincing argument that there are more similarities than differences among the proponents of the different camps.

Kleckner, T., Frank, L., Bland, C., Amendt, J. H., Bryant, R.dR. (1992). The myth of the unfeeling strategic therapist. *Journal of Marital and Family Therapy, 18,* 41–51.

This article addresses the belief that strategic therapists neglect clients' feelings in therapy. The authors provide a strong argument for the focusing on feelings in strategic therapy.

Madanes, C. (1981). *Strategic family therapy.* San Francisco: Jossey-Bass.

Madanes broadens the scope of strategic family therapy with her therapeutic use of pretending and her metaphoric formulations of the role of symptoms. Her case examples are particularly helpful.

Madanes, C. (1990). *Sex, love, and violence: Strategies for transformation*. New York: Norton.

Madanes divides family problems into four types: (1) to dominate and to control; (2) to be loved; (3) to love and protect; and (4) to repent and to forgive. She includes a 16-stage treatment model.

Madanes, C. (1991). Strategic family therapy. In A. S. Gurman & D. P. Kniskern (Eds.), *Handbook of family therapy* (Vol. 2). New York: Brunner/Mazel.

This chapter is a good introduction for those wishing to gain an initial understanding of Madanes's "sex, love, and violence" model.

Minuchin, S. (1974). *Families and family therapy*. Cambridge, MA: Harvard University Press.

Minuchin clarifies his theory through the use of verbatim therapy transcripts and parallel commentary. Also, his illustrative use of family mapping is particularly helpful. This is a key text in structural family therapy and an excellent place to begin reading.

Minuchin, S., & Fishman, H. C. (1982). *Techniques of family therapy*. Cambridge, MA: Harvard University Press.

The authors clearly discuss and illustrate the techniques of structural family therapy through verbatim excerpts from therapy. Techniques presented include joining, reframing, enactment, restructuring, unbalancing, and the use of paradox. This volume, however, is not simply a manual on the application of techniques; Minuchin and Fishman also articulate the spontaneous, artful side of family therapy.

Minuchin, S., Montalvo, B., Guerney, B. G., Rosman, B. L., & Schumer, F. (1967). *Families of the slums*. New York: Basic Books.

This is the first book to describe the theory and practice of structural family therapy. This volume grew out of the authors' work with disadvantaged children at the Wiltwyck School in New York.

Minuchin, S., & Nichols, M. P. (1993). *Family healing: Tales of hope and renewal from family therapy*. New York: Free Press.

This intriguing book includes an autobiographical section offering glimpses into the life of one of the founding fathers of family therapy. The remainder of the book uses case studies representing families at various stages of development to illustrate Minuchin's evolving technique. The reader learns about Minuchin's reactions to these families and his reflections about their progress in therapy.

Minuchin, S., Rosman, B. L., & Baker, L. (1978). *Psychosomatic families: Anorexia nervosa in context*. Cambridge, MA: Harvard University Press.

This important volume outlines the theory, research, and practice of structural family therapy with psychosomatic children and their families. Perhaps its greatest contribution is in the suggestions the authors present for dealing with the parental enmeshment characteristic of these families. The authors also outline important research with psychosomatic families.

Papp, P. (1980). The Greek chorus and other techniques of paradoxical therapy. *Family Process, 19,* 45–57.

In this classic paper, Papp describes the creative uses of a treatment team in family therapy. This paper has had a major impact in the development of team strategies and procedures of live supervision.

Papp, P. (1983). *The process of change.* New York: Guilford Press.

This is a well-written book by a creative master clinician. It grew out of Papp's work with the Ackerman Brief Therapy Project. Although the project was inspired by the Milan approach, the Ackerman group also integrates aspects of the work of Minuchin, Haley, and the MRI.

Penn, P. (1982). Circular questioning. *Family Process, 21,* 267–280.

Penn liberally draws from Bateson, Keeney, and others in describing circular questioning from the perspective of a cybernetic epistemology. Her categories of circular questions help to demystify the process, as does her fascinating case study (which includes an ongoing commentary/explanation).

Penn, P. (1985). Feed-forward: Future questions, future maps. *Family Process, 24,* 299–310.

This article extends the theory and practice of Milan-style future questions. Penn uses "feed-forward" in conjunction with positive connotation and encourages families to imagine possible patterns of the relationships in the future. She uses a case study to clearly underline the power of this procedure.

Prata, G. (1990). *A systemic harpoon into family games: Preventive interventions in therapy.* New York: Brunner/Mazel.

This is perhaps the best single source on the use of the invariant prescription. Prata is exceptionally frank in her discussions on the state of psychiatry and medication management, her theoretical orientation, and her practices in the therapy room.

Price, J. A., & Keim, J. (Eds.). (1993). Strategic humanism [Special issue]. *Journal of Systemic Family Therapy, 12*(4).

This important special issue provides a new conceptual core for Haley–Madanes strategic therapy, strategic humanism. Cloé Madanes provides an excellent chapter on the theory of systemic humanism, while Jay Haley offers a tongue-in-cheek view on how supervisors can continue to train therapists without knowing how to change anyone.

Segal, L. (1991). Brief therapy: The MRI approach. In A. S. Gurman & D. P. Kniskern (Eds.), *Handbook of family therapy* (Vol. 2). New York: Brunner/Mazel.

This chapter presents a brief overview of the concepts and techniques of the

MRI approach. Most notable is its discussion on why the MRI model is difficult to practice and how these ideas fit within the current constructivist paradigm.

Selvini Palazzoli, M. (1986). Towards a general model of psychotic family games. *Journal of Marital and Family Therapy, 12,* 339–349.

This article presents Selvini Palazzoli's 6-stage model for the development of psychotic families. Understanding this model led to her use of the invariant prescription. This article is both interesting and controversial.

Selvini Palazzoli, M., Boscolo, L., Cecchin, G., & Prata, G. (1978). *Paradox and counterparadox.* New York: Jason Aronson.

This classic volume outlines the original theory and practice of the Milan group. It provides detailed descriptions of their use of a treatment team in family therapy. Many of the concepts presented in this book are no longer used (e.g., paradoxical interventions) by members of the team; however, this book had quite an influence on the field.

Selvini Palazzoli, M., Boscolo, L., Cecchin, G., & Prata, G. (1980). Hypothesizing–circularity–neutrality: Three guidelines for the conductor of the session. *Family Process, 19,* 3–12.

Perhaps one of the most influential articles in the last 20 years, this paper presents the theoretical cornerstone of the Milan team's work, hypothesizing, circularity, and neutrality. It continues to be a major theoretical focus for the work of Boscolo and Cecchin and has had a major impact on the new epistemology and constructivist movements.

Selvini Palazzoli, M., Cirillo, S., Selvini, M., & Sorrentino, A. M. (1989). *Family Games: General models of psychotic processes in the family.* New York: Norton.

Written with Selvini Palazzoli's new team, this book presents the evolution and a detailed description of her "family games" model of family psychosis.

Tomm, K. (1987a). Interventive interviewing: Part I. Strategizing as a fourth guideline for the therapist. *Family Process, 26,* 3–13.

Tomm, K. (1987b). Interventive interviewing: Part II. Reflexive questioning as a means to enable self-healing. *Family Process, 26,* 167–183.

Tomm, K. (1988). Interventive interviewing: Part III. Intending to ask lineal, circular, strategic, or reflexive questions. *Family Process, 27,* 1–15.

These three articles expand on the ideas of hypothesizing, circularity, and neutrality, and the role of questioning as intervention in systemic therapy (Selvini Palazzoli et al., 1980). They include a fourth stance of strategizing and the role of reflexive questions. The author provides guidelines for the use of lineal, circular, reflexive, and strategic questions.

Watzlawick, P., Beavin, J. H., & Jackson, D. (1967). *Pragmatics of human communication: A study of interactional patterns, pathologies, and paradoxes.* New York: Norton.

The authors explain key aspects of communication and relate them to cybernetic and general systems concepts. This book is must reading, in that the authors outline the theoretical underpinnings of much of strategic family therapy.

Watzlawick, P., Weakland, J., & Fisch, R. (1974). *Change.* New York: Norton.

The authors outline the basic assumptions of the Palo Alto school and innovative interventions that are consistent with these assumptions. The authors bring to life the concepts of first- and second-order change, and the strategic use of paradox by using excellent examples from both within and outside family therapy.

Weakland, J. H., & Ray, W. A. (Eds.). (1995). *Propagations: Thirty years of influence from the Mental Research Institute.* Binghamton, NY: Haworth.

In this book, the editors present a compilation of papers from the thirtieth anniversary conference of the MRI. The book provides a fascinating look at how core theoretical ideas have evolved to fit various contexts and treatment populations.

REFERENCES

Aponte, H. J., & VanDeusen, J. M. (1981). Structural family therapy. In A. S. Gurman & D. P. Kniskern (Eds.), *Handbook of family therapy.* New York: Brunner/Mazel.

Bateson, G. (1972). *Steps to an ecology of mind.* New York: Ballantine.

Bateson, G., Jackson, D. D., Haley, J., & Weakland, J. (1956). Toward a theory of schizophrenia. *Behavioral Science, 1,* 251–264.

Boscolo, L., & Bertrando, P. (1993). *The times of time: A new perspective in systemic therapy and consultation.* New York: Norton.

Boscolo, L., Cecchin, G., Hoffman, L., & Penn, P. (1987). *Milan systemic family therapy: Conversations in theory and practice.* New York: Basic Books.

Bodin, A. B. (1981). An interactional view: Family therapy approaches of the Mental Research Institute. In A. S. Gurman & D. P. Kniskern (Eds.), *Handbook of family therapy.* New York: Brunner/Mazel.

Campbell, D., Draper, R., & Crutchley, E. (1991). The Milan approach to family therapy. In A. S. Gurman & D. P. Kniskern (Eds.), *Handbook of family therapy* (Vol. 2). New York: Brunner/Mazel.

Cecchin, G. (1987). Hypothesizing, circularity, and neutrality revisited: An invitation to curiosity. *Family Process, 26,* 405–413.

Colapinto, J. (1991). Structural family therapy. In A. S. Gurman & D. P. Kniskern (Eds.), *Handbook of family therapy* (Vol. 2). New York: Brunner/Mazel.

Fisch, R., Weakland, J. H., & Segal, L. (1983). *The tactics of change.* San Francisco: Jossey-Bass.

Fishman, H. C. (1993). *Intensive structural therapy: Treating families in their social context.* New York: Basic Books.

Fleuridas, C., Nelson, T., & Rosenthal, D. (1986). The evolution of circular questions: Training family therapists. *Journal of Marital and Family Therapy, 12,* 113–127.

Gurman, A. S., & Kniskern, D. P. (Eds.). (1991). *Handbook of family therapy* (Vol. 2). New York: Brunner/Mazel.

Haley, J. (1980). *Leaving home.* New York: McGraw-Hill.

Haley, J. (1987). *Problem-solving therapy* (2nd ed.). San Francisco: Jossey-Bass.

Hoffman, L. (1981). *Foundation of family therapy.* New York: Basic Books.

Madanes, C. (1980). Protection, paradox, and pretending. *Family Process, 19,* 73–85.

Madanes, C. (1981). *Strategic family therapy.* San Francisco: Jossey-Bass.

Madanes, C. (1990). *Sex, love, and violence: Strategies for transformation.* New York: Norton.

Madanes, C. (1991). Strategic family therapy. In A. S. Gurman & D. P. Kniskern (Eds.), *Handbook of family therapy* (Vol. 2). New York: Brunner/Mazel.

Madanes, C., & Haley, J. (1977). Dimensions of family therapy. *Journal of Nervous and Mental Disease, 165,* 88–98.

Minuchin, S. (1974). *Families and family therapy.* Cambridge, MA: Harvard University Press.

Minuchin, S., & Fishman, H. C. (1981). *Family therapy techniques.* Cambridge, MA: Harvard University Press.

Minuchin, S., Montalvo, B., Guerney, B. G., Rosman, B. L., & Schumer, F. (1967). *Families of the slums.* New York: Basic Books.

Minuchin, S., & Nichols, M. P. (1993). *Family healing: Tales of hope and renewal from family therapy.* New York: Free Press.

Minuchin, S., Rosman, B. L., & Baker, L. (1978). *Psychosomatic families: Anorexia nervosa in context.* Cambridge, MA: Harvard University Press.

Penn, P. (1982). Circular questioning. *Family Process, 21,* 267–280.

Penn, P. (1985). Feed-forward: Future questions, future maps. *Family Process, 24,* 299–310.

Piercy, F., & Sprenkle, D. (1984). The process of family therapy education. *Journal of Marital and Family Therapy, 10*(4), 399–407.

Prata, G. (1990). *A systemic harpoon into family games: Preventive interventions in therapy.* New York: Brunner/Mazel.

Raskin, D. E., & Klein, Z. E. (1976). Losing a symptom through keeping it: A review of paradoxical treatment techniques and rationale. *Archives of General Psychiatry, 33,* 548–555.

Segal, L. (1991). Brief therapy: The MRI approach. In A. S. Gurman & D. P. Kniskern (Eds.), *Handbook of family therapy* (Vol. 2). New York: Brunner/Mazel.

Selvini Palazzoli, M. (1986). Towards a general model of psychotic family games. *Journal of Marital and Family Therapy, 12,* 339–349.

Selvini Palazzoli, M., Boscolo, L., Cecchin, G., & Prata, G. (1978). *Paradox and counterparadox.* New York: Jason Aronson.

Selvini Palazzoli, M., Boscolo, L., Cecchin, G., & Prata, G. (1980). Hypothesizing–circularity–neutrality: Three guidelines for the conductor of the session. *Family Process, 19,* 3–12.

Selvini Palazzoli, M., Cirillo, S., Selvini, M., & Sorrentino, A. M. (1989). *Family games: General models of psychotic processes in the family.* New York: Norton.

Stanton, M. D. (1981). Strategic approaches to family therapy. In A. S. Gurman & D. P. Kniskern (Eds.), *Handbook of family therapy*. New York: Brunner/Mazel.

Stanton, M. D., Todd, T. C., & Associates. (1982). *The family therapy of drug abuse and addiction*. New York: Guilford Press.

Stone Fish, L., & Piercy, F. P. (1987). The theory and practice of structural and strategic family therapy: A Delphi study. *Journal of Marital and Family Therapy, 13*, 113–125.

Tomm, K. (1984a). One perspective on the Milan systemic approach: Part I. Overview of development, theory and practice. *Journal of Marital and Family Therapy*, 113–125.

Tomm, K. (1984b). One perspective on the Milan systemic approach: Part II. Description of session format, interviewing style and interventions. *Journal of Marital and Family Therapy, 10*, 253–271.

Tomm, K. (1987a). Interventive interviewing: Part I. Strategizing as a fourth guideline for the therapist. *Family Process, 26*, 3–13.

Tomm, K. (1987b). Interventive interviewing: Part II. Reflexive questioning as a means to enable self-healing. *Family Process, 26*, 167–183.

Tomm, K. (1988). Interventive interviewing: Part III. Intending to ask lineal, circular, strategic, or reflexive questions? *Family Process, 27*, 1–15.

Watzlawick, P., Weakland, J. H., & Fisch, R. (1974). *Change: Principles of problem formation and problem resolution*. New York: Norton.

Weakland, J. H., Fisch, R., Watzlawick, P., & Bodin, A. M. (1974). Brief therapy: Focused problem resolution. *Family Process, 13*, 141–168.

Weakland, J. H., & Ray, W. A. (1995). *Propagations: Thirty years of influence from the Mental Research Institute*. Binghamton, NY: Haworth.

Weeks, G. R., & L'Abate, L. (1979). A compilation of paradoxical methods. *American Journal of Family Therapy, 7*, 61–76.

4

Experiential Family Therapies

JOSEPH L. WETCHLER
FRED P. PIERCY

POPULAR HUMANISTIC, existential therapies of the 1960s, such as Gestalt therapy, psychodrama, client-centered therapy, logotherapy, and the encounter group movement, have all influenced the theory and technique of various experiential family therapies. And, like individual, humanistic psychotherapies, experiential family therapies challenge the reductionist tenets of some of the problem-focused schools of family therapy.

A founder and leading catalyst in the evolution of experiential family therapies is undoubtedly Virginia Satir. Satir (1983, 1988) blended Gestalt techniques, psychodrama, encounter techniques, and communications training into a dynamic family therapy that continues to influence the field.

Carl Whitaker was another charismatic and influential experiential family therapist (Napier & Whitaker, 1978; Neill & Kniskern, 1982; Whitaker & Bumberry, 1988; Whitaker & Keith, 1981; Whitaker & Ryan, 1989). In fact, Whitaker may have been the first to have used the term "experiential psychotherapy" (Whitaker & Malone, 1953). Although Whitaker's approach was unconventional and idiosyncratic, the basic assumptions underlying his therapy are largely consistent with existential, humanistic thought.

Other experiential family therapists include Walter Kempler (1973, 1981), a proponent of Gestalt family therapy; Fred and Bunny Duhl (Duhl, 1983, 1987; Duhl & Duhl, 1981; F. J. Duhl & Duhl, 1979), the developers of "integrative family therapy"; Ronald Levant (1978), who has proposed a client-centered family therapy approach; and Leslie Greenberg and Susan

Johnson (1985, 1988), whose "emotionally focused couple therapy" integrates experiential and systems-based models and is the first of these theories to develop a strong research base.

Each of these experiential family therapists conducts therapy in a uniquely different way; however, certain theoretical tenets are common to each. A discussion follows regarding several of the major theoretical assumptions held by most experiential family therapists.

PRIMACY OF EXPERIENCE

Sartre's (1946) classic philosophical assertion, "Existence precedes essence," is basic to experiential family therapy. Our thoughts and intellectualizations ("essence") are our attempts to decipher meaning from our experiences ("existence"), but the experience of living comes first.

A person who only lives intellectually is not in touch with or reflecting on his or her own life experience. Consequently, important nonrational experiential data are ignored. This person would not know him- or herself and thus would have no authentic self to offer others in relationships. As Whitaker (1976) suggests, such a person is "doing" to avoid the anxiety of nonbeing. Kempler (1973) describes it this way: "There is the risk of becoming the victims of our own logical minds, living lives guided, at best, by sensitive intelligence and practical reality. . . . Family is essential to sustaining, in the deepest sense, the happening we call living; and without whom life is reduced to an intelligent reflex arc" (p. 79).

Experiential family therapy succeeds in reminding us of the importance of firsthand experiential data, which is often underemphasized by other schools of family therapy. The experiential family therapist asserts that there is more to life than what can be observed and measured. The more is the human, creative, life-and-breath dimension of family. As B. S. Duhl and Duhl (1981) state, "It is hard to kiss a system" (p. 488).

Because experiential family therapists are interested in the direct experience of families, they employ a variety of procedures to facilitate here-and-now experiences, whether in the form of dreams, fantasies, feelings, or sensations.

AFFECT

Families not in touch with their present experiencing are thought to be emotionally dead. Experiential family therapists use evocative procedures to unblock honest emotional expression in such families. Their goal is to open individuals to their inner experience, thus helping them to be more fully human. In this sense, affect is, in itself, therapeutic and growth producing (Greenberg & Safran, 1989; Johnson & Greenberg, 1994). Experiential family therapy helps family members begin to feel, to experience each other as real people, and to directly attack the emotional sterility that has enveloped the family. As Carl Whitaker is fond of saying, "One hug from a family member is worth a hundred from a therapist."

THE PERSON OF THE THERAPIST

Experiential family therapists participate actively and personally in therapy sessions; they do not attempt to hide behind a therapeutic mask. This means at times being vulnerable with family members and at other times being angry or upset. If the therapist expects the family to have the courage to be real, the therapist must also demonstrate that courage (B.S. Duhl, 1987; Keith, 1987; Keith, Connell, & Whitaker, 1991; Satir, 1983; Whitaker & Ryan, 1989).

Such self-disclosure has therapeutic benefit for both family and therapist. The therapist's realness and present-centered encounters often stimulate expanded experience and intimate encounters within the family. Likewise, the therapist wants and needs real human contact during the therapy hour (Keith et al., 1991). Whitaker and Keith (1981) state that if the therapist gets nothing for himself/herself during therapy, chances are that the family members are not getting much either.

SPONTANEITY AND CREATIVITY

Since creative, nonrational experiencing is an important goal of experiential family therapy, spontaneity is desired for both therapist and family. In fact, Whitaker and Keith (1981) advocate craziness—nonrational, right-brain experiencing—as a measure of health in both therapist and family.

Any techniques that the experiential therapist might use are meant to foster creative experiencing. Techniques such as family sculpting (F. J. Duhl, Kantor, & Duhl, 1973), family art therapy (Geddes & Medway, 1977; Linesch, 1993), puppetry (B. S. Duhl & Duhl, 1981), family drawings (Bing, 1970; Burns, 1990), psychodramatic techniques (Satir, 1983; Satir & Baldwin, 1983), and Gestalt ground rules (Kempler, 1973, 1981) are all applied to free the family members to experience each other and life more creatively and personally.

Techniques, however, are not central to experiential family therapy. Whitaker, for example, believes that the best interventions, particularly in later sessions, are those that arise out of the therapist's own creativity in the moment, rather than any preplanned interventions (Neill & Kniskern, 1982). As Whitaker and Keith (1981) state, "The objective of all techniques is to eliminate techniques" (p. 218).

FREEDOM, HOLISM,
AND EXISTENTIAL ANXIETY

Experiential family therapists follow in the tradition of the existential philosophers, in that their views may be regarded as a sustained protest (Kaufman, 1956) against the reduction of human existence to mere behaviors, cognitions, or theories. Whitaker, for example, emphasizes many of the traditional themes of existentialism: freedom; not fate but choices; anxiety; and awareness of death (Napier & Whitaker, 1978). Whitaker emphasizes these themes in therapy, not because they are strategically useful, but because he believes that they are central to the experience of human living.

Experiential family therapists assume the personal freedom of the family members with which they work. But with freedom comes choice, and as Bunny Duhl (1983) states, "We are not accustomed to reaching inward for our answers" (p. 37). Whether through Gestalt techniques, evocative challenges, or silence, the therapist encourages self-responsibility within the family. As Whitaker (in Neill & Kniskern, 1982) states, "The integrity of the family must be respected. They must write their own destiny" (p. 329).

"I–THOU" RELATIONSHIP

Experiential family therapists want to do more than help family members experience their inner reality; they want to encourage an "I–Thou" (Buber, 1970) encounter among family members and perhaps with themselves. Such an existential encounter has sometimes been described as resulting in an "existential shift," a change in referent point, or a "carrying-forward effect" among family members, which leads to a change in how family members experience and relate to one another (Gendlin, 1973). Experiential family therapists believe in the healing nature of human relationships. I–Thou encounters have therapeutic value, in that they set into motion the growth potential of family members (Keith et al., 1991)

PRESENT-CENTEREDNESS

Immediate experiencing and person-to-person encounters can take place only in the present. When the past or future is discussed, family members are taken away from direct experience. Such intellectualizations, therefore, are typically seen as counterproductive to the experiential family therapist. As Whitaker states, "Life isn't mind over matter, it's present over past and present over future" (in Neill & Kniskern, 1982, p. 372).

GLOBAL VERSUS SPECIFIC GOALS

Experiential family therapists typically describe their goals in general terms, such as a heightened sense of competence, well-being, and self-esteem (B. S. Duhl & Duhl, 1981); role flexibility (Whitaker & Ryan, 1989; Whitaker & Keith, 1981); awareness and self-responsibility (Kempler, 1973, 1981); and "leveling" communication (Satir, 1988). Such vague, nonoperationalized goals have been criticized by many family therapy researchers; however, experiential family therapists, with the notable exception of Greenberg and Johnson (1988), give these criticisms relatively little weight, since, after all, internal experience is seen as infinitely more valid than external, intellectual, nonexperiential data.

SYMBOLIC–EXPERIENTIAL FAMILY THERAPY

Symbolic–experiential family therapy is associated with Carl Whitaker and colleagues (e.g., Napier, 1987a, 1987b; Roberto, 1991; Whitaker & Bumberry, 1988; Whitaker & Keith, 1981). It evolved from Whitaker's early work with both fighter pilots during the Second World War and with schizophrenics (Whitaker & Ryan, 1989). Many of his ideas, initially developed with colleagues Thomas Malone and John Warkentin (Whitaker & Malone, 1953; Whitaker, Warkentin, & Malone, 1959), shocked the psychotherapy establishment. They espoused a model of therapeutic encounter in which both the therapist and client regressed to where the therapist became a "parent imago" to the "child self" of the client. As the client's early issues were worked through this joint fantasy, the therapist and client could progress to an adult-to-adult, give-and-take relationship at termination (Whitaker & Malone, 1953). "By relating primarily on a symbolic level, the therapeutic relationship itself becomes an *interactional metaphor* (Connell, Mitten, & Whitaker, 1993, p. 244, italics in original)."

Over the years, Whitaker moved to a family perspective on treatment, based on the numerous failures he encountered. The relationship between the therapist and client was not strong enough to overcome the client's relationship with his or her own family (Neill & Kniskern, 1982; Whitaker & Ryan, 1989). This led to Whitaker's notion of the family as a key organizational unit.

> I found myself intrigued by the assumption that *there is no such thing as a person,* that *a person is merely the fragment of a family.* . . . This led to the obvious inference that marriage is not really a combination of two persons; rather it is the product of two families who send out a scapegoat to reproduce themselves. (Whitaker & Ryan, 1989, p. 116, italics in original)

This revelation led to his bringing whole families and multiple generations of families into the therapy room (Roberto, 1991; Whitaker & Keith, 1981). The therapeutic encounter now included the therapist and the whole family. It is through this encounter that Whitaker attempts to dislodge rigid feelings and patterns of interacting and, instead, develop flexibility and creativity in the family.

Whitaker defines himself as an "I" to the family's "Thou" by bringing his sense of personhood into the therapy room. With this comes his use of fantasy, feelings, and willingness to change his stance at the drop of a hat. The family then changes its own response to the therapist and eventually develops flexibility within itself.

Whitaker conducts therapy in a two-step process. First is the "battle for structure," in which the therapist tells the family who will attend and how therapy will be conducted. This places the therapist in the role of expert and blocks the family from invoking its typical patterns on the therapy (Whitaker & Keith, 1981; Whitaker & Ryan, 1989). Next, the therapist engages the family in the "battle for initiative," in which responsibility for work in the session is passed on to the family. This gives the family the message that although the therapist is an important figure in the therapy, the family members themselves are in charge of their own lives. Whitaker makes it clear that he is a coach and not a teammate of the family. At the same time, he is clear that it is the therapist's responsibility to provide the family with the expertise to help them achieve their goals (Roberto, 1991; Whitaker & Ryan, 1989).

Cotherapy is important to the process of symbolic–experiential therapy. In a therapy that is dependent on therapists modeling their own craziness and free associations, it is helpful to have a lifeline to another colleague. Furthermore, by developing a cotherapy relationship that is more important to the therapists than their relationship to the family, they can rely on their interpersonal intimacy to sustain them rather than expecting the client family to meet their needs (Napier & Whitaker, 1978).

Carl Whitaker, who died in 1995, gave the following tips for helping therapists stay emotionally alive (Whitaker, 1976, p. 164):

1. Relegate every significant other to second place.
2. Learn how to love. Flirt with any infant available. Unconditional . . . regard probably isn't present after the baby is three years old.
3. Develop a reverence for your own impulses, and be suspicious of your behavior sequences.
4. Enjoy your mate more than your kids, and be childish with your mate.
5. Fracture role structures at will and repeatedly.
6. Learn to retreat and advance from every position you take.
7. Guard your impotence as one of your most valuable weapons.
8. Build long-term relationships so you can be free to hate safely.
9. Face the fact that you must grow until you die. Develop a sense of the

absurdity of life—yours and those around you—and thus learn to transcend the world of experience. If we can abandon our missionary zeal we have less chance of being eaten by cannibals.

10. Develop your primary process living. Evolve a joint craziness with some one you are safe with. Structure a professional cuddle group so you won't abuse your mate with the garbage left over from the day's work.

11. As Plato said, "Practice dying."

VIRGINIA SATIR

Virginia Satir's work (e.g., 1983, 1988; Satir & Baldwin, 1983) is a hallmark of experiential family therapy. Her warmth, compassion, and genuineness were a model for many family therapists (Brothers, 1991a). Although some considered her ideas simplistic, others viewed her with almost mystical reverence. Brothers (1991a) states:

> Virginia was able to manifest and to *teach the manifestations of philosophies* taught by venerated thinkers and philosophers stretching out, through time, behind her. She designed processes which made available the experiencing of the Tao, of Teilhard's ultra-human, of Gandi's *ahimsa* (truth-force). If they were the theory, Virginia was the laboratory experience. (p. 4, italics in original)

Satir's ideas went beyond family treatment to encompass issues of spiritual growth and world peace (Brothers, 1991a; Satir, 1988). Her views on the importance of interconnectedness among humanity pervaded all aspects of her work.

Satir believed strongly in the importance of congruent communication both between others and within the self (Satir, 1983; Brothers, 1991b). This is a reciprocal process, because as individuals become more in touch with the messages within themselves, they are able to communicate more congruently with others. Furthermore, the development of honest communication facilitates all individuals engaged in the process to become more aware of themselves. Her "Parts Party" (Satir & Baldwin, 1983; Winter & Parker, 1991), in which others act out various aspects of a person's personality under his or her direction, served as a way to get in touch with the different "parts" of oneself and to share them with other members of the family.

The importance of communication goes far beyond family therapy and problem resolution. Satir (1988) states:

> I see communication as a huge umbrella that covers and affects all that goes on between human beings. Once a human being has arrived on this earth, *communication is the largest single factor determining what kinds of relationships she*

or he makes with others and what happens to each in the world. How we manage
survival, how we develop intimacy, how productive we are, how we make
sense, how we connect with our own divinity—all depend largely on our
communication skills. (p. 51, italics in original)

Also central to Satir's ideas is the concept of the triad (Satir & Baldwin,
1983). She viewed family triads as interconnected, with the "mother, father,
child triad" as being especially important (Baldwin, 1991). It is through this
triad that the child learns about the nature of parent-to-child and adult-to-
adult intimacy. Although triads can lead to dysfunctional processes in
families, they also serve as a path toward growth. Her technique of "family
reconstruction" (Satir & Baldwin, 1983) used psychodrama to help individuals experience the development of primary triads through several
generations. It is a powerful way of harnessing the curative aspects of the
family triad in personal development.

Satir strongly believed in the goodness of people. It was this basic
optimism that enabled her to touch the lives of so many clients, students,
and family therapists around the world.

EMOTIONALLY FOCUSED COUPLE THERAPY

Emotionally focused couple therapy (EFT; Greenberg & Johnson, 1985,
1986, 1988; Johnson & Greenberg, 1987) represents the new wave of
experiential family therapy. While holding true to many of its tenets, it
breaks with tradition by providing replicable procedures (Greenberg &
Johnson, 1985, 1988) and developing outcome studies to test its effectiveness
(Dandeneau & Johnson, 1994; Johnson & Greenberg, 1985a, 1985b).

EFT integrates aspects of family systems (Fisch, Weakland, & Segal,
1983; Watzlawick, Weakland, & Fisch, 1974) and experiential therapies.
It posits that due to problems with attachment (Bowlby, 1969), couples
will hide their "primary emotions" (actual emotions such as fear or need
for attachment) and instead exhibit "secondary reactive emotions" (defensive or coercive emotions). This leads to a "negative interaction," such
as pursue–distance or blame–withdraw, that serves as a defense against
exhibiting the more vulnerable primary emotions. The enactment of
these negative interaction patterns in a marriage, however serves to
heighten the fear that one's partner is not worthy of trust, which in turn
maintains the pattern and further buries primary emotions (Greenberg
& Johnson, 1986, 1988). The goal of therapy is to access these primary
emotions, enhance the emotional bond, and alter negative interactional
sequences (Greenberg & Safran, 1989; Johnson, 1986). Greenberg and
Johnson (1988) state:

The purpose of EFT can be described as attempting to change the interactional and emotional field so that individuals and interactions are reorganized to result in more functional relationships. A major goal of EFT is restructuring the emotional bond so as to promote a continually regenerative I-thou dialogue between partners. (pp. 41–42)

The experience of primary affect serves as a means for couples to reframe their relationship. This enables them to alter their negative interaction sequence and develop ways of solving their problems (Greenberg & Johnson, 1988; Johnson & Greenberg, 1994). For example, as Mary begins to see John's withdrawal as the fear of being emotionally hurt and John understands that her anger is due to her fear of being abandoned by him, they will begin to talk differently to each other and develop a more stable bond.

The therapist–client relationship is crucial in EFT for clients to access their primary emotions. Unconditional positive regard (Rogers, 1961) for each member of the couple creates a safe atmosphere to explore deep feelings. As EFT therapists often must work with one partner at a time in the presence of the other to access primary emotions, this relationship is crucial for the observing spouse to not feel sided against (Greenberg & Johnson, 1988).

Greenberg and Johnson (1985, 1988) propose a nine-step procedure for conducting EFT:

1. Delineate the issues presented by the couple and assess how these issues express core conflicts in the areas of separateness–connectedness and dependence–independence.
2. Identify the negative interaction cycle.
3. Access unacknowledged feelings underlying interactional positions.
4. Redefine the problem(s) in terms of the underlying feelings.
5. Promote identification with disowned needs and aspects of self.
6. Promote acceptance by each partner of the other partner's experience.
7. Facilitate the expression of needs and wants to restructure the interaction.
8. Establish the emergence of new solutions.
9. Consolidate new positions. (p. 66)

Many schools of family therapy have achieved prominence based on the personal charisma of their leaders (Broderick & Schrader, 1991). The experiential family therapies have suffered a severe blow with the deaths of Virginia Satir and Carl Whitaker. The emergence of EFT could not be more timely. Perhaps, with its emphasis on replicability and research, emotionally focused therapy will be the force that carries the experiential family therapies into the 21st century.

KEY CONCEPTS

Alienation. The condition of being shut off from one's true feelings. Most experiential therapists agree that dysfunctional family members are alienated, thus making family intimacy difficult to achieve.

Awareness. Considered by Kempler (1973) to be the "process of processes," which involves a "re-minding, a realization, a bringing into consciousness of the mind's own inherent mechanism for orienting" (p. 61). New awareness potentially leads to self-responsibility and growth. For example, if a person becomes aware of his or her need for support or independence, he or she is then better able to act on that need.

Battle for initiative. After the therapist has won the "battle for structure" (see next definition), Carl Whitaker (Whitaker & Keith, 1981) emphasizes the importance of allowing the family the freedom to determine the course of therapy. Although Whitaker is concerned and active, he is respectful of the family's right to choose its own destiny, both in the therapy room and in its life outside.

Battle for structure. Carl Whitaker's (Whitaker & Keith, 1981) term for the therapist's task of establishing workable administrative control with a family at the beginning of therapy. Whitaker does this, for example, by clearly being in charge of when the sessions will be held, who will come, and what the process will be.

Communication. The way in which people share meaning with one another. Direct, clear, person-centered communication is generally considered healthy by experiential family therapists, and is particularly emphasized by Satir (1983, 1988), Kempler (1973, 1981), and B. S. Duhl and Duhl (1981).

"Craziness." Whitaker's (e.g., Whitaker & Ryan, 1989) concept for nonrational, right-brain, creative functioning that he believes is appropriate and healthy for both therapist and family to be able to establish access and to engage in.

Existential shift. A change in referent point or "carrying forward" (Gendlin, 1973) that occurs in a relationship when two people have a moving, present-centered, person-to-person encounter. Such a powerful experience goes beyond one's ability to describe it and often results in a marked change in how one perceives and acts in the world.

Experience. According to Kempler (1973), experience is the "key to growth and regrowth and to the therapeutic process" (p. 62). By this, Kempler means intimate experience that brings with it new awareness. Gestalt experiential family therapy facilitates experiences that stimulate awareness, thus helping family members get in touch with and reintegrate parts of themselves, which in turn fosters greater self-responsibility.

Flight into health. The tendency of many families, according to Carl

Whitaker (e.g. Whitaker & Ryan, 1989), to terminate therapy prematurely when family stress is reduced. Whitaker defines this as a positive growth effort that should not be prevented. Moreover, if the family should again seek therapy at a later time, members are often more united and resolved to get the most out of therapy.

Negative interaction cycle. Defined by Greenberg and Johnson (1988) as a problem-maintaining sequence in couples that derives from and maintains the use of secondary reactive emotions such as anger listed to defend against the more vulnerable primary emotions of fear or emotional pain listed.

Primary emotions. Emotionally focused therapists (Greenberg & Johnson, 1988) view these emotions as expressing our core feelings. They attempt to access these during therapy to alter negative interaction cycles and promote bonding between partners. For example, a withdrawing husband would be encouraged to discuss how he is afraid that his wife will hurt him when she yells at him.

Primary family triad. Satir (Satir & Baldwin, 1983) saw the primary family therapy triad as being comprised of mother, father, and child. It is from this triad that the child learns about relationships, gender behavior, and communication. Although membership in a triad can serve to maintain problems, it also serves as the means for problem resolution and emotional growth.

Secondary reactive emotions. These are emotions that serve as defenses to protect the more vulnerable primary emotions. An example would be a husband who yells at his wife to mask the fact that he is hurt by her inattentiveness. Greenberg and Johnson (1988) believe that couples rely on secondary emotions when there is a lack of attachment and bonding in their relationship. Unfortunately, reliance on secondary reactive emotions serves also to maintain a couple's lack of trust.

Self-awareness. A goal of experiential family therapies (particularly Gestalt family therapy) in which the rigid cycles of automatic behaviors are unblocked. As a person becomes more self-aware by exploring his or her present experience, he or she moves to a position of recognizing choices and responsibility for behavior. Furthermore, self-awareness often brings about an integration of fragmented or "unfinished" aspects of the self that have been outside awareness.

Self-worth. The feelings (self-esteem) and ideas (self-concept) one has about one's self (Satir, 1988). Most experiential family therapists believe that increased self-worth is an important process and outcome of family therapy.

Unfinished business. A term coined by Fritz Perls (1973), the founder of Gestalt therapy, and frequently used by Gestalt family therapists such as Walter Kempler (1973, 1981) to mean unresolved feelings and/or disowned parts of one's self. Through present-centered Gestalt therapy, such unfinished business can come into awareness and be integrated and responsibly handled.

KEY CLINICAL SKILLS

Although the use of techniques is minimized in experiential family therapy, we have included here several ways in which experiential family therapists facilitate present-centered, person-focused contact with client families.

Accessing emotional experiences. This is the process that emotionally focused couple therapists engage in to access primary emotions in a couple. Greenberg and Johnson (1988) utilize empathic reflection, directing focus, enactments, and empathic interpretations to help couples access this information.

Changing interactional positions. Emotionally focused therapists utilize accessed primary emotions to help couples alter negative interaction sequences. Primary emotions serve to reframe a couples' behavior and motivate them to behave in new ways. This, in turn, serves to strengthen their emotional bond.

Encounter. A powerful personal experience, the encounter occurs when two people drop defenses and interact with one another honestly. Even when a therapist is being authentically angry with a family member, such a powerful personal encounter may encourage a potentially more caring, person-to-person relationship in the future.

Family drawing. An experiential family therapy technique, family drawing occurs when family members draw their conception of how their family is organized, in order to stimulate new learnings and insights (see Bing, 1970; Burns, 1990; Geddes & Medway, 1977; Linesch, 1993).

Family reconstruction. A technique of Virginia Satir (Satir & Baldwin, 1983), family reconstruction utilizes psychodrama to help individuals experience the key triads in their families of origin. Clients select individuals (or friends) to act out the roles of members of the primary triads in their families of origin. While experiencing participants acting out key family situations, clients gain new insights into their family and their own lives.

Gestalt techniques. These are a wide variety of techniques used by Gestalt family therapists to encourage present-centered family interaction and interpersonal awareness. For example, ground rules such as "No gossiping" and "Statements, not questions," as well as facilitative therapist responses such as "Tell *him* that, not me," encourage person-to-person communication and interpersonal awareness (cf. Kaplan & Kaplan, 1978; Kempler, 1973, 1981).

Parts party. This experiential technique of Virginia Satir (Satir & Baldwin, 1983; Winter & Parker, 1991) is designed to help clients experience the different parts of their personalities and enable them to see how they operate as an integrated whole. Individuals (or friends) are chosen to act out specific parts of the client's personality. The client then watches as these parts interact with each other to foster personal experience and insight.

Personal involvement. As stated earlier, personal involvement is a critical factor in the successes of experiential family therapy. The therapist must have the courage to be involved in a real, caring way with the client family. According to Whitaker, if the therapist is not personally involved, there is no real learning.

Sculpture (also known as "space sculpture," "family sculpture," "relationship sculpture," and "spatialization"). A technique developed initially by David Kantor, in which symbolic processes and events are portrayed through spatial analogies (e.g., distancing and posturing of various family members; Constantine, 1978; Duhl, 1983). Some family therapists use sculpture to disengage the clients from emotional experience and thus facilitate insight into the past and present situations (Constantine, 1978). Others (e.g., Satir, 1988) use sculpture to bring about an affective experience that will unblock unexpressed emotions.

Self-disclosure. The sharing of aspects of one's self with one's clients, in which virtually all experiential family therapists engage. Self-disclosure is thought to increase trust, provide alternatives through metaphor, facilitate person-to-person encounters, and allow the therapist to be known to the family as an accessible person rather than a distant professional.

Symbolic drawing of the family life space. An expressive activity initially developed by Damuta Mostwin, in which family members graphically represent emotional distance and communication patterns among one another through symbolic drawings on a blackboard. It is thought to be a nonthreatening task that facilitates meaningful family interaction and provides a wealth of information about the family in therapy (Geddes & Medway, 1977).

Temperature reading. A technique developed by Satir (1988), in which family members set aside a specific time each day to get in touch with each other. Discussion centers on expressing their appreciations of each other, complaints and recommendations, questions, hopes, and wishes.

TEACHING TOOLS AND TECHNIQUES

Family Sculpture

Consistent with the ideas discussed in Duhl, Kantor, and Duhl (1973), we believe it is important for students to *experience* the feeling of being in a family system. Family sculpture enables students to experience the interactional nature of families. Students can sculpt either a family they are currently working with or their own family of origin. It is most helpful to sculpt the family both as they perceive it now and as they would like it to be. Teachers should be aware that sculpting a student's family of origin may be a profound emotional experience for the student and his or her classmates. The experience should be voluntary, and plenty of time should be allotted to process the experience for all participants and observers.

As a Family Therapist . . .

This activity helps beginning clinicians identify the various emotional parts (Satir & Baldwin, 1983) of themselves as family therapists. It also helps them to recognize that many of their feelings are common among their peers as well. Students are instructed to complete a series of open-ended sentences and then discuss their responses in a small group. The sentences are as follows:

> As a family therapist I am proudest when . . .
> As a family therapist I am most scared when . . .
> As a family therapist I am angriest when . . .
> As a family therapist I am happiest when . . .
> As a family therapist I am saddest when . . .
> As a family therapist I am silliest when . . .
> As a family therapist I am most worried when . . .
> As a family therapist my greatest strength is . . .
> As a family therapist my greatest growth area is . . .
> As a family therapist my greatest hope is . . .

Small-Group Discussion:
Theoretical Tenets of Carl Whitaker

The class is broken down into small groups, with each group given a statement or question to discuss what Carl Whitaker has dealt with in his writings. After each group discusses personal opinions related to its respective statement, a spokesperson from each group summarizes the major issues of the group discussion to the entire class. After each summary, the instructor discusses with the class what Carl Whitaker has said about that particular topic (see Neill & Kniskern, 1982). Often lively discussions ensue. The following are questions used in this exercise, along with a summary of Whitaker's views on each particular issue.

1. *What results do you want in working with a family? Describe how you want the family to function at the end of therapy.* Whitaker emphasizes role flexibility, as well as an increased sense of unity and autonomy as appropriate

goals of therapy. Whitaker prizes the individuality of families and their freedom to determine their own lives. He does not want them to fit some therapist's narrow definition of "well functioning." By and large, he hopes that therapy will expand a family's options.

2. *We, as people helpers, are professional parents. Do you agree or disagree? Why?* Whitaker would agree with this. A therapist, like a parent, allows more and more responsibility as time progresses. The therapist also goes through stages with the families, analogous to family life-cycle stages (e.g., "terrible twos," psychosexual stages, rebellious adolescents, "empty nest" syndrome).

3. *The therapist must use power in his or her work with families. What are some specific ways of claiming your power during the therapy process?* Whitaker's "battle for structure" (Whitaker & Keith, 1981, p. 204) starts with the first phone call, when he tells all family members to come to the first session. He also decides when the session will be, who will speak, what the process will be, and so forth. As therapy proceeds and his administrative control is assured, he then supports the freedom and initiative of the family in setting the direction of therapy.

4. *If "love is not enough" and "techniques are not enough," what is? Discuss the basic ingredients in being an effective therapist. Include love and techniques in your discussion.* Whitaker would agree that both love and techniques (to a lesser extent) are important ingredients. According to Whitaker, the therapist should ideally care deeply about the client family. Although Whitaker emphasizes the therapeutic value of the therapist–client relationship, he also has identified various therapeutic techniques (cf. Whitaker & Keith, 1981; Whitaker & Napier, 1977). However, as Whitaker and Napier state, "The objective of technique is the development of . . . the therapist . . . beyond 'using' techniques" (p. 5).

5. *When cotherapy is used, should it involve a male and female?* Whitaker believes that it is not essential to have a male and female cotherapist so long as the cotherapists can establish themselves as symbiotic parents to the whole family. What really helps is that both are ageless and sexless, free "to play all the keys." Whitaker, for example, can be a tender mother and a tough grandfather.

6. *Families should not leave a session with confusion or unfinished feelings. Do you agree or disagree?* Whitaker would disagree. Confusion is good—the beginning of creativity. Napier and Whitaker (1978) tell families, "Don't try to sort it out. Let it cook in you, and don't talk about this 'stuff' at home. The things that are valuable will sort themselves out and begin to make sense to you as we go on" (p. 77).

7. *The therapist's contribution comes primarily out of his or her own person, not out of his or her professional skill. Do you agree or disagree?* Whitaker would agree. The therapist's intuitive and deeply personal involvement in a "reparenting" process characterizes his approach, as does his goal of establishing a caring, person-to-person relationship with the members of the

family. Through the therapist's allowing his or her own personhood into therapy, an existential shift can occur that results in positive family growth.

Read–Summarize–React Exercise: Provocative Statements of Carl Whitaker

Many of Carl Whitaker's provocative statements are included by Neill and Kniskern (1982) in a chapter entitled "Gatherings." Statements related to the therapeutic process and theoretical tenets of Whitaker are typed on separate 5″ × 7″ cards. Students are formed into groups of five, with 10 cards in the middle of each group. Students are instructed, in turn, to (1) take a card and silently read Whitaker's statement, (2) paraphrase the statement, (3) give their own reactions to it, and (4) allow any other member of the group to respond. This exercise, plus any discussion that follows, provides students opportunities to clarify their own theoretical suppositions as they learn more about those of Carl Whitaker.

Several examples of provocative statements made by Carl Whitaker include the following:

- "Professionalism can be a serious problem."
- "Insight is a by-product of growth or change rather than a precursor or a cause of growth or change."
- "My theory is that all theories are bad except for preliminary game playing with ourselves until we get the courage to give up theories and just live."
- "You can fall in love but you can't fall out."
- "Psychotherapy is like yearning to play the piano. How much, how long, how deeply depends on what you want as an experience—to play hymns or to play Bach or Beethoven."
- "You don't really know somebody until you know their parents."
- "Real hatred is probably never destructive—we don't want to lose the object of our hatred; hatred has a unifying effect."
- "The best way to avoid psychotherapy is to have regular interviews with a therapist."

Position Paper

The following assignment for a five-page position paper is made after a thorough reading of Kempler (1973, 1981). It should be noted that this assignment could be adapted easily to cover any experiential family therapy.

Kempler (1973) discusses Hegel's contention that any thought (thesis) implies its own equal and opposite thought (antithesis), and when these two specific points are confronted they unite (synthesis) to become a single point (thesis) in a new spiral of thesis–antithesis–synthesis. Based on your assigned readings, what major thoughts (theses) of Kempler are directly confronted by your own thinking (antithesis)? From this dialectic tension and resulting synthesis, what theses, if any, emerge for you?

Satir Communications Exercise

In many of her workshops, Virginia Satir employed an experiential activity that demonstrates the personal and interpersonal impact of five types of communication (Satir, 1988). This exercise may also be used as a training activity that familiarizes students/trainees with Satir's contentions related to these styles of communication. In the exercise, groups of four are formed into "families." A mother, a father, an oldest child, and a youngest child are chosen in each "family." Then the following five communications styles are presented in a minilecture (see Satir, 1988):

1. *Placating*—pacifying, smoothing over differences, being nice, being protective, defending others gently, covering up.
2. *Avoiding* (distracting)—being quiet, pretending not to understand, changing the subject, playing weak, playing helpless.
3. *Blaming*—judging, bullying, comparing, complaining.
4. *Computing*—using logic, lecturing, using outside authority.
5. *Leveling*—"real" responding (i.e., integrated, flowing, and alive; appropriate to the situation; verbally and nonverbally consistent).

After the minilecture, each family is instructed to "plan where you will go and what you will do on your vacation." Each of five 5-minute family discussions takes place in which family members act out one of Satir's communication styles. The assignment of styles we have employed is as follows:

	Mother	Father	Oldest child	Youngest child
Role play #1	3	4	1	2
Role play #2	1	3	2	4
Role play #3	2	1	4	3
Role play #4	(Student chooses his or her own role.)			
Role play #5	5	5	5	5

After each role play, there is an opportunity for each group to debrief. A large-group discussion typically follows the completion of the small-group exercises. It is our experience that students get very involved in these small-group exercises and that the personal insights shared are considerable.

TEACHING TOOLS AND TECHNIQUES

Films/Videotapes

The following representative films or videotapes provide useful examples of experiential family therapy:

- *AAMFT Master Series*. Available from AAMFT, 1133 15th Street, N.W., Suite 300, Washington, DC 20005-2710.
- *Virginia Satir Teaching Tapes*. Available from Golden Triad Films, Inc., 3312 Broadway, Kansas City, MO 64111.
- Menninger Video Productions. Exclusively distributed by Altschul Group Corporation, 1560 Sherman Avenue, Suite 100, Evanston, IL 60201.
- *Making the Invisible Visible* (family sculpture, with Peggy Papp). Available from Nathan W. Ackerman Institute for Family Therapy, 149 East 78th Street, New York, NY 10021.
- *Affinity* (with Carl Whitaker). Available from Philadelphia Child Guidance Clinic, Two Children's Center, 34th Street & Civic Center Boulevard, Philadelphia, PA 19104.
- *A Different Kind of Caring: Family Therapy with Carl Whitaker*. Available from Brunner/Mazel Publishers, 19 Union Square West, New York, NY 10003.
- *Emotionally Focused Therapy for Couples* (with Susan Johnson). Available from University of Ottawa, Department of Psychology, Psycho-logical Services, 11 Marie Curie, Ottawa, Ontario, Canada K1N 6N5.

RESEARCH ISSUES

Experiential family therapists are generally uninterested in empirical research, largely because any "objective" reality is considered to be, at best, an imperfect reflection of lived human experience. Also, global, nonspecific goals such as "growth," "self-responsibility," and "self-worth" are difficult to operationalize, and to operationalize any such concept as scores on a self-report test is felt to be taking a life-and-blood experience and reducing it to a sterile, intellectual concept far different from the experience itself.

Research is at best inferential, however. Just because the mystical aspects of the therapeutic experience cannot be completely comprehended or described by current research methodology does not mean that research should not be conducted on experiential family therapies. Not to examine therapeutic process is to allow experiential family therapy to develop as an unguided cult. We have much to learn about experiential family therapies at both the micro- and the macrolevels that could potentially lead to more effective therapy. The following are examples of possible research questions:

• With the notable exception of emotionally focused couple therapy (e.g., Dandeneau & Johnson, 1994; Johnson & Greenberg, 1985a, 1985b), the experiential family therapies have yet to prove their clinical effectiveness. How effective are experiential family therapies compared to no-treatment control groups? Furthermore, how effective are experiential family therapies compared to other family therapies (e.g., structural, strategic, Bowen Systems Theory)?

• Is the evocation of primary emotions necessary to alter negative-interaction cycles as Greenberg and Johnson (1988) suggest?

• What is the relationship between emotional experience and insight or behavior change?

• Does Gestalt experiential family therapy lead to more responsible behavior (e.g., more first-person pronouns, completion of personal goals) than does a more nondirective, client-centered experiential family therapy?

• What family behavior occurs immediately after certain experiential therapeutic interventions (e.g., Gestalt awareness exercises, therapist self-disclosure, therapist encounter)? What are the family members' reactions to these therapist interventions?

• Is there a correlation between the quality and quantity of therapist self-disclosure and family self-disclosure?

• Are the therapist's goals for family members consistent with the family members' goal for themselves? When the goals are not consistent, is therapy as effective as when they are?

• How does the personality of an experiential family therapist differ from the personalities of therapists from other schools of family therapy? Do certain personality traits of experiential family therapists successfully predict outcome?

• Are cotherapy teams more creative in therapy than solo family therapists (as suggested by Whitaker & Keith, 1981), and does this translate into more creativity on the part of client families?

• Is experiential family therapy best taught by the trainee experiencing therapy in a cotherapy relationship (as suggested by Whitaker & Keith, 1981), or can it better be taught through the use of step-by-step training manuals (as suggested by Greenberg & Johnson, 1988).

• What are the short- and long-term effects of therapist confrontation?

More specifically, what type of confrontation is beneficial for what type of family with what presenting problems? Furthermore, what are the rates of premature termination by clients in confrontive therapies versus less confrontive models?

• Is there a correlation between the therapist's psychological health and the extent of family improvement in family therapy (as suggested by Whitaker & Keith, 1981)?

KEY BOOKS, CHAPTERS, AND ARTICLES

Brothers, B. J. (Ed.). (1991). *Virginia Satir: Foundational ideas.* Binghamton, NY: Haworth.

This book presents foundational ideas and key techniques of Virginia Satir. The chapters are written by students of Satir and provide a scholarly, theoretical view of her work. The book is clearly a tribute to Satir and closes with reflections on her death. It is an excellent integration of scholarship and experience.

Constantine, L. (1978). Family sculpture and relationship mapping techniques. *Journal of Marriage and Family Counseling,* 4(2), 13–23.

This article provides an overview of family sculpture and a variety of illustrative ways it may be used. The examples of sculpture techniques should prove helpful to clinicians wishing to expand their use of spatialization procedures.

Duhl, B. S. (1983). *From the inside out and other metaphors: Creative and integrative approaches to training in systems thinking.* New York: Brunner/Mazel.

This is a book about teaching nonlinear concepts in a nonlinear manner. Duhl teaches through metaphor, movement, analogy, play, imitation, and more. She engagingly explains the process of learning through doing, experiencing, and debriefing, that is, learning from the inside out.

Duhl, F. J., Kantor, D., & Duhl, B. S. (1973). Learning, space, and action in family therapy: A primer of sculpture. In D. A. Bloch (Ed.), *Techniques of family psychotherapy: A primer.* New York: Grune & Stratton.

Family sculpting provides the kind of insight that makes it impossible to return to a previously implicit way of functioning, thereby encouraging new behavioral patterns. The association provided between sculpturing and learning is interesting. Instructions on debriefing are included.

Geddes, M., & Medway, J. (1977). The symbolic drawing of family life space. *Family Process, 16,* 219–228.

The authors review expressive techniques used by other family therapists and present the symbolic drawing of the family life space as a simple and effective activity for lowering anxiety and reducing blocks to communication. The activity involves family members' graphically representing emotional distances and communication patterns among one another through a drawing on a blackboard. Several examples are given.

Greenberg, L. S., & Johnson, S. M. (1988). *Emotionally focused therapy for couples.* New York: Guilford Press.

This excellent book provides an in-depth presentation of the emotionally focused therapy model. It provides a thorough discussion of the role of emotions in marital relationships and clinical change. It also presents a step-by-step guide to conducting this approach and is filled with excellent clinical examples. Furthermore, the authors provide empirical results demonstrating the efficacy of this approach. This book should serve as a model for future family therapy theoreticians wanting to present their work.

Johnson, S. M., & Greenberg, L. S. (Eds.). (1994). *The heart of the matter: Perspectives on emotion in marital therapy.* New York: Brunner/Mazel.

Johnson and Greenberg are intent on championing the cause for the inclusion of emotion in marital theory and therapy. This edited book presents numerous theoretical models underlining the importance of emotion in the change process. This book is an important recentering for a field that has become caught up in issues of pattern, structure, and narrative, and has forgotten the importance of feelings in marriage.

Johnson, S. M., & Greenberg, L. S. (1995). The emotionally focused approach to problems in adult attachment. In N. S. Jacobson & A. S. Gurman (Eds.), *Clinical handbook of couple therapy.* New York: Guilford Press.

This chapter provides a concise overview of emotionally focused couple therapy, an approach integrating experiential and systems-based family therapies. It presents a brief theoretical rationale, the nine steps of the model, and a discussion of clinical issues. It is a good introduction to this approach.

Kaplan, M. L., & Kaplan, N. R. (1978). Individual and family growth: A Gestalt approach. *Family Process, 17,* 195–205.

This article provides a good background to Gestalt family therapy. The authors discuss basic concepts and distinctions between Gestalt family therapy, and other experiential family therapies are clarified.

Kempler, W. (1973). *Principles of Gestalt family therapy.* Salt Lake City: Deseret Press.

Kempler illustrates many Gestalt family therapy principles in this short, crisply written, eminently readable book. His excellent use of self and ability to facilitate meaningful person-to-person communications are illustrated in a variety of fascinating examples.

Kempler, W. (1981). *Experiential psychotherapy with families.* New York: Brunner/Mazel.

This is Kempler's fullest explication of Gestalt experiential family therapy. As in his other works, Kempler makes excellent use of illustrative dialogue and emphasizes the powerful effects of person-to-person encounter, therapist involvement, and present-centered family interaction.

Levant, R. F. (1978). Family therapy: A client centered approach. *Journal of Marriage and Family Counseling, 4*(2), 35–42.

The author contrasts the pessimistic assumptions of psychodynamic and systems therapies to the growth orientation of a client-centered approach to family therapy. Theoretical assumptions of client-centered family therapy are clearly presented, but the author appears to sidestep the issue of how such a nondirective approach might deal with rigid, manipulative, and other difficult family systems.

Linesch, D. (Ed.). (1993). *Art therapy with families in crisis: Overcoming resistance through nonverbal expression.* New York: Brunner/Mazel.

This book not only shows how to use art therapy in family crisis situations, but it also serves as a good guide for utilizing art therapy with families in general. Both theoretically sound and loaded with examples, the chapters focus on the use of art therapy with a variety of problem situations. This book is a good guide for helping family therapists overcome their resistance to using art therapy.

Napier, A. Y. (1987). Early stages in experiential marital therapy. *Contemporary Family Therapy, 9,* 23–41.

Napier, A. Y. (1987). Later stages in experiential marital therapy. *Contemporary Family Therapy, 9,* 42–57.

This two-part article provides a detailed stage approach to the process of experiential marital therapy. It provides a more in-depth stage model than Whitaker's "Battle for Structure" and "Battle for Initiative." The articles contain goals and problems associated with each stage. These are important articles, in that they help to demystify the process of symbolic–experiential therapy that is often obfuscated in Whitaker's papers.

Napier, A. Y., & Whitaker, C. (1978). *The family crucible.* New York: Harper & Row.

This engaging book is about one family's struggles and growth in long-term therapy with Napier and Whitaker. The reader is given a rare bird's-eye view of how Carl Whitaker, a family therapy pioneer, conducted his brand of experiential family therapy from beginning to end. This book is an eminently readable "true story" novel.

Neill, J. R., & Kniskern, D. P. (Eds.). (1982). *From psyche to system: The evolving therapy of Carl Whitaker.* New York: Guilford Press.

This book presents the vintage writings of Carl Whitaker and is as provocative an experience as the experiential therapy he espouses. The first section provides a useful biographical sketch of the life experiences that contributed to his work. The writings span over 40 years, allowing the reader to examine Whitaker's evolution "from psyche to system." Those expecting an instruction manual will be disappointed, but Whitaker's writings are guaranteed to challenge basic assumptions about therapy, marriage, and life in general.

Roberto, L. G. (1991). Symbolic-experiential family therapy. In A. S. Gurman & D. P. Kniskern (Eds.), *Handbook of family therapy* (Vol. 2). New York: Brunner/Mazel.

Roberto is perhaps the finest interpreter of symbolic–experiential family therapy today. Her chapter provides an excellent understanding of this model and dispels several myths often associated with it. She further provides grist for the theoretical mill by developing a rationale for its inclusion as a transgenerational family therapy. As this chapter lacks some of the flavor of Whitaker's writing, it is best read in conjunction with Whitaker and Keith's (1981) chapter in the first volume of the *Handbook of Family Therapy* (listed).

Satir, V. (1983). *Conjoint family therapy* (3rd ed.). Palo Alto, CA: Science and Behavior Books.

In the third edition of this classic, Satir illustrates her approach to family therapy, which includes an integration of Gestalt, psychodramatic, communicational, and historical techniques. This book is helpful in its illustration of procedures she used to facilitate family communication and to unlock the affective resources of family members. It expands on earlier editions by including a subjective account of her process when meeting a person and how she worked with a team of therapists in a research project.

Satir, V. (1988). *The new peoplemaking.* Palo Alto, CA: Science and Behavior Books.

Satir, writing for a lay audience, discusses the basic concepts she believes are tied to individual and family health. Her discussions of self-esteem and communication styles are particularly clear and may be useful as reading assignments for certain client families. This revised edition includes issues of adolescence and the older years, and exemplifies her concerns regarding world peace and spirituality.

Satir, V., & Baldwin, M. (1983). *Satir step-by-step.* Palo Alto, CA: Science and Behavior Books.

This book is perhaps the best exemplification of Satir's work. The first part is a verbatim session transcript of her work with a family. The second part contains Michelle Baldwin's discussion of Satir's theory and technique. Although some readers may be put off by the book's use of large print and pictures, as in *Peoplemaking,* it is worthwhile in that it provides a more concise presentation of her theory and work than previous publications.

Whitaker, C. A., & Bumberry, W. M. (1988). *Dancing with the family: A symbolic–experiential approach.* New York: Brunner/Mazel.

This book allows readers to get inside the head of Carl Whitaker as he does therapy. It presents the verbatim session transcript of Whitaker working with a family in therapy and is punctuated by Whitaker's own commentary on what he was doing and why. The text is further advanced through a question-and-answer discussion between Whitaker and Bumberry at key points in each chapter over the preceding work.

Whitaker, C. A., & Keith, D. V. (1981). Symbolic–experiential family therapy. In A.

S. Gurman & D. P. Kniskern (Eds.), *Handbook of family therapy*. New York: Brunner/Mazel.

This is perhaps the most comprehensive, well-organized, and well-written chapter that Carl Whitaker has authored on his approach to family therapy. Although Whitaker's charm and "craziness" are reflected in certain case examples, the real contribution of this chapter is in its demystification of Whitaker's brand of experiential family therapy.

Whitaker, C. A., & Ryan, M. O. (1989). *Midnight musings of a family therapist*. New York: Brunner/Mazel.

This book condenses Whitaker's ideas from previous papers in an understandable whole. The first part of the book serves as an autobiography and places many of his ideas in historical content. The second part presents his views on families and family therapy. Unfortunately, this later presentation of his ideas lacks some of the bite of his earlier works. To fully appreciate the "Whitaker experience," we believe that trainees should read this book in conjunction with Neill and Kniskern (1982).

Woods, M. D., & Martin, D. (1984). The work of Virginia Satir: Understanding her theory and technique. *American Journal of Family Therapy, 11*(1), 35–46.

The authors do a fine job of summarizing the philosophical assumptions, principles, goals, and basic techniques of Virginia Satir. This is a good introductory source.

REFERENCES

Baldwin, M. (1991). The triadic concept in the work of Virginia Satir. In B. J. Brothers (Ed.), *Virginia Satir: Foundational ideas*. Binghamton, NY: Haworth.

Bing, E. (1970). The conjoint family drawing. *Family Process, 9*, 173–194.

Bowlby, J. (1969). *Attachment and loss: Vol. 1. Attachment*. New York: Basic Books.

Brothers, B. J. (1991a). Introduction. In B. J. Brothers (Ed.), *Virginia Satir: Foundational ideas*. Binghamton, NY: Haworth.

Brothers, B. J. (1991b). Methods for connectedness: Virginia Satir's contribution to the process of human communication. In B. J. Brothers (Ed.), *Virginia Satir: Foundational ideas*. Binghamton, NY: Haworth.

Broderick, C. B., & Schrader, S. S. (1991). The history of professional marriage and family therapy. In A. S. Gurman & D. P. Kniskern (Eds.), *Handbook of family therapy* (Vol. 2). New York: Brunner/Mazel.

Buber, M. (1970). *I and thou*. New York: Scribner's.

Burns, R. C. (1990). *Family-centered circle drawings*. New York: Brunner/Mazel.

Connell, G. M., Mitten, T. J., & Whitaker, C. A. (1993). Reshaping family symbols: A symbolic experiential approach. *Journal of Marital and Family Therapy, 19*, 245–251.

Constantine, L. (1978). Family sculpture and relationship mapping techniques. *Journal of Marriage and Family Counseling, 4*(2), 13–23.

Dandeneau, M. L., & Johnson, S. M. (1994). Facilitating intimacy: Interventions and effects. *Journal of Marital and Family Therapy, 20,* 17–33.

Duhl, B. S. (1983). *From the inside out and other metaphors: Creative and integrative approaches to training in systems thinking.* New York: Brunner/Mazel.

Duhl, B. S. (1987). Uses of self in integrated contextual systems therapy. *Journal of Psychotherapy and the Family, 3*(1), 71–84.

Duhl, B. S., & Duhl, F. J. (1981). Integrative family therapy. In A. S. Gurman & D. P. Kniskern (Eds.), *Handbook of family therapy.* New York: Brunner/Mazel.

Duhl, F. J., & Duhl, B. S. (1979). "Structured spontaneity": The thoughtful art of integrative family therapy at BFI. *Journal of Marital and Family Therapy, 5,* 59–76.

Duhl, F. J., Kantor, D., & Duhl, B. S. (1973). Learning, space and action in family therapy: A primer of sculpture. In D. A. Bloch (Ed.), *Techniques of family therapy: A primer.* New York: Grune & Stratton.

Fisch, R., Weakland, J. H., & Segal, L. (1983). *Tactics of change.* New York: Norton.

Geddes, M., & Medway, J. (1977). The symbolic drawing of family life space. *Family Process, 16,* 219–228.

Gendlin, E. T. (1973). Experiential psychotherapy. In R. Corsini (Ed.), *Current psychotherapies.* Itasca, IL: Peacock.

Greenberg, L. S., & Johnson, S. M. (1985). Emotionally focused couples therapy. In N. S. Jacobson & A. S. Gurman (Eds.), *Clinical handbook of marital therapy.* New York: Guilford Press.

Greenberg, L. S., & Johnson, S. M. (1986). Affect in marital therapy. *Journal of Marital and Family Therapy, 12,* 1–10.

Greenberg, L. S., & Johnson, S. M. (1988). *Emotionally focused therapy for couples.* New York: Guilford Press.

Greenberg, L. S., & Safran, J. D. (1989). Emotion in psychotherapy. *American Psychologist, 44,* 19–29.

Johnson, S. (1986). Bonds or bargains: Relationship paradigms and their significance for marital therapy. *Journal of Marital and Family Therapy, 12,* 259–267.

Johnson, S. M., & Greenberg, L. (1985a). The differential effects of experiential and problem solving interventions in resolving marital conflict. *Journal of Consulting and Clinical Psychology, 53,* 175–184.

Johnson, S. M., & Greenberg, L. S. (1985b). Emotionally focused marital therapy: An outcome study. *Journal of Marital and Family Therapy, 11,* 313–317.

Johnson, S. M., & Greenberg, L. S. (1987). Integration in marital therapy: Issues and progress. *International Journal of Eclectic Psychotherapy, 6,* 202–215.

Johnson, S. M., & Greenberg, L. S. (1994). Emotion in intimate relationships: Theory and implications for therapy. In S. M. Johnson & L. S. Greenberg (Eds.), *The heart of the matter: Perspectives on emotion in marital therapy.* New York: Brunner/Mazel.

Kaplan, M. L., & Kaplan, N. R. (1978). Individual and family growth: A Gestalt approach. *Family Process, 17*, 195–205.

Kaufman, W. (Ed.). (1956). *Existentialism from Dostoevsky to Sartre.* New York: World.

Keith, D. V. (1987). The self in family therapy: A field guide. *Journal of Psychotherapy and the Family, 3*(1), 61–70.

Keith, D. V., Connell, G. M., & Whitaker, C. A. (1991). A symbolic–experiential approach to the resolution of therapeutic obstacles in family therapy. *Journal of Family Psychotherapy, 2*(3), 41–56.

Kempler, W. (1973). *Principles of Gestalt family therapy.* Salt Lake City: Deseret Press.

Kempler, W. (1981). *Experiential psychotherapy with families.* New York: Brunner/Mazel.

Levant, R. F. (1978). Family therapy: A client-centered approach. *Journal of Marriage and Family Counseling, 4*(2), 35–42.

Linesch, D. (Ed.). (1993). *Art therapy with families in crisis: Overcoming resistance through nonverbal expression.* New York: Brunner/Mazel.

Napier, A. Y. (1987a). Early stages in experiential marital therapy. *Contemporary Family Therapy, 9,* 23–41.

Napier, A. Y. (1987b). Later stages in experiential marital therapy. *Contemporary Family Therapy, 9,* 42–57.

Napier, A. Y., & Whitaker, C. (1978). *The family crucible.* New York: Harper & Row.

Neill, J. R., & Kniskern, D. P. (Eds.). (1982). *From psyche to system: The evolving therapy of Carl Whitaker.* New York: Guilford Press.

Perls, F. (1973). *The Gestalt approach and eye witness to therapy.* Palo Alto, CA: Science and Behavior Books.

Roberto, L. G. (1991). Symbolic–experiential family therapy. In A. S. Gurman & D. P. Kniskern (Eds.), *Handbook of family therapy* (Vol. 2). New York: Brunner/Mazel.

Rogers, C. R. (1961). *On becoming a person.* Boston: Houghton Mifflin.

Sartre, J. P. (1946). *Existentialism and humanism.* London: Methuen.

Satir, V. (1983). *Conjoint family therapy* (3rd ed.). Palo Alto, CA: Science and Behavior Books.

Satir, V. (1988). *The new peoplemaking.* Palo Alto, CA: Science and Behavior Books.

Satir, V., & Baldwin, M. (1983). *Satir step-by-step.* Palo Alto, CA: Science and Behavior Books.

Watzlawick, P., Weakland, J. H., & Fisch, R. (1974). *Change: Principles of problem formation and problem resolution.* New York: Norton.

Whitaker, C. A. (1976). The hindrance of theory in clinical work. In P. J. Guerin, Jr. (Ed.), *Family therapy: Theory and practice.* New York: Gardner.

Whitaker, C. A., & Bumberry, W. M. (1988). *Dancing with the family: A symbolic–experiential approach.* New York: Brunner/Mazel.

Whitaker, C. A., & Keith, D. V. (1981). Symbolic–experiential family therapy. In A. S. Gurman & D. P. Kniskern (Eds.), *Handbook of family therapy.* New York: Brunner/Mazel.

Whitaker, C. A., & Malone, T. P. (1953). *The roots of psychotherapy.* New York: Blakiston.

Whitaker, C. A., & Napier, A. Y. (1977). Process techniques of family therapy. *Interaction, 1*(1), 4–19.

Whitaker, C. A., & Ryan, M. O. (1989). *Midnight musings of a family therapist.* New York: Norton.

Whitaker, C. A., Warkentin, J., & Malone, T. P. (1959). The involvement of the professional therapist. In A. Burton (Ed.), *Case studies in counseling and psychotherapy.* Englewood Cliffs, NJ: Prentice-Hall.

Winter, J. E., & Parker, L. R. E. (1991). Enhancing the marital relationship: Virginia Satir's parts party. In B. J. Brothers (Ed.), *Virginia Satir: Foundational ideas.* Binghamton, NY: Haworth.

5

Behavioral Family Therapies

JOSEPH L. WETCHLER
FRED P. PIERCY

BEHAVIOR MODIFICATION is associated with principles of learning derived from extensive laboratory research examining the effects of environmental events on the frequency of behavior. The discovery that behavior can be predictably increased or decreased by the manipulation of antecedent and consequent events (usually in the form of punishments and rewards) has led to a far-reaching behavioral technology that is evident in virtually every area of our lives. Predictably, behaviorists use the terminology of operant and classical conditioning to explain family dynamics. For example, marital satisfaction is sometimes defined as a relatively high rate of rewards to punishers. Supporting this view, researchers have found that distressed couples exchange relatively higher rates of displeasing behavior and lower rates of pleasing behavior than nondistressed couples (Gottman, Markman, & Notarius, 1977).

The concepts of coercion and reciprocity also are used frequently by behavioral family therapists. "Coercion" is the general use of negative events to control family interaction. "Reciprocity," on the other hand, involves partners' tendencies to reward and punish each other at approximately equal rates over time. Lederer and Jackson (1968) were referring to reciprocity when they stated that "nastiness begets nastiness" (p. 269); however, every interchange among couples is not reciprocal. Gottman et al. (1976) discuss a "bank account" model of marital exchange, in which a spouse's rewarding behavior may be considered an investment over time. This concept accounts for a husband responding to his sick wife's anger with a loving remark. Over the long haul, however, both partners expect an equitable rate of positive return on their positive investments.

Behavioral family therapists increasingly recognize the importance of cognitions (Baucom & Epstein, 1990; Falloon, 1991; Jacobson, 1991) as events mediating family interactions. For example, Patterson (1982) states that parents of aggressive children tend to attribute negative intentions to their children's behavior. Such attributions serve to maintain negative response cycles. Similarly, Jacobson and Margolin (1979) state that a spouse's overall feeling of marital satisfaction (i.e., a cognition) may influence his or her immediate response to his or her partner.

In summary, then, behavioral marital and family therapists generally assume that family interactions are maintained and changed by environmental events preceding and following each family member's behavior. These environmental events, or contingencies, along with mediating cognitions, influence the form and frequency of each family member's behaviors.

Although behavioral family therapies often are not considered systems therapies, they do take into consideration the interactive qualities of family relationships. Discussing marriage, Jacobson and Margolin (1979) state:

> Since each spouse is providing consequences for the other on a continuous basis, and since each partner exerts an important controlling influence on the other's behavior, the marital relationship is best thought of as a process of circular and reciprocal sequences of behavior and consequences, where each person's behavior is at once being affected by and influencing the other. (p. 13)

In other words, each family member's behavior is intertwined in various stimulus–response–reinforcement cycles. What is a response for one family member (e.g., a crying child) may be a reinforcement for another (i.e., a teasing sibling) and a stimulus for still another (i.e., a parent). Endless chains such as these make up what we call family interaction (Hahlweg, Baucom, & Markman, 1988). The interactional sequences typical of families with problems are often characterized by reciprocal patterns of coercion and pain control (Patterson, 1982).

The hallmark of the behavior therapies is the importance placed on conducting a detailed, continuous assessment of family functioning (Arrington, Sullaway, & Christiansen, 1988; Baucom & Epstein, 1990; Falloon, 1991). Interventions are evaluated in terms of the effectiveness within which they serve to diminish specific problem behaviors identified in the family assessment. Although specific change strategies have been associated with behaviorism, many techniques can be used, as long as they are subjected to experimental evaluation within the context of therapy (Falloon, 1991).

ROLE OF THE THERAPIST

The role of the behavioral marital or family therapist is that of a teacher who often employs instructions, coaching, modeling, and behavioral rehearsal in order to impart the skills necessary for couples or families to begin interacting more effectively. Generally, the therapist assesses the contingencies influencing problematic behaviors, then develops intervention strategies aimed at changing these contingencies. Popular interventions include parent skills training, problem-solving/communication skills training, contingency contracting, cognitive restructuring, assertion training, and home token economies. Also, behavioral marital and family therapists are increasingly emphasizing the importance of issues previously neglected by behaviorists, such as the therapist–client relationship (Alexander & Parsons, 1982; Birchler, 1988; Falloon, 1991) and the therapist's ability to establish a "collaborative set" with the couple or family (Holtzworth-Munroe & Jacobson, 1991; Jacobson & Margolin, 1979).

Behavioral family therapists tend to stress the importance of procedures such as charting, homework, and follow-up assessment, which promote and evaluate the maintenance and generalization of positive changes in therapy. The presumed necessity of long-term maintenance procedures in behavioral family therapies contrasts sharply with the assumption of strategic and structural therapies that homeostatic processes will maintain family behavior once it is changed.

BEHAVIORAL FAMILY THERAPY
AND PARENT SKILLS TRAINING

Behavioral family therapy owes much of its development to the work of Gerald Patterson (1971; Patterson, McNeil, Hawkins, & Phelps, 1967) with conduct-disordered boys and Robert Liberman (1970) with the adult mentally ill. Their approaches highlight the importance of teaching behavioral strategies to diminish problematic behaviors. Liberman's (e.g., Falloon & Liberman, 1983) work served as the basis for the psychoeducational approach toward acute mental illness and is presented in Chapter 11. Patterson's ideas were influential in the development of parent skills training, which is discussed here.

Parent skills training involves teaching behavioral skills to parents so that they can employ them with their own children. The initial focus of therapy is on the parents themselves, who learn how to apply behavior change procedures to increase the prosocial behavior and decrease problematic behavior of their children (McAuley, 1988; Sisson & Taylor, 1993). In essence, the behavioral parent trainer functions as a "consultant" to the parents, who then become the primary therapists or behavior change agents for their children (Tharp & Wetzel, 1969).

There are a variety of theoretical and practical arguments to support behavioral parent training (e.g., Cone & Sloop, 1974; Graziano, 1977; O'Dell, 1974). The simplicity and straightforwardness of specific learning theory principles (Gordon & Davidson, 1981) allow them to be taught economically, either to individual parents (Wiltz & Gordon, 1974) or groups (Gordon, Lerner, & Keefe, 1979). Generally, behavioral parent training involves (1) an introduction to social learning theory; (2) the pinpointing of problem behaviors; (3) an analysis of antecedent and consequent behaviors; (4) procedures for monitoring and recording behaviors (e.g., frequency counts, charts); (5) the collection of baseline data; and (6) the training of specific behavior change procedures. The procedures most often taught in behavioral parent training include the definition and enforcement of rules and the use of positive reinforcement, time-out, behavioral contracting, and home token economies (Gordon & Davidson, 1981).

Although research to date has been impressive (e.g., Fleischman, 1981; Graziano, 1974; Patterson, 1982), more needs to be learned about the effectiveness of behavioral parent training for different groups. For example, it appears that behavioral parent training is less effective in cases of marital disturbance and parental separation (Cox & Rutter, 1985; Wolkind & Rutter, 1985). Furthermore, McAuley (1988) cautions that individual constitutional factors such as child temperament and differing family styles may effect outcomes.

FROM BEHAVIORAL TO COGNITIVE-BEHAVIORAL MARITAL THERAPY

Behavioral marital therapy owes its origin to the pioneering efforts of Richard Stuart (1969), who began using contingency contracting to enhance reciprocal behaviors in couples. In part, Stuart helped distressed marital dyads to focus on positive patterns within their relationship rather than coercive processes. Specific interventions employed to increase positive interchanges between spouses include "caring days" (Stuart, 1980) and "love days" (Jacobson & Margolin, 1979). In both, spouses agree to engage on certain days in specific behaviors that their partners find rewarding.

Although positive reciprocity is important, the couple also must learn how to talk to each other. Behavioral couple therapists teach problem-solving/communication skills under the assumption that some communication patterns are more adaptive and useful than others (Holtzworth-Munroe & Jacobson, 1991). This assumption is supported by research on communication patterns of distressed and nondistressed couples and families (e.g., Alexander, 1973; Billings, 1979; Gottman, 1979; Robin & Weiss, 1980). The goals of problem-solving/communication skills training usually include (1) defining problems in a nonblaming way, (2) listening empathically, (3) formulating "I want" statements, (4) generating solutions, (5) deciding upon a solution, and (6) implementing the solution (see Jacobson & Margolin, 1979).

In an attempt to further refine behavioral marital therapy, Jacobson and colleagues (Christensen, Jacobson, & Babcock, 1995; Cordova & Jacobson, 1993; Jacobson, 1991, 1992) have integrated the concept of "couple acceptance" with their traditional focus on promoting change. Basically, they help the partners recognize that, since certain problems within their relationship cannot be resolved, they need to learn how to develop acceptance. The therapist frames their disagreement as an unsolvable problem and helps the couple pull together and support each other against the common enemy, the problem, which they must face together (Christensen et al., 1995; Cordova & Jacobson, 1993).

Cognitive-behavioral marital therapy arose from a belief that marital assessment and treatment was more complex than allowed for in a pure behavioral perspective (Epstein, Schlesinger, & Dryden, 1988). Some behaviorists began to integrate the cognitive theories of Beck (1976) and Ellis (1962) to develop a more complex model of marriage and marital therapy. Although there is less empirical evidence for cognitive-behavioral marital therapy than behavioral marital therapy, there is a growing body of support for the use of cognitive restructuring in marital therapy (e.g., Baucom & Lester, 1986; Emmelkamp et al., 1988; Huber & Milstein, 1985).

Cognitive-behaviorists believe that cognitions and affect serve a mediating function with behavior. Often the way individuals think or feel affects how they interact with others. Furthermore, individuals' thoughts and feelings serve as lenses for how they interpret their partners' behavior (Baucom & Epstein, 1990; Epstein, Baucom, & Rankin, 1993). Their interpretation of this outside behavior leads to their own behavioral response. Assessment and treatment of cognitions, emotions, and behaviors are central to this model. Baucom and Epstein (1990) state:

> Because behaviors, cognitions, and emotions are so intertwined in marital interaction, it is important that the assessment of a couple's problems include evaluations of all three types of factors, as well as the ways in which the factors influence each other. Furthermore, the complex interplay of behavior, cognition, and affect in influencing spouses' marital satisfaction necessitates that therapeutic interventions address each of the three areas. (p. 16)

FUNCTIONAL FAMILY THERAPY

Functional family therapy, originally identified as systems-behavioral family therapy, was initiated and refined through the work of James

Alexander and his colleagues (Alexander & Parsons, 1973, 1982; Barton & Alexander, 1981; Morris, Alexander, & Waldron, 1988). It integrates three models of human functioning: systems theory, behaviorism, and, more recently, cognitive therapy (Morris et al., 1988). As with other behavioral models, its claims are based on empirical support (e.g., Alexander & Parsons, 1973; Klein, Alexander, & Parsons, 1977).

Functional family therapy assesses the interactional sequences in which problems are embedded. It then identifies the end point, or *function,* of these behaviors. The interpersonal function of behaviors provides closeness, distance, or a vacillation between the two (midpointing) among family members (Alexander & Parsons, 1982). Specific functions are considered neither good nor bad; however, the way they are expressed can be problematic. For example, a father and son who exhibit closeness through engaging in a hobby together are very different from a father and son who are only able to achieve closeness after the son runs away from home.

Interspersed throughout the assessment process is the identification of cognitions that family members have about each other and the specific problem behaviors they exhibit. It is often the attributions that family members ascribe to each other that maintain specific problem sequences.

Functional family therapy is divided into two steps: (1) therapy, in which cognitive change is addressed; and (2) education, in which specific strategies are provided to bring about behavior change (Barton & Alexander, 1981). The goal of therapy is to provide new behavior patterns to meet individual functions of each family member. As symptoms are viewed as problematic ways of achieving functions, no attempt is made to change a specific function.

KEY CONCEPTS AND CLINICAL SKILLS

Because the key concepts in behavioral family therapies are inextricably linked to and often overlap with specific behavior intervention procedures, both are presented together in this section.

Affect. Individuals' feelings and emotions about themselves and their environment. Cognitive-behaviorists (e.g., Baucom & Epstein, 1990) believe that affect, cognitions, and behavior interact to affect marital quality. Any change in one may bring about change in the others.

Baseline. The initial recorded observations of behaviors that are intended to be changed once different treatment conditions are introduced. For example, a child's hitting behaviors between 4:00 P.M. and 6:00 P.M. may be counted for a week prior to initiating an intervention program, so that baseline data will be available to determine whether the intervention program, when it is begun, actually decreases the frequency of hits.

Behavioral exchange theory. A theory that explains relationship behaviors in terms of costs and benefits. A distressed relationship, for example, is one in which there is a scarcity of benefits or rewards relative to costs or aversive events. According to Jacobson and Margolin (1979), marital distress can be described both in terms of reduced reward–punishment ratios and increased reactivity to the partner's aversive behavior.

Caring days. A structured method of concurrently increasing the caring behaviors of spouses. Each spouse identifies various behaviors that the partner finds enjoyable and commits him- or herself to increasing these behaviors (Stuart, 1980). A daily record is kept by the couple of the extent to which each partner initiates caring behaviors for the other. In social exchange terms, the family therapist who uses caring days is attempting to increase the reward within the relationship, thus increasing the perceived value of the relationship.

Classical conditioning. The process by which a stimulus takes on the ability to elicit certain behaviors or emotions by being associated with a behavior-eliciting stimulus. For example, a song that was played at times a couple was romantic may eventually in and of itself elicit romantic emotions for the couple.

Coaching. The process of structuring interaction by providing verbal instructions. For example, a family therapist may coach a wife who is having trouble getting her husband's attention when she talks by saying, "This time when he turns his head away, I want you to squeeze his hand gently and tell him you really want him to listen."

Coercion. An interaction in which a person uses aversive stimuli or responses to control the behavior of others. Negative reinforcement explains the maintenance of coercive behavior; that is, the use of coercion to terminate an aversive stimulus increases the likelihood of the use of coercion in the future. For example, if a husband's shouting terminates a wife's nagging, the husband has used a coercive response that will probably be repeated in similar circumstances.

Cognitions. Individuals' thoughts and views about themselves and their environment. Cognitive-behavioral marital therapists (e.g., Baucom & Epstein, 1990) believe that cognitions interact with behaviors and emotions to affect the quality of marriage. Cognitive-behavioral marital therapists help clients alter cognitive distortions as well as learn new behaviors.

Contingency contract. A written agreement between spouses that specifies expectations of behavior and consequences for either meeting or not meeting those expectations. Contracts may be either quid pro quo, in which the behavior of one spouse is contingent on another, or parallel, in which one spouse's behavior is independent of another's (Jacobson & Margolin, 1979).

Discriminative stimulus (cue). A signal indicating that a likely and positive set of results will occur contingent upon a particular behavior being performed (Jacobson & Margolin, 1979). For example, if a mother and daughter have agreed that the daughter has 5 minutes to start her household chores once the mother holds up her five fingers as a cue (the discriminative stimulus), then the daughter knows she can avoid her mother's nagging if she begins to work within the 5-minute time frame.

Extinction. The procedure by which previously reinforced behaviors are no longer reinforced. For example, a father who has been attentive to his daughter only when she makes funny noises may start to ignore her antics. Since the funny noises are no longer reinforced by the father's attention, the daughter eventually stops making them (i.e., they are extinguished).

Functions. According to Alexander and Parsons (1982), symptoms typically serve the "function" or purpose of creating interpersonal closeness or distance (i.e., dependence or autonomy) relative to other family members. For example, a teenage girl's symptom of stealing may serve the function of bringing her "closer" to her parents through the lectures they give her (i.e., a "closeness" function) or may serve to isolate her from her parents (a "distance" function).

Home token economy. A contingency-contracting procedure in which secondary reinforcers (e.g., points, poker chips) are earned by accomplishing appropriate tasks. Home token economies can include both rewards and fines for behaviors, and are instituted in order to modify the contingencies and frequency of behaviors within the family.

Love days. A structured procedure in which on a given day one spouse noncontingently increases behavior that the other spouse finds pleasurable (Jacobson & Margolin, 1979). For instance, on an assigned day, one spouse may try to be especially pleasing to the other (regardless of the other's behavior) by offering breakfast in bed, a surprise gift, a shower of kisses, and other rewarding behaviors and comments.

Modeling. In social learning theory, a term for acquiring new behavior or strengthening–weakening previously learned responses on the basis of noticing rewarding or punishing consequences for observed behavior (Bandura, 1971). For example, if a young child observes that his older brother's whining behavior results in rewards, the younger child will be more likely also to engage in whining behavior in the future.

Negative reinforcement. The procedure by which a behavior is strengthened when it results in the removal of a certain stimulus (usually aversive). For example, if a child's lie stops a parent's angry questioning, lying behavior may increase in the future (i.e., it is "negatively reinforced" by the cessation of an aversive stimulus, the angry questioning). If telling the truth also results in a decrease of the parent's angry questioning, negative reinforcement still occurs (given that telling the truth increases in the future). In other words, the term "negative" refers to a taking away or decrease of a subsequent event and not to a negative valence of the preceding behavior.

Operant conditioning. The process by which the frequency of a behavior is altered by its consequences. Consequences may be variably introduced as either positively reinforcing, negatively reinforcing, or punishing.

Parallel (good faith) contract. A contingency contract in which the behavior of one spouse is independent of that of the other. For example, a husband may receive the reward of playing golf after doing the laundry, while the wife earns the reward of going shopping for herself after she vacuums the house.

Positive reinforcement. The procedure by which the appearance of an event strengthens the behavior that precedes it. For example, if a husband self-discloses more frequently when his self-disclosures are followed by appreciative statements from his wife, those appreciative statements are considered positive reinforcers.

Punishment. The procedure by which the appearance of a stimulus decreases the behavior that precedes it. For example, if (and only if) a child's misbehavior decreases after a spanking is the spanking considered a punishment.

Quid pro quo contract. A contingency contract in which the behavior of one person is contingent on that of another. For example, a husband may agree to do the dishes each evening in exchange for the wife taking the children to school and picking them up again. Likewise, her driving the children is contingent upon his doing the dishes.

Reciprocal inhibition (counterconditioning). A process in which specific behaviors may be weakened by establishing antagonistic behaviors. For example, a father's anxiety may be decreased by teaching him to be more assertive. Likewise, systematic desensitization, which teaches one to relax while imagining increasingly anxiety-provoking situations, is another example of reciprocal inhibition.

Reciprocity. The likelihood that two people will reinforce each other at approximately equitable rates over time.

Successive approximation (shaping). The reinforcement of gradual changes in behavior toward a desired goal. For example, the process of toilet training may be broken down into successively more complicated steps (e.g., walking to the potty, pulling down pants, sitting down, etc.). Completion of each step is rewarded in the step-by-step shaping of appropriate toileting behavior.

Time-out. A means of extinguishing inappropriate behavior by removing the reinforcing consequences of that behavior. Typically, in time-out, a child is immediately removed from a situation that reinforces unproductive behavior (e.g., a class of giggling children) and placed in a solitary location (e.g., an empty room) where the behavior is likely to decrease. Time-out procedures may be literally thought of as "time-out" from reinforcement.

TEACHING TOOLS AND TECHNIQUES

Minilecture: Similarities and Differences between Behavioral and Structural–Strategic Therapies

A short lecture comparing and contrasting behavioral and structural–strategic therapies can be given, based on the following points made by Foster and Hoier (1982). Those wishing to compare cognitive-behavioral family therapy with functional, structural–strategic, and psychoanalytic family therapies are referred to Epstein, Schlesinger, and Dryden (1988).

Similarities

1. The same behaviors and interpersonal interactions are monitored.
2. The focus is on behavioral sequences versus subjective experiences.
3. Problems are conceptualized interactionally within the environment or system, rather than in terms of individual pathology.
4. Problems serve some function.
5. Problems are maintained by family processes.
6. "Here and now" rather than past history is emphasized.
7. The focus is on changing target behaviors and/or behavioral sequences.
8. The goal of therapy is to restructure interactions via behavioral or cognitive change in order to change a presenting problem.
9. Instruction, cognitive restructuring (reframing), and coaching in sessions are employed.
10. Homework is assigned to generalize change.
11. Behavioral parent training is like restructuring family hierarchies.

Differences

Behavioral	*Structural–strategic*
The main interest is in observables, operationalizability, and a molecular view.	Systems descriptions are inferred from observables and represent motor constructs (e.g., enmeshment).
Therapy is more likely to engage in subsystem analysis.	Therapy begins with descriptions of family system.
Causal factors that can be tested are hypothesized.	Circular causality and homeostasis, which *are not* tested, are assumed.
Resistance is rejected.	Resistance is expected.
There is a concern with long-term maintenance.	The assumption is that homeostatic processes will maintain change.

Experiential Assignments

Students may be given assignments that encourage their firsthand application of behavioral principles. The following is such an assignment that our students have found particularly worthwhile.

> Jacobson and Margolin (1979) state that negative cycles of behavior "can be abated if spouses learn to maintain consistently high levels of pleasing behaviors" (p. 176). Similarly, they discuss the positive affects that may occur when one spouse independently increases his or her pleasing behaviors toward the other. Your task is to experientially examine the validity of independently increasing positive behaviors in a relationship. Without telling him or her about this assignment, choose a person you have sustained contact with and count the number of pleasing behaviors you emit toward that individual in a week's time. During the second week, at least double your reinforcing or pleasing behaviors toward this individual. Notice the results. Does the quality of his or her behaviors toward you change? And what about the quality of your relationship? Describe the effects of this experiment on both you and your chosen subject. What implications do your findings have for your practice of marital therapy? Also, how would you explain these results in behavioral terms?

Journal Days

The extensive literature related to behavioral marital and family interventions is overwhelming to assign to students in its totality. Students may be exposed to many of the key journal articles in behavioral marital and family therapy by scheduling occasional "journal days." On these days, each student summarizes and critiques for the class two articles assigned from an extensive bibliography. Many of these 5-minute summaries/critiques generate provocative discussions regarding the theory, research, and practices of the particular behavioral family therapy being studied. Students are also asked to write short annotations to their assigned articles. These annotations are later combined to form an annotated bibliography for the class. (This suggestion is taken from Piercy & Sprenkle, 1984.)

Practice Case Studies

Practice case studies may be assigned that will encourage students to grapple with behavioral concepts as they relate to assessment and therapy. Students can work in teams to assess and develop treatment plans or write individual papers. The following is an example for cognitive-behavioral marital therapy.

> Based on Baucom and Epstein (1990), design a cognitive-behavioral therapy for the following couple. Make sure you deal with issues of

behavior, cognition, and affect. What interventions would you use to produce change in these areas?

Sam and Shirley have come to you for marital therapy. They are distressed about their marriage and are considering divorce; however, they are committed to resolving their marital problems first. The couple claims that their marriage is dead. They do nothing together. Sam typically watches TV while Shirley reads books in the bedroom. Sam reports that he can't remember when Shirley last told him she loved him, and he has no idea what she wants from him. Shirley says that if Sam really loved her, he would know how to please her. Their days have become totally routine. The only time they see each other is at dinner. The couple reports that they have major arguments that escalate into blowups in which they scream at each other. Sam has occasionally broken a vase or punched a wall in his anger (The couple has not ever hit each other.) Shirley says these fights are the only time that Sam shows his feelings. Sam believes that men should not show their emotions and views himself as the strong, silent type. Shirley believes that if couples really love each other, they will share all of their feelings. Small disagreements usually end with one member of the couple giving in to the other. Shirley thinks that Sam is an insensitive clod who needs to open up to her. Sam thinks Shirley always bugs him and should treat him with more respect. Of course, both of them want you to fix the other.

Behavioral Rehearsal

When behavioral (as well as other) skills are taught, we attempt to follow sequential steps: (1) to discuss the skill's theoretical rationale; (2) to demonstrate the skills through a role play or videotape; (3) to provide simulated opportunities for skills practice; and (4) to provide instructor or peer feedback to encourage skills improvement. We have used this theoretical rationale–modeling–behavioral rehearsal–reinforcement paradigm to teach family therapy skills such as communication skills training (Jacobson & Margolin, 1979), positive connotation (Constantine, Stone Fish, & Piercy, 1984), and behavioral contracting (Piercy & Sprenkle, 1984).

Position Papers

The student is assigned to read certain articles by authors holding behavioral and nonbehavioral theoretical views on specific issues related to family therapy. Each position paper should reflect the student's own view on the issue in question, in light of the assigned articles and the student's own professional training and background. A position paper is typically three to five double-spaced, typewritten pages in length.

The following examples illustrate several possible assignments for position papers that contrast behavioral and nonbehavioral theoretical orientations (from Piercy & Sprenkle, 1984, pp. 401–402).

Minuchin (1974) includes as possible goals of family therapy the involvement of an uninvolved parent and the disengagement of an overinvolved parent. However, Alexander and Parsons (1982) would probably see the function of the uninvolved parent's behavior as distancing and the function of the overinvolved parent's behavior as merging, and would consequently not try to change these functions. Your question is: Can and should a therapist change the degree of involvement of family members, assuming that their behavior is serving a distancing or merging function? Give a rationale for your answer and examples, if appropriate.

Jacobson and Margolin's (1979) approach to behavioral marital therapy emphasizes the importance of clear, straightforward communications among married couples. Consequently, they teach communications skills as part of their therapy. Carl Whitaker, on the other hand, contends that marriage should be an intense relationship where normal rules of social interaction are suspended. According to Whitaker, couples are not fair or polite to one another, nor should they try to be. As Whitaker is fond of saying, "Telephones are great, but they shouldn't be expected to heat the house!" (See Neill & Kniskern, 1982.) React to this statement and outline the role and importance you give to communications training in your own approach to marital therapy.

Films and Videocassettes

Several films and videocassettes on behavioral marital and family therapies are available from the following sources:

- *AAMFT Master Series,* AAMFT, 1133 15th Street, N.W., Suite 300, Washington, DC 20005-2710
- Research Press, 2612 N. Mattis Avenue, Champaign, IL 61821

RESEARCH ISSUES

More methodologically sound research has been conducted on behavioral marital and family therapies than on other family therapies, perhaps because of their emphasis on operationalization of treatment components and assessment of change. However, many questions regarding efficacy and the assumptions underlying behavioral interventions with couples and families remain to be answered. The following are some examples:

- Does "egalitarian" behavioral contracting subtly support the more powerful or articulate spouse at the expense of the other (as suggested by Jacobson, 1983)?
- What are the most effective components of communication skills training in bringing about change in couples?
- What sequence of interventions for specific behavioral family therapies will produce the most favorable outcome? (This question should be addressed for different subject populations and different presenting problems.)
- Should behavioral marital therapy, if indicated, precede behavioral parent training or vice versa? Do concurrent treatments improve effectiveness?
- Do certain types of clients benefit more from behavioral family therapies than others? What are the critical client variables?
- To what extent does behavioral parent training positively affect marital adjustment? Conversely, to what extent does behavioral marital therapy affect parent–child relationships?
- To what extent do the effects of behavioral family therapies generalize to behaviors not targeted in treatment? For example, what generalization occurs to the sibling of an identified patient?
- Some approaches to behavioral parent training have employed "refresher courses." How effective are these additional treatments in increasing and/or maintaining treatment effects?
- What factors contribute to attrition in behavioral family therapies?
- To what extent do elaborate assessment procedures contribute to change in couples and/or families (above and beyond the treatment itself?)
- To what extent are behavioral family therapies effective relative to specific nonbehavioral family therapies (see Jacobson & Weiss, 1978, p. 158)?
- Does adding the component of "acceptance" to behavioral marital therapy (Jacobson, 1992) significantly improve treatment outcomes at posttest and follow-up?
- Does cognitive-behavioral marital therapy (Baucom & Epstein, 1990) provide significantly better outcome results than standard behavioral marital therapy? Is it more effective with specific populations?
- Can cognitions and affect be operationalized for measurement and observation by cognitive behaviorists, or must they remain nonobservable phenomena (Holtzworth-Munroe & Jacobson, 1991)?
- Do closeness and distancing functions of interpersonal behavior change with behavioral and/or nonbehavioral family therapies? Is it more effective to attempt to change function in therapy, or, as

suggested by Alexander and Parsons (1982), to change behavior in ways consistent with family members' present interpersonal functions?

- To what extent do therapists' conceptual set, relationship skills, and structuring skills predict family change on a variety of outcome measures?

KEY BOOKS, CHAPTERS, AND ARTICLES

Alexander, J. F., & Barton, C. (1980). Systems-behavioral intervention with delinquent families: Clinical, methodological, and conceptual considerations. In J. D. Vincent, (Ed.), *Advances in family assessment and theory* (Vol. 1). Greenwich, CT: JAI Press.

This chapter outlines the research supporting the functional family therapy of Alexander and his associates. The outcome results are compelling. The authors also draw tentative conclusions about the effect of therapists' abilities and characteristics on the outcome of therapy.

Alexander, J. F., & Parsons, B. V. (1982). *Functional family therapy.* Monterey, CA: Brooks/Cole.

This book provides a detailed description of the functional family therapy model. The first part presents the specific skills used in the model, while the second discusses clinical issues involved in practice. This is a very good book for those wanting to learn and practice this model.

Atkeson, B. M., & Forehand, R. (1978). Parent behavioral training for problem children: An examination of studies using multiple outcome measures. *Journal of Abnormal Child Psychology, 6,* 449–460.

This article is a review of 24 studies that utilized three outcome measures: (1) independent observer–collected data, (2) parent-collected data, and (3) parent-completed questionnaire data. The data from the three outcomes were compared. All yielded positive results, but parent-collected data and parent-completed questionnaire data were associated with more positive outcome results than the independently collected data.

Barton, C., & Alexander, J. F. (1981). Functional family therapy. In A. S. Gurman & D. P. Kniskern (Eds.), *Handbook of family therapy.* New York: Brunner/Mazel.

This excellent chapter presents a concise overview of functional family therapy. It covers the issues of theory, assessment, and intervention. Detailed discussion is presented on the role of functions in families and therapy.

Baucom, D. H., & Epstein, N. (1990). *Cognitive-behavioral marital therapy.* New York: Brunner/Mazel.

This book is the single best source to date on cognitive-behavioral marital therapy. The authors provide an overview of the model, as well as strategies for assessment and treatment of cognitions, affect, and behavior. The credibility of the model is enhanced through numerous citations of supportive research.

Berkowitz, B. P., & Graziano, A. M. (1972). Training parents as behaviour therapists: A review. *Behaviour Research and Therapy, 10,* 297–317.

This article is a critical review of 34 studies ranging from single-case studies to large-scale, multifamily training programs. Of primary concern is the nature of family involvement and the responsibility the family has in planning and implementing the intervention program. The sophistication of research methods is also critically analyzed.

Christensen, A., Jacobson, N. S., & Babcock, J. C. (1995). Integrative behavioral couple therapy. In N. S. Jacobson & A. S. Gurman (Eds.), *Clinical handbook of couple therapy.* New York: Guilford Press.

This is the most complete summary to date of Jacobson's couple model. It integrates behavioral technology with the concept of acceptance.

Epstein, N., Baucom, D. H., & Rankin, L. A. (1993). Treatment of marital conflict: A cognitive-behavioral approach. *Clinical Psychology Review, 13,* 45–57.

This article discusses specific cognitions and behavioral patterns that exacerbate marital conflict. Representative cognitive-behavioral strategies are presented for altering couples' cognitions and modifying their conflict cycles.

Epstein, N., Schlesinger, S. E., & Dryden, W. (Eds.). (1988). *Cognitive-behavioral therapy with families.* New York: Brunner/Mazel.

This edited book provides a fine overview of cognitive-behavioral family therapy with a variety of treatment populations. Especially interesting are chapters comparing cognitive-behavioral with systems models of family therapy.

Falloon, I. R. H. (Ed.). (1988). *Handbook of behavioral family therapy.* New York: Guilford Press.

This highly recommended book addresses many of the important concerns currently facing behavioral family therapy, as well as specific applications. Traditional ideas are updated to deal with issues of assessment, resistance, theory, and treatment. This is an excellent source for the reader wishing to get a current view of behavioral theory and practice.

Falloon, I. R. H. (1991). Behavioral family therapy. In A. S. Gurman & D. P. Kniskern (Eds.), *Handbook of family therapy* (Vol. 2). New York: Brunner/Mazel.

This chapter provides a concise overview of behavioral family therapy. Included are brief discussions on historical development of the model, assessment issues, and treatment techniques. It argues that the hallmark of behavioral family therapy is the willingness to *assess the effectiveness* of a variety of change strategies rather than the reliance on operant conditioning and communication training.

Forehand, R., & Atkeson, B. M. (1977). Generality of treatment effects with parents as therapists: A review of assessment and implementation procedures. *Behavior Therapy, 8,* 575–593.

This review focuses on studies in which parents are trained to generalize treatment of a child's behavior over time, across settings, to other behaviors, and to other siblings. Generally, although parent training has been found effective with targeted behaviors, its effect on generalization has yet to be impressive. One exception is the contagion effect of one child's improvement on that of siblings. The authors concede that many of the studies cited are weak in methodology, and assert that studies examining methods for implementing generalization are needed.

Gordon, S. B., & Davidson, N. (1981). Behavioral parent training. In A. S. Gurman & D. P. Kniskern (Eds.), *Handbook of family therapy.* New York: Brunner/Mazel.

This excellent review includes a rationale and procedures for behavioral parent training. Its major strength, however, is in the distillation of the large body of literature in this area. The authors also do a fine job of identifying important issues related to research, training, and future directions for behavioral parent training.

Gottman, J. M. (1979). *Marital interaction: Experimental investigations.* New York: Academic Press.

This volume pulls together the theory and research of the author, drawing upon previous works from sociological, family systems, social learning, and developmental theories. The book is noteworthy for its analysis of patterns and sequence in marital interaction and is must reading for those interested in process research in couple communication. The culmination of the author's work is in the Couples Interaction Scoring System (CISS). The procedure is thorough but expensive and likely to be more practical for researchers than clinicians.

Graziano, A. M. (1977). Parents as behavior therapists. In M. Hersen, R. M. Eisler, & P. M. Miller (Eds.), *Progress in behavior modification* (Vol. 4). New York: Academic Press.

The author's compendium of literature regarding parents as behavior modifiers is extended to these child problem categories: somatic symptoms, mental deficiency or disturbance, aggressive behaviors, fears, language and speech disorders, and behavioral problems in the home. In addition, methods of training parents and evaluating change in a child's performance are identified. An extensive and useful set of references follows this chapter.

Gurman, A. S., & Knudson, R. M. (1978). Behavioral marriage therapy: I. A psychodynamic-systems analysis and critique. *Family Process, 17,* 121–138.

The authors list and critically examine five major clusters of implicit assumptions in behavioral marital therapy (e.g., "Repression is good for your marital mental health"), and this touches off a heated debate with Jacobson and Weiss, proponents of behavioral marital therapy in this issue of *Family Process.* The lively interchange that ensues raises important issues and makes for interesting reading.

Holtzworth-Munroe, A., & Jacobson, N. S. (1991). Behavioral marital therapy. In A. S. Gurman & D. P. Kniskern (Eds.), *Handbook of family therapy* (Vol. 2). New York: Brunner/Mazel.

This chapter provides a concise overview of behavioral marital therapy prior to incorporating the concept of "acceptance." It provides good, brief discussions of assessment and treatment procedures. It also provides an interesting comparison of behavioral marital therapy with cognitive-behavioral marital therapy.

Jacobson, N. S. (1991). Toward enhancing the efficacy of marital therapy and marital therapy research. *Journal of Family Psychology, 4,* 373–393.

This provocative article presents ideas for enhancing behavioral marital therapy and marital therapy research. Jacobson makes a strong case for more rigorous measures in outcome studies, especially in the design of treatment manuals. Furthermore, he discusses the concept of "partner acceptance" as an adjunct to behavioral marital therapy.

Jacobson, N. S. (1992). Behavioral couple therapy: A new beginning. *Behavior Therapy, 23,* 493–506.

This important article presents the theoretical change from Jacobson's original model of "Behavioral Marital Therapy" to his new approach, "Integrative-Behavior Couple Therapy." He discusses the strengths and limitations of the traditional approach and provides a theoretical rational for the inclusion of "acceptance of partner" to his model.

Jacobson, N. S., & Margolin, G. (1979). *Marital therapy: Strategies based on social learning and behavioral exchange principles.* New York: Brunner/Mazel.

This is a clear and comprehensive presentation of the authors' social learning approach to couple therapy. Its strength is in its detail regarding the initial interview, increasing couples' positive exchanges, communication and problem-solving training, and contingency contracting. The authors also discuss at length the importance of such intangibles as persuasion and the "collaborative set."

Liberman, R. P. (1970). Behavioral approaches to family and couple therapy. *American Journal of Orthopsychiatry, 40*(1), 106–118.

This classic article explains how social reinforcement employed in families balances aversive behavior from one family member with gratifying consequences for all members involved. Changing the contingencies by which attention and concern are shared is considered the crucial determinant for success in treatment. The reading is historically pivotal, in that it brought social learning theory to the treatment of whole families, rather than using it to target and treat deviant individuals.

Morris, S. B., Alexander, J. F., & Waldron, H. (1988). Functional family therapy. In I. R. H. Falloon (Ed.), *Handbook of behavioral family therapy.* New York: Guilford Press.

This chapter presents an up-to-date overview of functional family therapy. It is especially noteworthy for the amount of discussion paid to the role of cognitions in this model.

O'Dell, S. (1974). Training parents in behavior modification: A review. *Psychological Bulletin, 81,* 418–433.

This article reviews 70 studies of parents trained to apply behavioral principles to the discipline of their children, dating back to 1965. The author's conclusion notes that most of the studies have focused on changes in the children while ignoring the necessary phases of maintenance and generalization of the parent's behavior. This is a hefty and useful resource for early articles on behavioral parent training.

Patterson, G. R. (1975). *Families: Applications of social learning to family life.* Champaign, IL: Research Press.

Although this book was first published in 1971, it is still an excellent source for helping parents learn to apply social learning theory to family problems. Patterson's presentations of contracting and time-out are particularly clear and well illustrated with a variety of examples.

Patterson, G. R. (1983). *Coercive family process.* Eugene, OR: Castalia.

In this large volume, Patterson presents a wealth of empirical data and clinical observations that undergird an evolving coercion theory based upon the observed behavior of antisocial children and their families. This book is more descriptive and databased than his earlier "how-to" books for parents. As a comprehensive integration of research findings, it stands alone in its thoroughness in clarifying the dynamics of coercive families from a social learning theory perspective.

Patterson, G. R., Reid, J. B., Jones, R. R., & Conger, R. E. (1975). *A social learning approach to family intervention: Vol. 1. Families with aggressive children.* Eugene, OR: Castalia.

This treatment manual, based on the work of the Oregon Research Institute, reports on the noncoercive behavioral methods used to reduce aggressive behavior in children. A child's behavior is controlled primarily through behavioral contracting and time-out, not only by parents but also by school personnel who are regularly involved with the child. The author's attention to procedural details and to databased assessment makes this a particularly useful volume.

Peters, R. DeV., & McMahon, R.J. (Eds.). (1988). *Social learning and systems approaches to marriage and the family.* New York: Brunner/Mazel.

This edited book presents chapters by the participants of the 1985 Banff International Conference on Behavioral Sciences. The focus is on the integration of behavioral and family systems approaches to the understanding of family process and the treatment of a variety of disorders.

Robin, A. L., & Foster, S. L. (1989). *Negotiating parent–adolescent conflict: A behavioral-family systems approach.* New York: Guilford Press.

The authors present their model, which integrates cognitive-behavioral and family systems approaches to the treatment of adolescent difficulties. They discuss behavioral, cognitive, and systemic assessment and intervention with this population and include clinical examples and full-length case studies.

Sanders, M. R., & Dadds, M. R. (1993). *Behavioral family intervention*. Boston: Allyn & Bacon.

This book is written with clinicians in mind. It presents a treatment manual for conducting behavioral therapy with child-focused problems. It provides a brief empirical and theoretical overview of behavioral family therapy, with detailed procedures for assessing and treating childhood disorders. A chapter is included on adjunctive assessment and treatment of related marital problems for the parents.

Spinks, S. H., & Birchler, G. B. (1982). Behavioral systems marital therapy: Dealing with resistance. *Family Process, 21,* 169–183.

A behavioral systems marital therapy approach is presented as an integrative therapeutic model. The authors state that it is sometimes necessary to depart from the behavioral marital therapy model when resistance is not due to the design, timing, or appropriateness of assignment. Six basic options for interventions are presented, with a rationale for the departure from the behavioral framework.

Stuart, R. B. (1969). Operant interpersonal treatment for marital discord. *Journal of Consulting and Clinical Psychology, 33,* 675–682.

This classic article represents the first published application of a behavioral change contract to marital problems.

Stuart, R. B. (1980). *Helping couples change: A social learning approach to marital therapy.* New York: Guilford Press.

This well-documented book outlines a structured program for couples consistent with learning theory principles. Stuart's role as scholar/clinician is evident throughout. His specific descriptions of contracting, caring days, and procedures for containing conflict will be particularly useful to the practicing family therapist.

REFERENCES

Alexander, J. F. (1973). Defensive and supportive communications in normal and deviant families. *Journal of Consulting and Clinical Psychology, 40,* 223–231.

Alexander, J. F., & Parsons, B. V. (1973). Short-term behavioral intervention with delinquent families. *Journal of Abnormal Psychology, 81,* 219–225.

Alexander, J. F., & Parsons, B. V. (1982). *Functional family therapy.* Monterey, CA: Brooks/Cole.

Arrington, A., Sullaway, M., & Christensen, A. (1988). Behavioral family assessment. In I. R. H. Falloon (Ed.), *Handbook of behavioral family therapy.* New York: Guilford Press.

Bandura, A. (1971). *Psychological modeling: Conflicting theories.* Chicago: Aldine/Atherton.

Barton, A., & Alexander, J. F. (1981). Functional family therapy. In A. S. Gurman & D. P. Kniskern (Eds.), *Handbook of family therapy*. New York: Brunner/Mazel.

Baucom, D. H., & Epstein, N. (1990). *Cognitive-behavioral marital therapy*. New York: Brunner/Mazel.

Baucom, D. H., & Lester, G. W. (1986). The usefulness of cognitive restructuring as an adjunct to behavioral marital therapy. *Behavior Therapy, 17*, 385–403.

Beck, A. T. (1976). *Cognitive therapy and the emotional disorders*. New York: International Universities.

Billings, A. (1979). Conflict resolution in distressed and nondistressed married couples. *Journal of Consulting and Clinical Psychology, 47*, 368–376.

Birchler, G. R. (1988). Handling resistance to change. In I. R. H. Falloon (Ed.), *Handbook of behavioral family therapy*. New York: Guilford Press.

Christensen, A., Jacobson, N. S., & Babcock, J. C. (1995). Integrative behavioral couple therapy. In N. S. Jacobson & A. S. Gurman (Eds.), *Clinical handbook of couple therapy*. New York: Guilford Press.

Cone, J. D., & Sloop, E. W. (1974). Parents as agents of change. In W. W. Spradlin & A. Jacobs (Eds.), *The group as agent of change*. New York: Behavioral Publications.

Constantine, J., Stone Fish, L. S., & Piercy, F. (1984). A procedure for teaching positive connotation. *Journal of Marital and Family Therapy, 10*, 313–316.

Cordova, J. V., & Jacobson, N. S. (1993). Couple distress. In D. H. Barlow (Ed.), *Clinical handbook of psychological disorders: A step-by-step treatment manual*. New York: Guilford Press.

Cox, A., & Rutter, M. (1985). Diagnostic appraisal and interviewing. In M. Rutter & L. Hersov (Eds.), *Child and adolescent psychiatry: Modern approaches*. Oxford: Blackwell.

Ellis, A. (1962). *Reason and emotion in psychotherapy*. New York: Lyle Stuart.

Emmelkamp, P. M. G., van Linden van den Heuvell, C., Ruphan, M., Sanderman, R., Scholing, A., & Stroink, F. (1988). Cognitive and behavioral interventions: A comparative evaluation with clinically distressed couples. *Journal of Family Psychology, 1*, 365–377.

Epstein, N., Baucom, D. H., & Rankin, L. A. (1993). Treatment of marital conflict: A cognitive-behavioral approach. *Clinical Psychology Review, 13*, 45–57.

Epstein, N., Schlesinger, S. E., & Dryden, W. (1988). Concepts and methods of cognitive-behavioral family treatment. In N. Epstein, S. E. Schlessinger, & W. Dryden (Eds.), *Cognitive-behavioral therapy with families*. New York: Brunner/Mazel.

Falloon, I. R. H. (1991). Behavioral family therapy. In A. S. Gurman & D. P. Kniskern (Eds.), *Handbook of family therapy* (Vol. 2). New York: Brunner/Mazel.

Falloon, I. R. H., & Liberman, R. P. (1983). Behavioral family interventions in the management of chronic schizophrenia. In W. R. McFarlane (Ed.), *Family therapy in schizophrenia*. New York: Guilford Press.

Fleischman, M. J. (1981). A replication of Patterson's "Intervention for boys with conduct problems." *Journal of Consulting and Clinical Psychology, 49*, 342–351.

Foster, S. L., & Hoier, T. S. (1982). Behavioral and systems family therapies: A comparison of theoretical assumptions. *American Journal of Family Therapy*, *10*(3), 13–23.

Gordon, S. B., & Davidson, N. (1981). Behavioral parent training. In A. S. Gurman & D. P. Kniskern (Eds.), *Handbook of family therapy*. New York: Brunner/Mazel.

Gordon, S. B., Lerner, L. L., & Keefe, F. J. (1979). Responsive parenting: An approach to training parents of problem children. *American Journal of Community Psychology*, *7*, 45–56.

Gottman, J. M. (1979). *Marital interaction: Experimental investigations*. New York: Academic Press.

Gottman, J. M., Markman, H., & Notarius, C. (1977). The topography of marital conflict: A sequential analysis of verbal and nonverbal behavior. *Journal of Marriage and the Family*, *39*, 461–477.

Gottman, J. M., Notarius, C., Markman, H., Bank, S., Yoppi, B., & Rubin, M. (1976). Behavior exchange theory and marital decision making. *Journal of Personality and Social Psychology*, *34*, 14–23.

Graziano, A. M. (1974). *Child without tomorrow*. New York: Pergamon Press.

Graziano, A. M. (1977). Parents as behavior therapists. In M. Hersen, R. M. Eisler, & P. M. Miller (Eds.), *Progress in behavior modification*. New York: Academic Press.

Hahlweg, K., Baucom, D.H., & Markman, H. (1988). Recent advances in therapy and prevention. In I. R. H. Falloon (Ed.), *Handbook of behavioral family therapy*. New York: Guilford Press.

Holtzworth-Munroe, A., & Jacobson, N. S. (1991). Behavioral marital therapy. In A. S. Gurman, & D. P. Kniskern (Eds.), *Handbook of family therapy*. New York: Brunner/Mazel.

Huber, C. H., & Milstein, B. (1985). Cognitive restructuring and a collaborative set in couples' work. *American Journal of Family Therapy*, *13*(2), 17–27.

Jacobson, N. S. (1983). Beyond empiricism: The politics of marital therapy. *American Journal of Family Therapy*, *11*, 11–24.

Jacobson, N. S. (1991). Toward enhancing the efficacy of marital therapy and marital therapy research. *Journal of Family Psychology*, *4*, 373–393.

Jacobson, N. S. (1992). Behavioral couple therapy: A new beginning. *Behavior Therapy*, *23*, 493–506.

Jacobson, N. S., & Margolin, G. (1979). *Marital therapy*. New York: Brunner/Mazel.

Jacobson, N. S., & Weiss, R. L. (1978). Behavioral marriage therapy: III. The contents of Gurman *et al.* may be hazardous to our health. *Family Process*, *12*, 149–164.

Klein, N. C., Alexander, J. F., & Parsons, B. V. (1977). Impact of family systems intervention on recidivism and sibling delinquency: A model of primary prevention and program evaluation. *Journal of Consulting and Clinical Psychology*, *45*, 469–474.

Lederer, W. J., & Jackson, D. D. (1968). *Mirages of marriage*. New York: Norton.

Liberman, R. P. (1970). Behavioral approaches to family and couple therapy. *American Journal of Orthopsychiatry*, *40*, 106–118.

McAuley, R. (1988). Parent training: Clinical application. In I. R. H. Falloon (Ed.), *Handbook of behavioral family therapy*. New York: Guilford Press.

Minuchin, S. (1974). *Families and family therapy*. Cambridge, MA: Harvard University Press.

Morris, S. B., Alexander, J. F., & Waldron, H. (1988). Functional family therapy. In I. R. H. Falloon (Ed.), *Handbook of behavioral family therapy*. New York: Guilford Press.

Neill, J. R., & Kniskern, D. P. (Eds.). (1982). *From psyche to system: The evolving therapy of Carl Whitaker*. New York: Guilford Press.

O'Dell, S. (1974). Training parents in behavior modification: A review. *Psychological Bulletin, 81*, 418–433.

Patterson, G. R. (1971). *Families: Applications of social learning to family life*. Champaign, IL: Research Press.

Patterson, G. R. (1982). *Coercive family process*. Eugene, OR: Castalia.

Patterson, G. R., McNeil, S., Hawkins, N., & Phelps, R. (1967). Reprogramming the social environment. *Journal of Child Psychology and Psychiatry, 8*, 181–195.

Piercy, F., & Sprenkle, D. (1984). The process of family therapy education. *Journal of Marital and Family Therapy, 10*(4), 399–407.

Robin, A. L., & Weiss, J. G. (1980). The criterion-related validity of observational and self-report measures of problem-solving communications skills in distressed and nondistressed parent–adolescent dyads. *Behavioral Assessment, 2*, 339–353.

Sisson, L. A., & Taylor, J. C. (1993). Parent training. In A. S. Bellack & M. Herson (Eds.), *Handbook of behavior therapy in the psychiatric setting*. New York: Plenum Press.

Stuart, R. B. (1969). Operant interpersonal treatment for marital discord. *Journal of Consulting and Clinical Psychology, 33*, 675–682.

Stuart, R. B. (1980). *Helping couples change: A social learning approach to marital therapy*. New York: Guilford Press.

Tharp, R. G., & Wetzel, R. J. (1969). *Behavior modification in the natural environment*. New York: Academic Press.

Wiltz, N. A., & Gordon, S. B. (1974). Parental modification of a child's behavior in an experimental residence. *Journal of Behavior Therapy and Experimental Psychiatry, 5*, 107–109.

Wolkind, S., & Rutter, M. (1985). Separation, loss and family relationships. In M. Rutter & L. Hersov (Eds.), *Child and adolescent psychiatry: Modern approaches*. Oxford: Blackwell.

6

Social Constructionist Family Therapies

JOSEPH L. WETCHLER

SOCIAL CONSTRUCTIONIST family therapy refers to a loose grouping of therapies based on the concept that reality is an intersubjective phenomenon, constructed in conversation among people. These theories have at times been called constructivist, postmodern, narrative, reflexive, and second-order cybernetic. Although different theoretical ideas are associated with these terms (Hoffman, 1990), we have listed them under the heading "social constructionism" for ease of categorization. Social constructionist family therapies are based on the writings of Bateson (1972, 1979), Bruner (1986), Foucault (1965, 1980), Geertz (1983), Gergen (1982), Kelly (1963), Maturana and Varela (1980, 1987), Piaget (1952), von Foerster (1981), Wittgenstein (1958, 1968), and others.

Social constructionist theories arose in response to positivist, deterministic models. Although family therapy challenged the notion of individual pathology, some theorists believe that family therapy had simply moved the diagnosis from the individual to the family (Anderson & Goolishian, 1988; Hoffman, 1991; White, 1995). Prominent social constructionist family therapists include Tom Andersen (1987, 1991), Harlene Anderson and Harold Goolishian (1988, 1992), Steve de Shazer (1985, 1991), Insoo Berg (1993; Berg & Miller, 1992), Michael Durrant (1993, 1995), Lynn Hoffman (1990, 1991), Alan Parry and Robert Doan

(1994), and Michael White and David Epston (Epston & White, 1992; White & Epston, 1990).

Although each of these theorists has their own unique style of practice, several ideas are common to all of them. Some of the principle tenets of social constructionist family therapies are discussed here.

REALITY IS CONSTRUCTED IN CONVERSATION

Perhaps the foremost concept in social constructionist family therapy is that what we perceive as "real" is often due to dominant beliefs within ourselves and society (Parry & Doan, 1994; White, 1995). For example, a social constructionist would say that we cannot accurately observe a family because what we see is colored by our previous beliefs and interactions with the family. Parry and Doan (1994) state: "The introduction of the narrative dimension into family therapy . . . emphasizes that whether the viewer is a person, a family, a community, or a people, the world is unavoidably viewed through the lens of a succession of stories—not only a personal story, but gender, community, class, and cultural stories" (p. 24).

Social constructionists believe that not only is it impossible to be an accurate observer, but statements about normality are also flawed. For example, Anderson, Goolishian, and Windermand (1986) state that "diagnosis and treatment are fundamentally social creations that are created in language through dialogue; they are the invention of social communicative exchange" (p. 6).

Hoffman (1991) proposes that social constructionism presents six challenges to traditional views of therapy and research:

1. As the observer cannot be separated from the observed, there is no such thing as objective social research.
2. The concept of the "self" is socially constructed rather than being an observable, stable entity.
3. There is no universal standard of "normal development," as context plays a major role in how humans develop.
4. Emotions are context determined rather than internal, stable states.
5. There is no underlying meaning for communication, as what is defined as context is often subjective.
6. Therapists are not blessed with special insights into individuals or families, but rather are participants in constructing a reality with their clients.

Similarly, de Shazer (1994) says that often we are reduced to guessing when we attempt to find the deep structure within a clients behavior.

REJECTION OF THE SYSTEMS METAPHOR
FOR DESCRIBING FAMILIES

How we have viewed the family has undergone radical change in the past several years (Carter & McGoldrick, 1988). For example, our concepts of normality are constantly being challenged with the recognition of single-parent families, two-paycheck families, remarried families, and homosexual families. It becomes harder and harder for professionals to identify what is functional behavior. Social constructionists challenge the ability of therapists to objectively diagnose families. They also challenge the use of the systems metaphor. White (1995) states that "the metaphors of system and pattern encourage therapists to assume objectivity, and to step into a formal vocabulary of language that emphasizes a posture of spectatorship and impartiality" (p. 215).

The concept of systems originally was used as a metaphor for describing families. Over time, therapists began to view families as actually possessing those concepts borrowed from cybernetics and general system theory. It is de Shazer's (1991) belief that "this sort of misreading reifies concepts and moves the entire discourse into speculations about causation similar in kind to an explanation for behavior that attributes the behavior to 'poor ego strength.' Like the ego, the system is nowhere because it does not exist" (p. 26).

Some social constructionists have gone beyond rejecting the systems metaphor to challenge the very concept of family. Anderson et al. (1986) state:

> We must be cautious lest we think that there are entities called the family. If a family exists only in language (through description), there is a different family for everyone observing the family, including the members themselves. The family that we see and experience is no more than just one other reality of the many realities that are possible through the operation of distinctions called observation. In light of the foregoing, we must begin to wonder about our descriptive concept of family and family therapy. (p. 9)

THERAPIST EXPERTISE HOLDS NO MORE
PROMINENCE THAN CLIENT EXPERTISE

Social constructionist family therapists are concerned about placing therapist expertise at a higher level than client knowledge (Andersen, 1991, 1992; Anderson & Goolishian, 1988, 1992; Epston & White, 1992; White, 1995). Psychological knowledge and diagnosis often reproduce dominant cultural values that serve to marginalize the wisdom of those who are viewed as outsiders (White, 1995; White & Epston, 1990). By placing therapist knowledge above client knowledge, we not only further objectify and demean our clients, but we also close the door to new and possibly unique ways of viewing and solving client problems. White (1995) poses the following challenge to members of the mental health profession:

> It is impossible for us to arrive at a vantage point from outside of culture—and therefore outside of language and known ways of life—by which we might review our culture. However, this fact does not condemn us to blindly reproducing culture, without any hope of refusing or protesting those aspects which we experience as problematic. It does not restrict us to the role of accomplice to this modern system of power—we can assist persons to challenge certain practices of power. . . . We do not have to be entirely complicit with dominant culture—in fact, I think that we should make it our business to ensure that we are not so. (p. 45)

THERAPY IS CO-CONSTRUCTED BETWEEN THERAPIST AND CLIENT

The leveling of therapist and client knowledge makes social constructionist therapy a joint venture. Rather than clinicians giving directives, therapists and clients work together to co-construct outcomes (Andersen, 1987; Parry & Doan, 1994). The role of the therapist becomes one of opening doors for clients to explore new meanings in their lives. This means engaging them in a slightly different conversation than the ones they usually have around the problem (Andersen, 1991). It is through this joint conversation that clients develop new ways of looking at their situation and subsequently new outcomes for resolving their difficulties. Anderson and Goolishian (1988) state:

> In this framework, the therapist does not enter with an overarching map of psychological and social theory regarding human nature and human diffi-culties, a map on which to fit the clinical data and, thus, the client. Rather, therapist and client create the maps together—the therapeutic realities. From the initial contact and throughout the therapeutic relationship, the therapist and client are engaged in collaboratively creating descriptions and stories. (p. 384)

These comprise the major tenets of social constructionist family therapy. The following sections discuss four of the major theoretician/schools within this paradigm: Michael White and David Epston—narrative therapy; Harlene Anderson and Harry Goolishian—collaborative language systems approach; Tom Andersen—reflecting team; and Steve de Shazer and Insoo Berg—solution-focused therapy.

MICHAEL WHITE AND DAVID EPSTON:
NARRATIVE THERAPY

Michael White and David Epston's theory (Epston & White, 1992; White & Epston, 1990) commonly referred to as narrative therapy, developed in Australia and New Zealand, respectively. Their ideas were heavily influenced by the work of Michel Foucault (1965, 1980), who proposed that constructed ideas have the power to shape people's lives. From Foucault, White and Epston became concerned with how dominant stories affect client families (White & Epston, 1990).

Treatment families often view problems as if they were a reified, stable state (e.g., "John is depressed" or "We have a problem marriage"). In maintaining a dominant story of their problem, family members fail to see those times when they do not have the problem. White and Epston (1990) refer to this as a problem-saturated description of family life. Periods of success with the problem become subjugated stories, banished to the periphery of awareness (White, 1986; Epston, White, & Murray, 1992). White and Epston (1990) state: "The structuring of a narrative requires recourse to a selective process in which we prune, from our experience, those events that do not fit with the dominant evolving stories that we and others have about us. Thus, over time and of necessity, much of our stock of lived experience goes unstoried and is never 'told' or expressed" (pp. 11–12).

White and Epston loosen the hold of the dominant story by externalizing the problem from the individual (White & Epston, 1990; White, 1995). Rather than discuss the problem as "John's depression," they begin to talk about "when the depression takes charge of John." By viewing the problem as an external entity, they free the family to challenge its influence on their lives (White, 1995). After narrative therapists have externalized the problem, they ask the family to identify unique outcomes, times when they successfully fought off the influence of the problem. They accomplish this through the use of "landscape-of-action" questions that enable clients to situate unique outcomes within their past stories, and "landscape-of-experience" questions that promote reflection on the meaning of this new story in their lives (White, 1993).

White and Epston (1990) often write letters to families, discussing the family's efforts to ward off the influence of the problem as a means of rewriting the once subjugated story into a dominant one. This new story is further developed by having their clients share their success with others and develop certificates verifying their success (Epston & White, 1992; White & Epston, 1990).

Narrative therapy is more than a problem-focused approach. It is a process for helping people rewrite descriptions of their lives. Rather than objectifying or marginalizing people through diagnosing them, narrative therapists help them develop successful life stories as problem solvers (White, 1995). Through the therapist's questions, the family develops new stories about themselves and the ways they resolve their problems (Epston & White, 1992).

Narrative therapy, then, views therapy as a political process and is concerned with the role of therapist power at clients' expense (White, 1995). Narrative therapists stress the importance of leveling the playing field between therapist and client to allow clients a voice in the process of their treatment. As part of keeping themselves honest and their clients empowered, White and Epston have jointly written case notes with their families (White, 1995; White & Epston, 1990), used clients as consultants to their therapy (Epston & White, 1992; Epston, White, & "Ben," 1995), and have had clients observe and comment on the therapist's process on other cases through the use of a reflecting team (White, 1995).

HARLENE ANDERSON AND HARRY GOOLISHIAN: COLLABORATIVE LANGUAGE SYSTEMS APPROACH

The collaborative language systems approach of Harlene Anderson and the late Harold Goolishian is based on the premise that problems are maintained in language by a problem-determined system and subsequently are dissolved through conversation (Anderson & Goolishian, 1988; Goolishian & Anderson, 1987). Therapists take a "not-knowing stance" in which they subsume their expertise and allow room for their clients' knowledge to come forward (Anderson & Goolishian, 1992). They believe that conversation generates meaning, both for clients' systems and in their relationship with their therapist (Anderson & Goolishian, 1988, 1992).

Rather than focus on the family as maintaining a problem, Anderson and Goolishian focus on those individuals who view the situation as a problem, the problem-determined system (Anderson et al., 1986). This can be a family, an individual, certain members of a family, or family members and other members of the community. People are members of a problem-determined system if they are involved in a conversation that a problem exists. Particularly germane to a problem-determined system is a view of the problem that has impeded any successful means of resolution.

Anderson and Goolishian (Anderson, 1993; Anderson & Goolishian, 1988; Anderson et al., 1986) espouse a collaborative approach in which the therapist asks questions that stimulate clients to view the problem in a new light. Different from the Milan associates (Selvini Palazzoli, Boscolo, Cecchin, & Prata, 1980; see Chapter 3), Anderson and Goolishian (1992) avoid having specific therapist hypotheses dominate the conversation for fear of limiting more fruitful discourse. The problem-determined system eventually dissolves as clients and therapists generate new meanings about the problem and clients take new actions to resolve it (Anderson et al., 1986; Goolishian & Anderson, 1987). Anderson (1993) states:

> Implicit in this way of working is that each client, each problem, each therapy session, and each course of therapy is seen as unique. The approach does not rely on preconceived knowledge such as commonalities of problems or on across-the-board skills and techniques. This does not mean that "anything goes" or that this conversational therapeutic process unfolds simply by maintaining an atmosphere of nondirective and empathetic conversation. Instead, the process becomes a source for a wide range of thinking and action that is distinctive to the people involved and the issues at hand. Nor does it mean that therapists do not know anything and enter the room as a *tabula rasa*; quite naturally, they bring with them who they are and all that that entails. It means that the therapist's pre-experiences and pre-knowledges do not lead. In this process both the therapist's and the client's expertise are engaged to dissolve the problem. (p. 325)

TOM ANDERSEN: THE REFLECTING TEAM

Norwegian family therapist Tom Andersen (1987, 1991, 1995) demystified the process of the team behind the one-way mirror through his use of reflecting teams. Andersen was uncomfortable with the way traditional strategic and Milan teams (see Chapter 3) pathologized families and promoted therapist beliefs over client knowledge (Andersen, 1992). Having team members share their hypotheses in the presence of the family made therapy more transparent and less hierarchical. Andersen (1995) states:

> When we finally began to use this mode we were surprised at how easy it was to talk without using nasty or hurtful words. Later it became evident that how we talk depends on the context in which we talk. If we choose to speak about the families without them present, we easily speak "professionally," in a detached manner. If we choose to speak about them in their presence, we naturally use everyday language and speak in a friendly manner. (p. 16)

Although there now exist many versions of the reflecting team (e.g., Friedman, 1995; White, 1995), the basic process is for the interviewing therapist to engage in a conversation with the stuck system while the rest of the team quietly observes behind the mirror. At a certain point, the clients are asked if they want to hear comments from the team. The clients and interviewing therapist then observe the team have a conversation among themselves about their observations and thoughts *based on that particular session*. This is then followed by the stuck system discussing their reflections on the team's conversation (Andersen, 1987).

Andersen (1987, 1991, 1993) believes that individuals engage in two types of conversations: an external one in which they actively participate in sharing their ideas with others as they talk, and an internal one in which they talk to themselves as they listen to others. Individuals engage in both types of conversations as they talk with the interviewing therapist and listen to the reflecting team. Influenced by Norwegian physiotherapist Aadel Bulow-Hansen, Andersen (1991, 1992) believes that interviewers should ask questions that are moderately unusual from the clients' perspectives to facilitate internal and external conversation. Those questions that are too similar produce no new conversation, whereas those that are too discrepant inhibit the conversation.

Relatively few studies have been done on social constructionist family therapies; however, recent qualitative studies have found that clients and therapists find the reflecting team process beneficial (Sells, Smith, Coe, Yoshioka, & Robbins, 1994; Smith, Sells, & Clevenger, 1994).

STEVE DE SHAZER AND INSOO BERG: SOLUTION-FOCUSED THERAPY

Solution-focused therapy (de Shazer, 1985, 1991; de Shazer & Berg, 1992) is a brief, pragmatic treatment that integrates a problem focus with a social constructionist perspective. Rather than assessing the problem-maintaining system, solution-focused therapists help clients identify exceptions to the time the problem exists (de Shazer et al., 1986). This perspective is influenced by both the indirect approach of Milton Erickson (1954) and the poststructuralism of Ludwig Wittgenstein (1958). It developed from the theoretical expertise of Steve de Shazer (1985, 1991, 1994) and clinical wizardry of Insoo Berg (Berg, 1993; Berg & Miller, 1992).

Solution-focused therapists believe that patient diagnosis (de Shazer, 1991, 1994; de Shazer & Berg, 1992) and client resistance (de Shazer, 1984, 1988) exist only in the minds of therapists. Rather than engage in traditional diagnosis and treatment, they help clients solve their own problems by identifying and repeating those behaviors they were engaged in when the problem did not exist. Clients maintain their problems because they are unable to see the times in which they resolve them. Identifying these exceptions enables clients to repeat these behaviors and take control of their problems. Problems are deconstructed and resolved through a solution-focused conversation between therapist and client (de Shazer, 1988). In 1991, de Shazer states:

> The therapeutic relationship is a negotiated, consensual, and cooperative endeavor in which the solution-focused therapist and client jointly produce various language games focused on (a) exceptions, (b) goals, and (c) solutions. . . . All of these are negotiated and produced as therapists and clients

misunderstand together, make sense of, and give meaning to otherwise ambiguous events, feelings, and relationships. In doing so, therapists and clients jointly assign meaning to aspects of clients' lives and justify actions intended to develop a solution. (p. 74).

In generating a solution-focused conversation, therapists need to assess the category of the therapist–client relationship: visitor, complainant, or customer. The therapist then engages in the appropriate level of conversation, which is dependent on the category of the therapist–client relationship (de Shazer, 1988). For example, the therapist will take a more active role in helping the client look for exceptions if the client is a customer rather than just a visitor. Typically, the therapist uses specific assignments and questions. For example, in the "formula first-session task," the therapist instructs clients to focus on what aspects of their lives they wish to continue (de Shazer, 1985). In the "miracle question," the therapist asks clients to picture what they might notice if a miracle happened and the problem no longer existed (de Shazer, 1988).

KEY CONCEPTS

Complainant. In 1988, de Shazer used the term complainant to refer to a type of therapist–client relationship that is identified by the client describing a complaint but being currently unwilling to resolve it. This is not a diagnosis of the client but reflects the current state of the therapeutic relationship. The therapist's role in this relationship is to engage in solution-focused conversation with the client, compliment the client, and possibly give an assignment to observe when exceptions happen. By respecting this relationship and not pushing for change, the relationship may evolve into one in which the client is a "customer" (listed).

Customer. This refers to a therapist–client relationship in which the client describes a problem and is motivated to resolve it. The therapist's role in this relationship is to engage in solution-focused conversation, compliment the client, and assign tasks to reproduce those behaviors that are exceptions to the problem.

Exception. In 1985, de Shazer (1985) considered an exception to be when the client is either not engaged in the problem or briefly resolves it. A solution focused therapist focuses on exceptions to help clients alter their perceptions and develop solutions to their problems.

Dominant story. White and Epston (1990) use the term dominant story to describe one's principal view of the world. Dominant stories can be either helpful or hindering. They are problematic when clients view themselves as unable to resolve their problems. If a family's dominant story is that Mary is bad, they may not be able to observe those times when she behaves appropriately or when they are successful in getting her to behave. Helping the family see subjugated stories (listed) enables them to feel more powerful and exert more control over their problem.

Language games. Based on the ideas of Wittgenstein, de Shazer (1991) uses the term "language games" to refer to conversations that individuals engage in to determine reality. It also refers to those conversations that therapists and clients engage in as they deconstruct the perceived reality and develop a more viable worldview.

Languaging. Languaging, as used by Anderson and Goolishian (1988), refers to the process of conversation in which the meaning of a situation emerges. A system engaged in language, for example, can decide if Mary's behavior is a sign of genius or a sign of pathology.

Multiversa. Andersen (1991) uses this term to refer to the multitude of ideas that potentially exist. Systems become stuck when they limit the number of views they hold about a problem.

Objectification. Diagnoses categorize individuals by their labels. They become stable objects rather than developing beings. White (1995) separates the label from the individual to enhance the process of problem resolution.

Problem-determined system. Goolishian and Anderson (1987) use this term for those individuals who, through conversation, agree that a problem exists. This can be an individual, a family, a subsystem of the family, or a larger system. This system's dominant view serves to maintain the problem. The problem-determined system can also include the therapist.

Problem-organizing, problem-dis-solving system. Anderson and Goolishian (1988) use this term to describe the therapeutic system. This system is organized by the belief in a problem and dis-solves the problem through conversation. Dissolution of the problem also leads to dis-solving the therapeutic system.

Stuck system (also referred to as "standstill system"). The term "stuck system" is used by Tom Andersen (1991) to describe a client system that is unable to resolve its problem.

Subjugated story. White and Epston (1990) use this term to identify alternate stories of success, alternative options, or different ways of viewing a problem that are obscured by the dominant story. There are potentially an infinite number of subjugated stories to describe a situation. Some of them have the potential to be helpful, and some do not.

Unique outcome. "Unique outcomes" are those situations in the past when clients have resolved their problems but had not previously been aware that they had done so. In White and Epston's (1990) words, clients discover through narrative therapy that they have successfully withstood their "dominant story."

Visitor. This is the third type of therapist–client relationship identified by de Shazer (1991). A "visitor" client does not wish to be a part of therapy, does not have a complaint, and does not wish to work on anything. The therapist's role in this relationship is to engage in solution-focused conversation and simply compliment the client. The therapist hopes that this respectful stance will allow the relationship to move forward into a customer relationship or provide the freedom for the therapeutic relationship to end if there is no desire to move forward.

KEY CLINICAL SKILLS

Co-construction. "Co-construction" refers to the therapist and client jointly developing an alternate view of a situation. As they develop new meanings, clients also develop new ways of resolving their problems. This process differs from reframing (see Chapter 3), in that a co-constructed meaning is established jointly between therapist and client rather than being introduced by the therapist to bring about change.

Collaborative case notes. Narrative therapists (White, 1995) often collaboratively write their case notes with their clients to jointly construct the meaning of the session. Therapist ideas do not take precedence over those of the client. This blocks the therapist from objectifying the client through diagnosis and levels the discrepancy between therapist and client power.

Compliment. Compliments are used by solution-focused therapists (de Shazer, 1985) to establish a positive, hopeful atmosphere within the therapeutic relationship. The therapist's compliments are genuine and emerge during the process of the session.

Deconstruction. This refers to a global technique in which the therapist-client conversation diminishes the client's problem-maintaining, dominant view so that the client can recognize alternate views.

Externalization. White and Epston (1990) use externalization to separate the client from the symptom. Rather than viewing Johnny as depressed, they might discuss the times when depression takes control of Johnny. By externalizing the problem, the family stops viewing Johnny as existing in a stable state of depression. This enables him, and those around him, to discover times when he has fought off his depression.

Formula first-session task. Solution-focused therapists (de Shazer, 1985) use this end-of-session technique as a standard part of the first session. Clients are asked to think about what they *do not want to change* about their lives as a result of therapy. This focuses them on the strengths in their lives and begins the solution-generating process.

Landscape-of-action questions. White (1993) uses "landscape-of-action" questions to identify situations (unique outcomes) in his clients' past when they successfully withstood their problems. This is part of the process of deconstructing the client's dominant story.

Landscape-of-meaning questions. After White (1993) uses landscape-of-action questions to discover unique outcomes, he uses "landscape-of-meaning questions" to help clients begin seeing themselves differently. For example, after the therapist asks Johnny about the times he has fought off depression, the therapist might ask questions such as "How did you decide that you needed to take that first step to lessen the effects of depression?" "What does this say about you, that you successfully blocked the depression from taking control of you?"

More-of-the-same assignments. After an exception to a problem has been found, de Shazer (1985) instructs the client to practice this behavior at home. If Bill finds that his marriage goes better on days that he makes breakfast for Mary, the therapist would encourage him to make more breakfasts for her.

Miracle question. The miracle question asks clients to imagine how they would know that the problem was resolved if they woke up the next morning and it was gone. Solution-focused therapists (de Shazer, 1988) use the miracle question to help clients identify operational goals and potential solutions.

Not-knowing approach. Anderson and Goolishian (1992) discourage therapists from taking an expert stance (through using diagnoses or giving directives). They believe that therapist hypotheses tend to limit the ways a conversation may evolve and thus may limit potential solutions. In the "not-knowing approach," therapist join clients in a discovery of meanings and options in which any number of solutions may evolve from the therapeutic conversation.

Reflecting team. Developed by Tom Andersen (1987), the "reflecting team" is a process in which team members observe the therapy interview and then discuss their observations and thoughts in front of the therapist and clients. The therapist and family then discuss the team's conversation among themselves. This process enables clients to actively engage in both conversation and reflection about their situation.

Scaling questions. Solution-focused therapists use scaling questions to identify exceptions and to build a positive mind-set (de Shazer, 1988). Clients are asked, for example, on a scale of 1 to 10, how much they want to resolve this problem (1 being low and 10 being high), how bad the problem is, how much better the problem is, or why the problem is better at one time than another. These numbers are then used to construct a positive mind-set. For example, if a client says the problem is a 4, the therapist can ask questions about how the problem was a 4 and not a 1 or 2. The therapist can also ask what the client might do to move the problem from a 4 to a 5. Similarly, if a client responds that a problem was a 5 and is now a 7, the therapist can focus on how things have improved.

Therapeutic certificates. White and Epston (1990) have their clients create certificates to announce the resolution of their problems. Clients enhance their sense of accomplishment by showing these certificates to others and block relapses by viewing them when they feel themselves slipping.

Therapeutic letters. White and Epston (1990) write their clients therapeutic letters based on their sessions. They acknowledge unique outcomes and give life to their clients' subjugated stories of success or mastery over their problems and the oppressive dominant stories that keep their problems in place. This letter serves as a concrete reminder of the emerging subjugated story of personal success. It is much harder for clients to dismiss this new idea when it is in writing.

TEACHING TOOLS AND TECHNIQUES

Training Videotapes

Several excellent demonstration videotapes are available on social constructionist family therapies. Specific titles and places to obtain lists for purchase follow:

- *AAMFT Master Series,* AAMFT, 1133 15th Street, N.W., Suite 300, Washington, DC 20005-2710
- Brief Family Therapy Center, 13965 West Burleigh Road, Brookfield, WI, 53005
- Houston–Galveston Institute, 3316 Mount Vernon, Houston, TX 77006
- *Irreconcilable Differences* (Insoo Berg, therapist), W. W. Norton & Company, 500 Fifth Avenue, New York, NY 10110
- *I'd Hear Laughter* (Insoo Berg, therapist), W. W. Norton & Company, 500 Fifth Avenue, New York, NY 10110

Developing a Social Constructionist Classroom

Two major components in social constructionist theory are (1) the reduction of the hierarchy between therapist and client, and (2) the assumption that there is no such thing as an objective viewpoint. A social constructionist classroom embraces the concept of collaborative discovery. Although instructors may wish to incorporate only some of these suggestions, they are as follows:

1. Drop grading criteria. Either make the course pass–fail or agree to give every student an "A." This lessens the belief that the professor has a greater knowledge of what constitutes understanding of the material than the students and also lessens the power differential between professor and students.
2. Move to a discussion format rather than rely on lectures. The former encourages group interaction and a sharing of knowledge, whereas the latter reifies professor knowledge, diminishes student contribution and sense of

efficacy, and limits the number of ideas that are generated around the material.

3. Share in the creation of the syllabus by having students add favorite books and articles to the reading list.

4. Develop a seminar format that promotes joint leadership of the course. In each class, either the professor or a different student is in charge of the discussion. This promotes a shared ownership of the class and the materials covered (In fact, several of the techniques that follow were developed by students in this format.)

5. Develop a spirit of course evaluation in which students and professor are free to openly discuss the strengths and growth areas of the course in a group format.

Reflecting Papers

"Reflecting papers" are modeled after the reflecting team concept of Tom Andersen (1987). Rather than providing students with a specific topic for a process paper, Students are asked to write a two- or three-page paper based on their thoughts after completing the readings. These papers then become part, or all, of the assigned reading for the next class. Students come to the next class prepared to discuss their new thoughts after reading each other's papers. This exercise establishes the importance of individual students' ideas and raises their contributions for discussion.

Theory Question Grab Bag

This class activity, adapted from Maria Bermudez, is an enjoyable way to develop theoretical knowledge and promote class discussion. The instructor develops a list of questions based on the theory he or she is currently teaching. The instructor writes these questions on separate pieces of paper and places them in a bag. The instructor then passes the bag around the class, one student at a time. Each student takes a slip of paper and responds to the question written on the slip. After the student responds and the class discusses the student's answer, the bag is passed to the next student. Questions can be knowledge based, applied, or promote personal growth, depending on one's goals. The following sample questions are based on narrative therapy (White & Epston, 1990).

Do personal stories reflect a person's reality?

What is your position on externalizing the problem versus taking responsibility for it?

What do people do to organize their lived experience to give it meaning and make sense of their lives?

Are power and knowledge inseparable, as Foucault proclaims?

In your opinion, is externalizing a problem, finding unique outcomes, and rewriting personal narrative enough to bring about long-term change?

How could one do narrative therapy with a client who is illiterate? Would their stories be more or less powerful?

Which is more powerful, the written or spoken language?

Will you share with us your dominant story?

What is a lived experience of your own that falls outside of your dominant story?

Reflecting Team Role Plays

In this exercise, students conduct a clinical role play based on the reflecting team format (Andersen, 1987). Several students role-play a family while one classmate interviews them. The rest of the class observes the session, then discusses their hypotheses while the role-play family and therapist observe. The therapist then interviews the family on their thoughts following the team's discussion. The exercise ends with the whole class discussing their reflections on the overall process. Similarly, the instructor may wish to set up reflecting teams when he or she is showing videotapes of master therapists. At some point in the middle of the session, the instructor turns off the video and has the class, or the designated reflecting team, simulate a reflecting team conversation.

Writing Therapeutic Letters

This exercise, adapted from Mary Bartram and David Schmidt, is based on White and Epston's (1990) technique of writing letters to families to emphasize the new narrative generated in the previous session. Students are divided into groups of two or three and given the summary of a previous session. They are then assigned to develop a letter that elevates the family's alternative story. Students then present their letters in class. An example of a session summary follows.

Juanita, age 13, and her mother Maria came to family therapy, because Juanita had been arrested that weekend for shoplifting a large quantity of merchandise at a mall with her girlfriends. She was placed overnight in juvenile lockup and is now on house arrest. Additionally, in the past year Juanita had been in several fights at school, and her grades had slipped. Maria is concerned that her daughter is hanging out with the wrong crowd. The family is Hispanic and lives in a relatively dangerous area in Chicago. Maria reported that her husband (Juanita's father) is unsupportive of therapy, does not get along well with Juanita, and is unwilling to attend the sessions. Juanita wants to be a model and is currently "dude" crazy.

In the first session, Juanita and her mother educated the therapist about the conditions of house arrest. The conditions include not leaving the house without the mother and without informing the probation officer by phone, receiving no phone calls, going no farther than the front porch, and having no visits from friends. Failure to comply with house arrest would lead to Juanita again being placed in juvenile lockup. The therapist and family discussed how difficult it would be for Juanita to resist "cabin fever" and for her mother to help her to comply with the rules.

In the second session, the therapist learned that the house arrest had been relatively problem free. Maria, while at times irritated by the hassle, had held to her role of monitoring Juanita. Juanita had not acted out, despite her feeling that she "wanted to punch the wall." She spent most of her time in her room, thinking about how she could resist peer pressure.

Writing Therapeutic Certificates

White and Epston (1990) often use certificates to acknowledge successful alternative stories that have emerged in their clients' lives. This activity, adapted from Tom Carlson, involves asking students currently in practicum to think about a client family that is showing improvement and to develop a certificate for them. Students then present their certificate to the class and discuss how the family has improved. This also serves as a means of building student self-esteem, as they get to share their clinical success stories with their peers. With modern computer programs, instructors can easily create blank certificates to make the activity more fun.

Big Name in the Field (BNIF)

In this activity, students play the role of a well-known social constructionist therapist. For example, a student might be assigned to be Steve de Shazer (1985, 1988, 1991). The student reads several of the BNIF's books and articles and makes a presentation on his work for the class. The class then engages in a question–and–answer period in which the student responds as de Shazer might.

Constructing Different Meanings for Objects

This activity, adapted from Julie Hawley and Walter Lowe, is a good way to demonstrate how multiple meanings can be attached to individual phenomena. The instructor displays several objects, one at a time, and asks the class to write down their personal meaning for each object. Objects can include lipstick, baby diapers, a picture of a horse, a dollar bill, a picture of a teenager, or anything else the instructor wishes. Then the instructor goes around the room and has the students share their responses to each object. Students are often surprised at the different meanings their classmates have given to objects that they believed had universal meaning.

RESEARCH ISSUES

Relatively little research exists on social constructionist family therapies. Many social constructionists have eschewed research, because they believe it supports the illusion of an objective reality. They fear that "objective research" marginalizes alternative ideas and limits creative growth. Although these are legitimate concerns, ethical responsibility requires that we develop means of assessing the theories and techniques we use with clients. Furthermore, many of the ideas espoused by social constructionists lend themselves quite well to both quantitative and qualitative inquiry. The following are some ideas for future research:

- How effective are social constructionist therapies at posttest and follow-up? What outcomes are most affected?
- How do social constructionist therapies compare to more directive therapies in terms of outcome?
- What do client families who engage in successful social constructionist therapy believe are the important components of their treatment?
- Anderson and Goolishian (1988) and White (1995) believe that social constructionist therapies empower families more than the more positivist directive therapies. How do families in social constructionist therapies experience personal empowerment and efficacy compared to those families receiving more directive therapies?
- A major concept in social constructionist therapies is the lessening of hierarchy between therapist and client (Andersen, 1991; Anderson & Goolishian, 1988; White, 1995). Is the perceived degree of therapist hierarchy related to client outcome?
- Do clients engaged in Andersen's (1987) open reflecting team process have different experiences than those clients involved in the more closed Milan team format (Selvini Palazzoli et al., 1980)?
- How do reflecting teams compare to the Milan team in terms of therapeutic outcome?
- Are social constructionist family therapies more effectively utilized on a short-term or long-term basis?
- Although solution-focused and narrative therapies share many similarities, a major difference is the problem focus of de Shazer (1985, 1991) versus altering personal stories by White and Epston (1990). Are there differences in outcome and clients' feelings of personal empowerment and efficacy in a problem-focused versus personal narrative-focused therapy?

KEY BOOKS, CHAPTERS, AND ARTICLES

Andersen, T. (1987). The reflecting team: Dialogue and meta-dialogue in clinical work. *Family Process, 26,* 415–428.

This is the key article that started the move toward using reflecting teams. This article describes the use and underlying theory of the reflecting team.

Andersen, T. (Ed.). (1991). *The reflecting team: Dialogues and dialogues about the dialogues.* New York: Norton.

The first five chapters of this book are written by Tom Andersen, with the remaining three written by other practitioners of this method. It provides theoretical discussion of the role of conversation and reflection in therapy, as well as the pragmatics of using the reflecting team.

Anderson, H., & Goolishian, H. A. (1988). Human systems as linguistic systems: Preliminary and evolving ideas about the implications for clinical theory. *Family Process, 27,* 371–393.

Anderson and Goolishian have had a major impact on social constructionist thinking around the world. This article is possibly their key achievement. It is their most thorough presentation of human systems as linguistic systems and is must reading for those interested in understanding social constructionist therapy.

Anderson, H., Goolishian, H. A., & Windermand, L. (1986). Problem determined systems: Towards transformation in family therapy. *Journal of Strategic and Systemic Therapies, 5*(4), 1–13.

This powerful article presents the key premises of Anderson and Goolishian's collaborative language approach. It challenges the traditional view of social structure that underlies psychotherapy theory. The authors support a move away from seeing families in therapy to working with the problem–determined system.

Berg, I. K. (1993). *Family based services: A solution-focused approach.* New York: Norton.

Whereas de Shazer has focused on the theoretical concepts in solution-focused therapy, Berg has dealt primarily with clinical issues. This book applies the solution-focused format to cases involving child welfare and family service specialists. It is an important and useful book for those working in the welfare system.

de Shazer, S. (1985). *Keys to solution in brief therapy.* New York: Norton.

This important book presents the key ideas of solution-focused therapy. It challenges the need to diagnose or even understand the problem to promote change. It presents the solution-focused model, several solution-focused tasks, and good case studies.

de Shazer, S. (1988). *Clues: Investigating solutions in brief therapy.* New York: Norton.

This fascinating book describes the process of solution-focused therapy. Through observing several proponents of solution-focused therapy and developing a computer program based on their behavior, de Shazer distills the commonalities within this approach. This book succeeds in presenting the various types of therapy situations and subsequent therapist responses that comprise solution-focused therapy.

de Shazer, S. (1991). *Putting difference to work*. New York: Norton.

Prior to this book, solution-focused therapy was often placed in the strategic therapy camp. Here de Shazer explains the social constructionist underpinnings of his approach through Wittgenstein's "language games." This is a crucial book for those wishing to understand solution-focused therapy.

de Shazer, S. (1994). *Words were originally magic*. New York: Norton.

This delightful book expands on the ideas presented in *Putting Difference to Work*. It challenges the structuralist beliefs in an objective reality and the ability to determine deeper levels of meaning in behavior.

de Shazer, S., & Berg, I. K. (1992). Doing therapy: A post-structural re-vision. *Journal of Marital and Family Therapy, 18,* 71–81.

de Shazer and Berg make their definitive statement that solution-focused therapy is a social constructionist model. Based on Wittgenstein's "language games," they challenge the structuralist models of doing therapy. They use a single-session example to exemplify their stance.

de Shazer, S., Berg, I. K., Lipchik, E., Nunnally, E., Molnar, A., Gingerich, W., & Weiner-Davis, M. (1986). *Brief therapy: Focused solution development, 25,* 207–221.

This pioneering article presents the key assumptions of solution-focused therapy. It challenges the concept of problems being maintained by interactional sequences and presents the idea of helping clients find exceptions to their problems and do more of the same.

Durrant, M. (1993). *Residential treatment: A cooperative, competency-based approach to therapy and program design.* New York: Norton.

Australian psychologist, Michael Durrant, presents a solution-focused approach to residential treatment. Durrant gently pushes those who work in these settings to focus on enhancing patient strengths rather than promoting the unit program at the expense of patient development.

Durrant, M. (1995). *Creative strategies for school problems: Solutions for psychologists and teachers.* New York: Norton.

This practical, how-to book takes a solution-focused approach to school problems. It is relevant to family therapists, teachers, and school counselors. Durrant includes particularly good case examples.

Efran, J. S., Lukens, M. D., & Lukens, R. J. (1990). *Language, structure, and change: Frameworks for meaning in psychotherapy.* New York: Norton.

This excellent book is one of the few in the field to apply Maturanan constructivism to therapy. This theoretically sound volume discusses constructivist thought in relation to living our lives, client symptomatology, ethical responsibility in relationships, and conducting therapy. The authors deserve high praise for their ability to present many of Maturana's difficult ideas in an easily understandable manner.

Epston, D., & White, M. (1992). *Experience, contradiction, narrative and imagination: Selected papers of David Epston and Michael White 1989–1991.* Adelaide, South Australia: Dulwich Centre Publications.

This collection of Epston and White's papers is especially noteworthy for David Epston's case studies. The book showcases the clinical aspect of their model and provides a study of 45 cases of childhood stealing that assess the effectiveness of the narrative approach.

Friedman, S. (Ed.). (1993). *The new language of change: Constructive collaboration in psychotherapy.* New York: Guilford Press.

This edited volume is especially noteworthy for providing a clinical focus to a largely theoretical domain. Each chapter, by a leading proponent of the social constructionist movement, contains a brief theory presentation, a verbatim case example, and a question and answer section between the editor and the author over the theory and its application.

Friedman, S. (Ed.). (1995). *The reflecting team in action: Collaborative practice in family therapy.* New York: Guilford Press.

The idea of the reflecting team has had phenomenal growth since Tom Andersen's (1987) original article. This edited volume presents a variety of different uses for the approach, as well as its application to different treatment populations.

Gilligan, S., & Price, R. (Eds.). (1993). *Therapeutic conversations.* New York: Norton.

This book presents the papers presented at the 1990 Tulsa Conference on Therapeutic Conversations. Several current ideas are discussed. This book has the added bonus of a different conference participant providing a commentary on each paper.

Goolishian, H., & Anderson, H. (1987). Language systems and therapy: An evolving idea. *Psychotherapy, 24,* 529–538.

In this article, Goolishian and Anderson focus on the concept of human systems as engaged in language rather than based on social organization. The authors proclaim that the systems view of families has failed and offer the language system model as an alternative.

Hoffman, L. (1990). Constructing realities: An art of lenses. *Family Process, 29,* 1–12.

Lynn Hoffman is one of the foremost teachers of family therapy. This excellent article describes her movement away from the systems model of family therapy to one based on social constructionism and gender. In the process, she beautifully describes the differences and implications of these approaches. This is a good first article for those wanting to understand the ideas inherent in the social constructionist movement.

Hoffman, L. (1991). A reflexive stance for family therapy. *Journal of Strategic and Systemic Therapies, 10*(3–4), 4–17.

In this provocative article, Hoffman shows how postmodern thought challenges the accepted assumptions of the mental health profession. She also shows how maintaining a systems metaphor distances family therapists from their clients. She proposes a collaborative partnership as an alternative.

McNamee, S., & Gergen, K. J. (Eds.). (1992). *Therapy as social construction.* Newbury Park, CA: Sage.

Kenneth Gergen has had a strong influence on the social constructionist movement in family therapy. In this edited volume, he and Sheila McNamee present a series of excellent essays by people such as Lynn Hoffman, Anderson and Goolishian, Tom Andersen, Epston and White, William O'Hanlon, and Gianfranco Cecchin. We recommend this collection.

Parry, A., & Doan, R. E. (1994). *Story Re-Visions: Narrative therapy in the postmodern world.* New York: Guilford Press.

This is an excellent source for those wishing to deepen their understanding of narrative therapy. It is a theoretically strong book that places narrative therapy in the context of a changing, postmodern world. The book also provides unique clinical techniques and strong case examples.

Real, T. (1990). The therapeutic use of self in constructionist systemic therapy. *Family Process, 29,* 255–272.

The author traces the steps from strategic to constructionist family therapy. Five stances are presented for how therapists position themselves when conducting constructionist therapy. This is a good article for understanding how therapists practice constructionist therapy.

Walter, J., & Peller, J. (1992). *Becoming solution-focused in brief therapy.* New York: Brunner/Mazel.

This may be one of the best books available for learning solution-focused therapy. Although not breaking any theoretically new ground, it is a book that trainees will appreciate as they struggle with the nuances of this approach.

White, M. (1986). Negative explanation, restraint, and double description: A template for family therapy. *Family Process, 25,* 169–184.

This foundational article was written prior to the influence of Foucault on White's work; however, the core of many of White's ideas can still be found here. White discusses the limitations of systems in recognizing alternative options and how therapy leads to the discovery of new solutions. He also discusses the need for families to discuss the relative influence of the problem on their lives and their relative influence over the problem.

White, M. (1995). *Re-authoring lives: Interviews and essays.* Adelaide, South Australia: Dulwich Centre Publications.

Michael White's ideas continue to change as the years progress. He expands on his views on the politics of traditional therapy and diagnosis and promotes narrative therapy as a possible alternative to the objectification and marginalization of clients. In this book, White includes provocative ideas on the treatment of abuse, the use of reflecting teams, using clients as consultants, and the comparison of the systems metaphor to the narrative metaphor.

White, M., & Epston, D. (1990). *Narrative means to therapeutic ends.* New York: Norton.

This important book presents the core assumptions of the narrative approach. The theoretical influences of Michel Foucault abound as the authors discuss how a positivist orientation encourages individuals to comply with their own subjugation. They explain the use of externalization to separate individuals from their problems and encourage the discovery of unique outcomes to rewrite their personal narrative. The book is also noteworthy for its extensive discussion and examples of therapeutic letters and documents.

REFERENCES

Andersen, T. (1987). The reflecting team: Dialogue and meta-dialogue in clinical work. *Family Process, 26,* 415–428.

Andersen, T. (Ed.). (1991). *The reflecting team: Dialogues and dialogues about the dialogues.* New York: Norton.

Andersen, T. (1992). Relationship, language and pre-understanding in the reflecting process. *Australian and New Zealand Journal of Family Therapy, 13,* 87–91.

Andersen, T. (1993). See and hear, and be seen and heard. In S. Friedman (Ed.), *The new language of change: Constructive collaboration in psychotherapy.* New York: Guilford Press.

Andersen, T. (1995). Reflecting processes; acts of informing and forming: You can borrow my eyes, but you must not take them away from me! In S. Friedman (Ed.), *The reflecting team in action: Collaborative practice in family therapy.* New York: Guilford Press.

Anderson, H. (1993). On a roller coaster: A collaborative language systems approach to therapy. In S. Friedman (Ed.), *The new language of change: Constructive collaboration in psychotherapy.* New York: Guilford Press.

Anderson, H., & Goolishian, H. A. (1988). Human systems as linguistic systems: Preliminary and evolving ideas about the implications for clinical theory. *Family Process, 27,* 371–393.

Anderson, H., & Goolishian, H. A. (1992). The client is the expert: A not-knowing approach to therapy. In S. McNamee & K. J. Gergen (Eds.), *Therapy as social construction.* Newbury Park, CA: Sage.

Anderson, H., Goolishian, H. A., & Windermand, L. (1986). Problem determined systems: Towards transformation in family therapy. *Journal of Strategic and Systemic Therapies, 5*(4), 1–13.

Bateson, G. (1972). *Steps to an ecology of mind.* New York: Ballantine.

Bateson, G. (1979). *Mind and nature.* New York: Bantam.

Berg, I. K. (1993). *Family-based services: A solution-focused approach.* New York: Norton.

Berg, I. K., & Miller, S. D. (1992). *Working with the problem drinker: A solution-focused approach.* New York: Norton.

Bruner, J. (1986). *Actual minds, possible worlds.* Cambridge, MA: Harvard University Press.

Carter, B., & McGoldrick, M. (Eds.). (1988). *The changing family life cycle: A framework for family therapy* (2nd ed.). New York: Gardner.

de Shazer, S. (1984). The death of resistance. *Family Process, 23,* 11–21.

de Shazer, S. (1985). *Keys to solution in brief therapy.* New York: Norton.

de Shazer, S. (1988). *Clues: Investigating solutions in brief therapy.* New York: Norton.

de Shazer, S. (1991). *Putting difference to work.* New York: Norton.

de Shazer, S. (1994). *Words were originally magic.* New York: Norton.

de Shazer, S., & Berg, I. K. (1992). Doing therapy: A post-structural re-vision. *Journal of Marital and Family Therapy, 18,* 71–81.

de Shazer, S., Berg, I. K., Lipchik, E., Nunnally, E., Molnar, A., Gingerich, W., & Weiner-Davis, M. (1986). Brief therapy: Focused solution development. *Family Process, 25,* 207–221.

Durrant, M. (1993). *Residential treatment: A cooperative, competency-based approach to therapy and program design.* New York: Norton.

Durrant, M. (1995). *Creative strategies for school problems: Solutions for psychologists and teachers.* New York: Norton.

Erickson, M. (1954). Pseudo-orientation in time as a hypnotic procedure. *Journal of Clinical and Experimental Hypnosis, 2,* 261–283.

Epston, D., & White, M. (1992). *Experience, contradiction, narrative, and imagination.* Adelaide, South Australia: Dulwich Centre Publications.

Epston, D., White, M., & "Ben." (1995). Consulting your consultants: A means to the co-construction of alternative knowledges. In S. Friedman (Ed.), *The reflecting team in action: Collaborative practice in family therapy.* New York: Guilford Press.

Epston, D., White, M., & Murray, K. (1992). A proposal for re-authoring therapy: Rose's revisioning of her life and a commentary. In S. McNamee & K. J. Gergen (Eds.), *Therapy as social construction.* Newbury Park, CA: Sage.

Foucault, M. (1965). *Madness and civilization: A history of insanity in the age of reason.* New York: Random House.

Foucault, M. (1980). *Power/knowledge: Selected interviews and other writings.* New York: Pantheon Books.

Friedman, S. (Ed.). (1995). *The reflecting team in action: Collaborative practice in family therapy.* New York: Guilford Press.

Geertz, C. (1983). *Local knowledge: Further essays in interpretive anthropology.* New York: Basic Books.

Gergen, K. J. (1982). *Toward transformation in social knowledge.* New York: Springer-Verlag.

Goolishian, H. A., & Anderson, H. (1987). Language systems and therapy: An evolving idea. *Psychotherapy, 24,* 529–538.

Hoffman, L. (1990). Constructing realities: An art of lenses. *Family Process, 29,* 1–12.

Hoffman, L. (1991). A reflexive stance for family therapy. *Journal of Strategic and Systemic Therapies, 10*(3–4), 4–17.

Kelly, G. A. (1963). *A theory of personality: The psychology of personal constructs.* New York: Norton.

Maturana, H. R., & Varela, F. J. (Eds.). (1980). *Autopoiesis and cognition: The realization of the living.* Boston: Reidel.

Maturana, H. R., & Varela, F. J. (1987). *The tree of knowledge: The biological roots of human understanding.* Boston: Shambhala.

Parry, A., & Doan, R.E. (1994). *Story Re-Visions: Narrative therapy in the postmodern world.* New York: Guilford Press.

Piaget, J. (1952). *The origins of intelligence in children.* New York: Norton.

Sells, S. P., Smith, T. E., Coe, M. J., Yoshioka, M., & Robbins, J. (1994). An ethnography of couple and therapist experiences in reflecting team practice. *Journal of Marital and Family Therapy, 20,* 247–266.

Selvini Palazzoli, M., Boscolo, L., Cecchin, G., & Prata, G. (1980). Hypothesizing–circularity–neutrality: Three guidelines for the conductor of the session. *Family Process, 19,* 3–12.

Smith, T. E., Sells, S. P., & Clevenger, T. (1994). Ethnographic content analysis of couple and therapist perceptions in a reflecting team setting. *Journal of Marital and Family Therapy, 20,* 267–286.

von Foerster, H. (1981). *Observing systems.* Seaside, CA: Intersystems.

White, M. (1986). Negative explanation, restraint, and double description: A template for family therapy. *Family Process, 25,* 169–184.

White, M. (1993). Deconstruction and therapy. In S. Gilligan & R. Price (Eds.), *Therapeutic conversations.* New York: Norton.

White, M. (1995). *Re-authoring lives: Interviews and essays.* Adelaide, South Australia: Dulwich Centre Publications.

White, M., & Epston, D. (1990). *Narrative means to therapeutic ends.* New York: Norton.

Wittgenstein, L. (1958). *The blue and brown books.* New York: Harper & Row.

Wittgenstein, L. (1968). *Culture and value.* Chicago: University of Chicago Press.

7

Sex Therapy

JAMES E. BURG
DOUGLAS H. SPRENKLE

P_{RIOR} TO 1970, people with sexual concerns relied primarily on folk cures or saw psychodynamically oriented therapists who offered long-term insight-oriented treatment with questionable results (Heiman, LoPiccolo, & LoPiccolo, 1981). Over the past century, the field of sex therapy has changed from primarily psychodynamic to cognitive-behavioral, and currently several authors are applying systemic–relational models of therapy.

The scope of sex-related issues is quite broad. This chapter will focus primarily on the development and status of sex therapy for sexual dysfunctions with individuals and heterosexual couples. The use of the term "dysfunction" in this chapter is for literary consistency, since the field of sex therapy has only recently begun to examine the role of culture in the expectations and definitions of sexual behavior. Several areas related to sex therapy are not covered in this chapter, such as sexual abuse (see Chapter 12), compulsive sexual behavior (Coleman, 1995), and counseling same-sex couples (Carl, 1990; Gonsiorek, 1982; Nichols, 1989).

EARLY PIONEERS

The current field of sex therapy owes a considerable intellectual debt to its pioneers. Sex therapy is generally considered to have come of age with the publication of Masters and Johnson's *Human Sexual Inadequacy* in 1970. Although certainly not the first work in this area, it did a great deal to establish the legitimacy of this form of intervention and helped spur the rapid growth of a variety of sex clinics and programs (Annon, 1975, 1976; Fisher & Gochros, 1977; Hartman & Fithian, 1972; Kaplan, 1974, 1979; Maddock, 1976).

Masters and Johnson's behavioral–learning–cognitive approach was predated by the application of systematic desensitization to sexual problems (Wolpe, 1958), assertiveness training (Lazarus, 1965), and cognitive restructuring (Ellis, 1962). LoPiccolo (1978) has written about the "quiet revolution in American psychotherapy," beginning in the late 1950s, which emphasized short-term techniques based on learning theory and present-centered direct retraining of behavior. Two earlier sex therapists deserve special note: James Semans developed an effective, direct behavioral method for the treatment of premature ejaculation in the mid-1950s (Semans, 1956), and Donald Hastings (1963) described programs to retrain couples to function better sexually, such as using direct clitoral stimulation for female anorgasmia (Heiman et al., 1981). The monumental sex research of Alfred Kinsey (Kinsey, Pomeroy, & Martin, 1948; Kinsey, Pomeroy, Martin, & Gebhard, 1953) also created a climate in which Masters and Johnson's work could be carried out and accepted. Kinsey and his University of Indiana associates also observed male and female responses in the laboratory during coitus and masturbation, even though they remained much more circumspect than Masters and Johnson concerning how such data were obtained.

MASTERS AND JOHNSON

Although not totally original, Masters and Johnson's work has nonetheless been monumental. Their contributions include the following:

1. The duo's clinical work was based upon the previous laboratory observation of the sexual response of 694 individuals, including 75 married couples. In *Human Sexual Response* (1966), they delineated four phases of sexual response (excitement, plateau, orgasm, and resolution) and clarified the parallel nature of male and female response by describing the analogous changes in each sex in each phase. The understanding of female sexuality was also enhanced by their attention to the multiorgasmic capacity of many women, and especially by their refutation of the physiological distinction between vaginal and clitoral orgasms (Freud asserted that a mark of female maturity was having vaginal, as opposed to the more infantile clitoral orgasms). This finding relieved women of the stigma of the labels of "immature" or "inadequate" because they were not able to have orgasms through vaginal intercourse alone. Another myth that was exploded in this

work is the alleged importance of having a large penis for female sexual pleasure.

2. Masters and Johnson stressed the importance of learning, both in the etiology and the remediation of dysfunction. They established how the ordinary processes of socialization (upbringing, role models, experiences, information–misinformation), and not just neurotic conflict, contributed substantially to an individual's capacity to perform in a sexual situation. They also showed that simple information (e.g., direct clitoral stimulation may be necessary) and the relearning that is the by-product of new experiences (e.g., sensate focus exercises) are often curative.

3. Masters and Johnson demonstrated that direct behavioral techniques can often be effective even in the absence of much attention to etiology or "underlying causes." For example, their treatment for premature ejaculation, the "squeeze technique," proved to be generally effective in brief, present-centered, problem-focused treatment.

4. Masters and Johnson also emphasized the role of anxiety in dysfunction and demonstrated that anxiety need not be related to remote or historical causes of dysfunctions. Simple "performance anxiety," which leads to "spectatoring" (anxiously watching one's own sexual performance), may be a significant contributing factor (performance anxiety can also be a by-product of dysfunction). The development of their sensate focus program (to be described) did a great deal to provide couples with an atmosphere in which performance demands were minimized.

5. Finally, Masters and Johnson stressed the systemic nature of dysfunction and emphasized that there is no such thing as an uninvolved party. For this reason, they stressed conjoint treatment, and for a time, they utilized surrogate sex partners when a patient was not in an ongoing relationship. While the relational component of dysfunction is something generally accepted today, it was quite innovative when it was introduced. Masters and Johnson were able to grasp, in a profoundly humane way, the interpersonal and emotional components of sexual interaction and capitalized on this in their treatment approaches. Their use of a dual sex therapy team and their emphasis on a couple's interaction helped to defocus the identified patient and to diminish the emphasis on blame.

Like all clinical research, Masters and Johnson's work received criticism. Zilbergeld and Evans (1980) vigorously attacked the methodological "inadequacy" of Masters and Johnson's *Human Sexual Inadequacy*. The interest of critics was piqued when they began to notice that other therapists did not seem to get results as good as those claimed by the St. Louis researchers. They also asserted that Masters and Johnson withheld, or presented in unclear ways, important information on their patient population, as well as on the criteria and measures used to assess treatment effects initially and at follow-up.

Kolodny (1981), the training director at the Masters and Johnson Institute, offered a defense in which he documented that few cases were screened out. He also operationalized treatment "failure" in a more careful way than was done in *Human Sexual Inadequacy*. In addition, Kolodny presented new data that supported the outcome claims of the basic volume. Kolodny also argued that unless other researchers went to the expense of truly replicating Masters and Johnson's procedures (e.g., dual-gender teams, intensive residential experience), they should not so readily criticize the St. Louis outcomes.

HELEN SINGER KAPLAN

Following Masters and Johnson, the next "giant" in the field was Helen Singer Kaplan. Her work can be seen in part as an answer to the question "What is sex therapy and how is it different from and similar to other forms of therapy?" Kaplan argued that sex therapy cannot be reduced to a series of techniques to be practiced by persons untrained in intrapsychic or interpersonal dynamics. On the other hand, she also rejected the notion that these dynamics must necessarily play a role in progress or cure.

Rejecting strict behavioral and psychodynamic orientations, Kaplan integrated these approaches, along with an emphasis on interpersonal processes, into what she called "psychosexual therapy." Like most behaviorists, she was concerned with symptomatic relief and used sexual and communication tasks as an integral part of treatment; however, in many cases she believed that the use of these methods alone would not produce adequate results.

Kaplan conceptualized several dysfunctions as psychosomatic (excluding those with an organic cause) problems. She proposed that at one level they were caused by a single factor—anxiety. This anxiety might be due to causes that were immediate or remote, mild or serious, intrapsychic or interpersonal. She called this the concept of "multicausal levels."

In treating a dysfunction, she felt it was necessary to attack the "specific immediate cause," which is similar for most individuals with the same dysfunction. Premature ejaculators, for example, regardless of whatever else may have caused their problem, experienced high anxiety during times of intense sexual arousal and suppress or repress their erotic sensations, which are sufficient cues to control ejaculation. Premature ejaculators could be taught to control anxiety through methods such as the "stop–start" procedure (see "Key Concepts" section).

What varied was the extent to which there were other causes and whether addressing these causes was necessary. Certain dysfunctions (especially desire disorders) generally had more serious and remote causes, and Kaplan believed that success was unlikely unless these causes were uncovered through longer term insight-oriented therapy. Mild anxieties, such as performance anxiety, overconcern for the partner, and anxieties related to unrealistic expectations could typically be dealt with through standard sex therapy procedures. Midlevel anxieties included success and pleasure anxieties, and fears of intimacy and commitment, all of which were less amenable to simple behavioral interventions. The most serious causes included hostile and neurotic relationship patterns, as well as "Oedipal" conflicts. These were unconscious and deeply threatening, and were not responsive to nonpsychodynamic sex therapy.

Kaplan's focus in therapy was on what was necessary to obtain relief for the presenting problem. Following initial assessment (a client's responses to interventions are a part of ongoing assessment), she introduced behavioristic interventions such as sensate focus. As sessions progressed, she helped clients to have an awareness of the immediate cause of the problem and of relationship patterns that affected or were influenced by the problem. To the extent she deemed necessary, or the clients requested it, she explored more serious or remote causes. Her techniques were an eclectic blend of Masters-and-Johnson-type strategies, family systems interventions, miscellaneous behavioral prescriptions, and psychodynamic psychotherapy. Unlike Masters and Johnson, she believed that a single therapist could work effectively with sexual dysfunctions on an outpatient basis.

Kaplan's other major contributions include the following:

1. She developed a triphasic concept of sexual response (Kaplan, 1979), which supplanted her earlier biphasic concept of "excitement" and "orgasm." She added the "desire" phase in response to the numbers of persons presenting with desire problems and nonresponsiveness to treatment.

2. Her concern with disorders of desire generated two significant books on this theme (Kaplan, 1979, 1995a).

3. Kaplan alerted the therapeutic community to the problem of phobic avoidance of sex, which could be distinct from disorders of desire, excitement, or orgasm (there might be nothing wrong with the client's sexual response). She demonstrated that if panic accompanied the phobia, 80–85% of such patients would improve if antipanic medication was included in the treatment (Kaplan, 1983).

4. She developed a systematic plan for assessment and evaluation (Kaplan, 1983) and gave special attention to the organic basis of many disorders. Although at one time it was believed that 95% of all sexual disorders had a psychological base, Kaplan believed that estimation was too high. For clients over the age of 40, illness and drugs must be ruled out, especially for those disorders that carry a high risk of organicity (Kaplan, 1983). In support of Kaplan's ideas, Rosen and Leiblum (1995) have noted the trend toward the "medicalization" of sex therapy. Much has been written about surgical, mechanical, or medical treatments for erectile

disorder, as well as pharmacological treatments for desire disorders and premature ejaculation.

RELATIONAL AND SYSTEMIC FOCUSES

As the field has moved toward relational or systemic ideas, there has been criticism for placing an undue emphasis on the physiological component of sexual response. Kinsey, for example, used female orgasm as the primary indicator of female sexual satisfaction. Masters and Johnson's response cycle was composed of physiological stages, and they tended to emphasize physical intensity of orgasm at the expense of more qualitative indices.

Since the 1980s there has been a shift from narrow notions of performance to broader models that emphasize psychological and experiential components. Early examples of this shift are reflected in the emphasis on cognitive models of sexual functioning (Ellis, 1980; Lazarus, 1980; Walen, 1980) and in the attention to attribution in sexual experience. Examples of the latter include Zilbergeld's (1980) attention to the role of labeling and relabeling of internal experience as a curative factor in treatment. Another important indicator of the shift is reflected by sex therapy researchers' concern for qualitative dependent variables in outcome research (Levine, 1980), such as a person's ability to enjoy sex and a couple's ability to enjoy sex together.

Masters and Johnson and Kaplan gave serious attention to interpersonal factors in the etiology and treatment of dysfunction. More recently, authors have taken a more radically ecosystemic view by developing models that give proportionately less attention to intrapsychic and personal-history variables and more emphasis to the role of one's current relationship contexts. Early examples of relation ideas include Regas and Sprenkle's (1983) discussion of how "inhibited sexual desire" (hypoactive sexual desire) often serves important functions in the current relationship context, and Fish, Fish, and Sprenkle's (1984) utilization of structural family therapy with inhibited sexual desire.

Atwood and Dershowitz (1992) discuss therapy through social constructionism theory, explaining how sexual-meaning systems and scripts can be used in an integrated model of marital and sexual therapy. Other models of relational and systemic approaches to sexual dysfunctions are offered in the edited works by Leiblum and Rosen (1989), Rosen and Leiblum (1995), and Weeks and Hof (1987).

Schnarch's (1991) "Sexual Crucible" provides a good example of a systemic conceptual framework that stands in contrast to the behavioristic and biological models. The "Crucible" model does not focus on the resolution of symptomatology or use cognitive-behavioral interventions. Instead, this model focuses on sexual potential and intimacy. The theoretical model is based on an integration of object relations and Bowenian theories. The therapeutic process is designed to resolve past personal or relational issues by increasing the individual's level of differentiation.

There has also been considerable attention recently given to working with couples with a partner who has been sexually abused. As with most sexual difficulties, these call for sensitive attention to the complex interplay of individual, relational, and larger system dynamics (see Chapter 12, this book; Maddock & Larson, 1995; Trepper & Barrett, 1989).

OTHER DEVELOPMENTS IN SEX THERAPY

Biological/Medical Perspectives

Although the field of sex therapy appears to moving toward an integration of biological, psychological, and relational perspectives, much of the research and writing is still compartmentalized by the different fields. One medical area that is showing positive results is the pharmacology of sexual dysfunctions. For example, the introduction of selective serotonergic reuptake inhibitors (SSRIs) in the treatment of depression have been associated with sexually related side effects (Jacobsen, 1992; Patterson, 1993). In the case of Prozac (fluoxetine), it tends to retard ejaculation and is being used as a treatment for premature ejaculation (Kaplan, 1994). Significant advances have also been made in the use of intracavernosal injections for treating erectile disorder (Eid & Pearce, 1993; Wagner & Kaplan, 1993).

There have also been important developments in the area of chronic illness and other organic causes of sexual dysfunction. Schover and Jensen (1988) provide an excellent book on working with chronically ill clients.

The Feminist Challenge

The feminist challenge to traditional sex therapy has provided the field with a larger perspective on sexual relationships (Nichols, 1995). One of the major criticisms has been the field's use of a universal sexual response cycle (e.g., desire, excitement, orgasm, and resolution) in classification and diagnosis (Tavris, 1992). The biologically (genital) based sexual response cycle has been applied universally to both sexes. Tiefer (1995) noted that this definition of healthy sexuality has focused on orgasm and has not reflected the importance of emotions, relationships, and contextual issues.

Tiefer (1995) has challenged Masters and Johnson's work as biased in several areas and suggests it does not make sense that the sexual response cycle has been held as the norm for everyone; however, Masters and Johnson's research findings have been applied by sexologists as the basis for what is "normal" sexual activity (Tiefer, 1995). Sex is more than a function of body parts, yet the DSM-IV focuses primarily on genital dysfunctions;

thus, sexual behaviors that could have been considered a satisfying sexual experience have been labeled as foreplay and discounted as only preparatory to the "real" sexual act of intercourse (Nichols, 1989).

The concept of sexual desire has also been a focus in feminist writing. The existence of hypoactive sexual desire is an example of social bias in the DSM-IV. There is an assumption that all people must experience sexual desire to be "normal" (Tiefer, 1995). This is further supported, in that there is not a diagnosis for hyperactive sexual desire. For many clients, the most beneficial route may not be through resolving the physical or desire "dysfunction" but to assist them in discovering their own understanding of sexual pleasure and of relationships (Nichols, 1995). The feminist critique challenges clinicians to move toward definitions of healthy sexual relationships that incorporate spiritual connection and sensual touch instead of a definition based on genitals and orgasm (Nichols, 1995; Tavris, 1992; Tiefer, 1995).

Self-Help Procedures

Couples sometimes turn to books and popular magazines for sexual advice and counsel. The phenomenal success of Alex Comfort's (1972) original *The Joy of Sex* and the sexual and marital "aids" industry (offering a smorgasbord of products through glossy catalogues and even boutiques in the local mall) attest to the continuing demand for such material. Reputable and noted sex therapists have produced materials designed to be used with limited therapeutic assistance. Examples include sexual growth programs for women (Heiman & LoPiccolo, 1988), help for impotence (Goldstein & Rothstein, 1990), and treatment for premature ejaculation (Kaplan, 1989). Althof and Kingsberg (1992) provide a listing of books clinicians have found helpful to clients with sexual problems. The degree to which people comply with these programs and reports of their efficacy are, with few exceptions, largely unknown.

Group Therapy

The group therapy format has been used successfully to treat a variety of dysfunctions for quite some time (Zilbergeld, 1980). Metz and Weiss (1992) offer an example of combining the treatment of marital and sexual dysfunctions in a group format. For both financial and therapeutic reasons, therapists and researchers are beginning to reevaluate the utility of group formats.

Assessment Instruments

Assessment has been done through direct observation of sexual behavior and clinical history taking (see "sex history" in the "Key Clinical Skills" section), or through assessment instruments, predominantly of the paper-and-pencil variety. The development of empirically reliable and valid instruments has been part of the trend (to be discussed) to emphasize accountability through research. Ideally, measures should assess change from multiple perspectives (client, therapist, partner). Instruments should also address both the presenting sexual problem and individual and the couple's more general functioning and satisfaction. Among paper-and-pencil instruments, the Marital Satisfaction Inventory (Snyder, 1981) and Prepare–Enrich (Olson, 1982) are examples of general marital instruments that have sexual satisfaction subscales. Among the instruments that specifically target sexual functioning are the Sexual Interaction Inventory (LoPiccolo & Steger, 1974), which focuses on 17 specific activities and asks each partner questions about frequency and enjoyment, as well as perceptions of their partner's responses to these activities, and the Derogatis Sexual Functioning Inventory (Derogatis & Melisaratos, 1979), a 245-item questionnaire that measures individual functioning in the areas of information, experience, drive, attitudes, symptoms, affect, gender-role definition, fantasy, body image, and satisfaction. The reader may also find valuable a compendium of instruments used in the assessment of sexual function and marital interaction found in Schiavi, Derogatis, Kuriansky, O'Connor, and Sharpe (1979). Other valuable resources include the books of instruments by Fischer and Corcoran (1994) and Talmadge and Talmadge's (1990) review of sexuality assessment measures.

KEY TERMS AND CONCEPTS

Acquired type (secondary dysfunction). A classification of the fourth edition of the *Diagnostic and Statistical Manual of Mental Disorders* (DSM-IV; American Psychiatric Association, 1994) for a dysfunction that follows a period of normal functioning. The antonym of lifelong or primary dysfunction.

Anorgasmia. See Female orgasmic disorder.

Compulsive sexual behavior. The past decade witnessed an enormous interest in "out of control," hyperactive sexual behavior that may be driven more by anxiety-reduction mechanisms than by sexual desire (Coleman, 1995). There is considerable debate as to whether this constitutes an "addiction." In fact, the DSM-IV does not classify hyperactive sexual behavior as a dysfunction. Some of this behavior is paraphilic (see Paraphilias) and some is nonparaphilic. Current treatment programs frequently rely on group modalities (including twelve-step programs) and the use of serotonin reuptake inhibitors such as Prozac.

Dyspareunia. DSM-IV restricts dyspareunia (302.76) to "recurrent or persistent genital pain associated with sexual intercourse in either the male or female" (p. 513). The term is derived from the Greek terms for "bad" or "painful" (dys) and for "lying in bed" (pareunia). It may be caused by a collection of dysfunctional conditions that have painful intercourse as the final common symptomatic presentation (Kaplan, 1983).

Emission. The contraction of the smooth muscles (contained in the walls of the internal male reproductive organs) that collects ejaculate in the posterior urethra (Kaplan, 1983). The sensation experienced may be perceived as the sensation of ejaculatory inevitability.

Excitement phase disorder. A term referring to male erectile disorder and female sexual arousal disorder. It is due to deficiencies in genital vasocongestion (see Vasocongestion, Female sexual arousal disorder, and Male erectile disorder).

Female orgasmic disorder (inhibited female orgasm, impaired female orgasm, orgasmic or orgastic dysfunction, or anorgasmia). The DSM-IV definition of female orgasmic disorder (302.73) is a

> persistent or recurrent delay in, or absence of, orgasm following a normal sexual excitement phase. Women exhibit wide variability in the type or intensity of stimulation that triggers orgasm. The diagnosis of Female Orgasmic Disorder should be based on the clinician's judgment that the woman's orgasmic capacity is less than would be reasonable for her age, sexual experience, and the adequacy of sexual stimulation she receives. (p. 505)

Kaplan (1974) says that 8–10% of women never experience orgasm under any circumstances and that perhaps 50% do not experience orgasm in coitus without additional stimulation. Hence, not having orgasm in coitus should be considered a common sexual variant and not a dysfunction. The incidence of secondary or situational anorgasmia is difficult to determine, since there are types of partners, types of stimulation, and certain settings that may lead to difficulties for perhaps half of all women (Munjack & Oziel, 1980). Immediate causes include obsessive observation during sex, the inability to relax, and insufficient stimulation (Kaplan, 1983).

Female sexual arousal disorder (inhibited sexual excitement in females). The DSM-IV definition of female sexual arousal disorder (302.72) is "a persistent or recurrent inability to attain, or to maintain until completion of the sexual activity, an adequate lubrication–swelling response of sexual excitement" (p. 502). It is relatively uncommon as an isolated clinical syndrome (if there is sufficient stimulation) except as a result of physiological factors such as estrogen deficiency. Having sex with a dry and nondistended vagina may lead to secondary inhibition of desire. The immediate cause is unknown, other than any emotional state that interferes with the dilating of the genital vasculature in response to a sexual stimulus (Kaplan, 1983).

Generalized type (absolute or global dysfunction). A DSM-IV classification term for dysfunction experienced in all situations with all partners. The antonym of acquired type or situational dysfunction.

Hypoactive sexual desire (inhibited sexual desire). DSM-IV states that hypoactive sexual desire (302.71) is a "persistently or recurrently deficient (or absent) sexual fantasies and desire for sexual activity. The judgment of deficiency or absence is made by the clinician, taking into account factors that affect sexual functioning such as age and the context of the persons life" (p. 498). This dysfunction is common in both males and females; it is described extensively by Kaplan (1979, 1995a) and has been summarized earlier in this chapter. Hypoactive sexual desire has several organic causes (e.g., diabetes) that should be addressed during assessment. Interestingly, DSM-IV offers no diagnosis for very high (hyperactive) sexual desire. This may reflect a social bias that only low sexual desire is dysfunctional.

Lifelong type (primary dysfunction). A DSM-IV classification for a dysfunction that has always been present; that is, there has never been a time of adequate functioning. The antonym of acquired type or secondary dysfunction.

Male erectile disorder (impotence, inhibited sexual excitement in males). The DSM-IV definition of male erectile disorder (302.72) is the "Persistent or recurrent inability to attain, or maintain until completion of the sexual activity, an adequate erection" (p. 504). Masters and Johnson (1970) included the condition of failing in more than 25% of one's attempts at intercourse. Kaplan (1974) says that about one-half of the male population has experienced at least occasional, transient episodes of impotence. The immediate causes include performance anxiety, pressure from the partner, and an overconcern with pleasing the partner (Kaplan, 1983). It is the dysfunction most likely to have an organic basis.

Male orgasmic disorder (retarded ejaculation, inhibited male orgasm, ejaculatory incompetence). The DSM-IV definition of male orgasmic disorder (302.74) is a "persistent or recurrent delay in, or absence of, orgasm following a normal sexual excitement phase" (p. 507). The immediate causes often include obsessive self-observation during sex and the inability to "let go" (Kaplan, 1983). In addition, secondary retarded ejaculation carries a significant risk of organicity.

Orgasm. In the male, the 0.8-second contractions of the striated perineal muscles that propel semen out of the urethra; in the female, the 0.8-second contractions of striated perineal muscles (Kaplan, 1983).

Orgasm phase disorders. A term referring to premature, retarded, or partially retarded ejaculation in males and to inhibited, delayed, or absent orgasm in females.

Paraphilias (perversions, deviations, variations). DSM-IV states, "The essential features of a Paraphilia are recurrent, intense sexually arousing fantasies, sexual urges, or behaviors generally involving (1) nonhuman objects, (2) the suffering or humiliation of oneself or one's partner, or (3) children or other nonconsenting persons, that occur over a period of at least six months" (p. 522). Common paraphilias include fetishism (use of nonliving objects for sexual excitement), transvestism (cross-dressing), pedophilia (use of prepubertal children), exhibitionism (exposing the genitals), voyeurism ("peeping"), masochism (being made to suffer), and sadism (sexual excitement from the suffering of others). These disorders are reported almost exclusively among males.

Partially retarded ejaculation. A relatively rare variation of retarded ejaculation in which the emission phase of the ejaculatory response is normal but the pleasant ejaculatory phase is inhibited. Semen seeps out, but there are neither contractions nor pleasure (Kaplan, 1983).

Performance anxiety. The anxiety that accompanies concern about performance. It is most often related to fear of failure, partner's demand for performance, or the excessive need to please one's partner.

Premature ejaculation. DSM-IV states that premature ejaculation (302.75) "is the persistent or recurrent onset of orgasm and ejaculation with minimal sexual stimulation before, on, or shortly after penetration and before the person wishes it" (p. 509). Premature ejaculation is the most common dysfunction among men and is especially common among the sexually inexperienced. The immediate cause is the suppression of preejaculatory sensations during periods of high sexual excitement (Kaplan, 1983).

Response cycle. The psychophysiological phases through which an individual progresses during the sex act. Masters and Johnson (1966) have posited a fourfold cycle of excitement, plateau, orgasm, and resolution. Kaplan (1974), because of conceptual difficulties with the plateau and resolution stages, developed a biphasic concept of excitement and orgasm. In a later book (1979), she posited a triphasic model that adds desire. Other authors (e.g., Walen, 1980; Zilbergeld & Ellison, 1980) have proposed more complex schemes that include more cognitive and subjective variables.

Retrograde ejaculation. A "dry orgasm" due to semen entering the urinary bladder rather than the urethra following the ejaculatory response. This is always due to organic causes. It should not be confused with retarded ejaculation, in which the physiological process of ejaculation itself is inhibited.

Sexual aversion disorders (phobias). The essential feature of a sexual aversion disorder is the aversion to and active avoidance of genital sexual contact with a sexual partner. The distinction between "simple" sexual phobia and phobia associated with panic disorder is of the utmost importance, since panic disorders are not amenable to psychological therapies alone. Antianxiety or antipanic medication is usually necessary (Kaplan, 1983, 1995b). Kaplan, Fyer, and Novick (1982) describe the difficulties in distinguishing between true inhibited sexual desire and the phobic avoidance of sex.

Situational type. A DSM-IV classification for a dysfunction experienced with certain partners and/or under certain circumstances (antonym of generalized type or global dysfunction). This distinction is important in making a differential diagnosis; if the symptom is clearly situational, psychogenicity is typically established and disease and drugs can usually be ruled out as causative factors (Kaplan, 1983).

Spectatoring. The tendency to watch oneself and monitor one's own sexual performance. It both causes and is caused by performance anxiety.

Testosterone. The primary sex ("libido") hormone for both genders. Testosterone levels are affected by mood. High anxiety or depression will lower levels of the hormone, and it may be best to postpone sex therapy until these conditions are remedied (Kaplan, 1974).

Vaginismus. According to DSM-IV, vaginismus (306.51) "is the recurrent and persistent involuntary contraction of the perineal muscles surrounding the outer third of the vagina when vaginal penetration with penis, finger, tampon, or speculum is attempted" (p. 513). The contractions are usually painful, and the woman is typically unable to have intercourse, even though she may be aroused, may lubricate, or may even experience multiple orgasms. In milder forms, it may cause dyspareunia rather than prevent intercourse. The immediate cause is a fear reaction evoked by vaginal penetration (Kaplan, 1979).

Vasocongestion. In the male, the dilation of penile arteries, which increases the inflow of blood while the outflow is diminished. It creates a high-pressure system in the cavernous sinuses of the penis, which produces erection. In the female this term describes the diffuse dilation of blood vessels in the labia and around the vagina, which produces genital swelling and vaginal lubrication (Kaplan, 1983).

KEY CLINICAL SKILLS

Bridge maneuvers. Maneuvers that are utilized for stimulation of the clitoris during intercourse when the female is unable to have orgasm during intercourse alone. Kaplan (1974) offers illustrations of these techniques to "bridge" manual stimulation of the clitoris and coitus. If these are successful, direct stimulation should cease progressively earlier before orgasm.

Coital alignment technique (CAT). The CAT (Eichel & Nobile, 1992; Eichel, Eichel, & Kule, 1988) is a sexual intercourse technique that involves a slow, rhythmic, gliding, back-and-forth rocking motion during coitus and orgasm. With the man on top, in a "high ride" position, the couple maintains full body contact throughout intercourse and orgasm. With this alignment, the penis and clitoris stimulate each other. Eichel and Nobile (1992) state that this technique improves the quality of sexual pleasure and orgasm in men and women and is an effective treatment for female coital anorgasmia. Although Kaplan and her staff (1992) were unable to replicate Eichel's report in their "pilot study," Hurlbert and Apt (1995) found significant improvements in orgasmic strength and consistency when CAT was used alone and in combination with directed masturbation.

Desensitization. Some means of gradually reducing anxiety-arousing stimuli. Since anxiety is associated with almost all forms of sexual dysfunction, treatment typically includes some type of desensitization. This may take the form of imagining progressively more anxiety-arousing situations or of experiencing them *in vivo* while remaining relaxed. The very structure of sex therapy itself, which typically begins with low-anxiety tasks and progressively moves to more threatening ones, is based on the principle of desensitization (Heiman et al., 1981).

Differential diagnosis. The term used to describe the differentiation between organicity (caused by genetics, disease, or drugs) and pychogenicity (caused by psychological impairment) of a sexual dysfunction. If a dysfunction has already been determined to be situational, one can usually rule out organicity.

Dilators. A series of objects of increasing size, inserted under the females's control into the her vagina for the purpose of gradual desensitization. Masters and Johnson (1970) pioneered the use of dilators in the treatment of vaginismus. Kaplan utilizes the finger instead, beginning with the female's own, followed by her partner's.

Homework assignments. See Structured sexual tasks or SIGS.

Masturbation or self-stimulation (as a part of treatment). The most widely used and effective method for the treatment of lifelong inhibited female orgasm (anorgasmia). It may be preceded by genital self-examination, various types of body awareness, use of erotic stimuli, and so forth. The client often uses lubrication or a vibrator as an aid. Self-stimulation in the presence of a partner may be used as a step preceding manual stimulation by the partner. For clients with coital anorgasmia, self-stimulation during intercourse may be recommended.

Orgasmic reconditioning. A process in which therapists direct clients' fantasies in conjunction with masturbation in order to modify the types of stimuli that are associated with arousal (Leiblum & Rosen, 1989). It has been used to treat concerns about object choice, such as fetishes or homosexuality; it is also used to enhance attraction in heterosexual relations (e.g., thinking about one's partner prior to orgasm). A classical conditioning paradigm is often used to explain the results.

Organicity. See Differential diagnosis.

Pause technique. See Stop–start.

Psychosexual evaluation. Kaplan's (1983) term for an evaluation that integrates the psychological and medical aspects of diagnosis of dysfunction. A cornerstone of this approach is the "sexual status examination" (listed).

Sensate focus. A procedure originally developed by Masters and Johnson to create an atmosphere whereby performance anxiety and spectatoring can be minimized. Couples are initially encouraged to be sensual (rather than sexual) through body exploration/massage of each other. While one person receives, the other massages/explores, encouraging feedback from the former concerning what feels good. The "giver" is also asked to get in touch with his or her own sensations. The process is designed to interrupt the current destructive sexual system of anxiety, expectation, and pressure, and couples are initially informed not to caress genitals or breasts in Sensate Focus I. In Sensate Focus II, partners may also pleasure each other's primary erotic areas but not to the point of orgasm. In Sensate Focus III, orgasm may be included.

Sex history. Many sex therapists believe that an in-depth history of clients' behavior is important, as well as knowledge of current attitudes and behaviors. Masters and Johnson advocated extensive interviews lasting about 7 hours, with male and female partners separated and interviewed by a same-sex therapist for the majority of the time. Other authorities (e.g., Annon, 1976) advocate a simpler approach. The efficacy of extensive history taking has not been empirically validated.

Sexual status examination. Kaplan's (1983) term for an important aspect of her psychosexual evaluation. It is a highly detailed description of the couple's current sexual experience through their self-reports. It is the closest one can ethically get to observing the couple and has the advantage of offering information about subjective experience and cognitive processes.

Stop–start. A method (the alternative to the "squeeze technique") pioneered by James Semans (1956) for the treatment of premature ejaculation. The client's partner is asked to stimulate his penis until he begins to feel premonitory sensations of orgasm. He then instructs her to stop, and the cycle is repeated. The method encourages concentrating on preorgasmic sensations rather than suppressing them (Kaplan, 1989). This procedure is used in a series of graduated sexual assignments culminating in intercourse.

Structured sexual tasks or SIGS. The specific behavioral strategies assigned by the therapist to modify the specific and immediate causes of the various dysfunctions. These differ, since the immediate causes of the dysfunctions differ. An excellent brief summary of these SIGS is found in Kaplan (1979, Chap. 3). Most involve the client couple in some form of gradual, *in vivo,* systematic desensitization procedure. Many begin with or include sensate focus.

Squeeze technique. A method pioneered by Masters and Johnson (1970) for the treatment of premature ejaculation. The client's partner is asked to stimulate his penis until he begins to feel premonitory sensations of orgasm. He then cues her to grasp his penis between the thumb and first finger of both hands and to squeeze the shaft just below the coronal ridge for about 3–4 seconds. Although most authorities now prefer the stop–start method, the advantage of the squeeze is that it more rapidly diminishes erection and therefore the potential for ejaculation. Like the stop–start method, this technique is used in a series of graduated sexual assignments culminating in intercourse.

TEACHING TOOLS AND TECHNIQUES

Class "Icebreakers" and Introductions

If the class is small, this exercise can be done individually. If large, it can be carried out in dyads. Each class member introduces him- or herself through describing the sex socialization and education he or she received in his or her family of origin. These issues are generally far enough removed from the present to make this task relatively unthreatening, yet the exercise also sets the tone for openness in the class.

What Is Sexual "Health"?

The class is divided into triads. The groups are asked, "Given that this is a course on sexual dysfunction, is there some kind of standard or 'ideal' from which one is dysfunctional?" Alternately, one can prepare a handout or overhead display on "sexual health" based on Maddock's (1976) definition. This suggests that a sexually healthy individual has, first, a certain amount of cognitive knowledge about sexual phenomena; second, a degree of self-awareness about his or her own attitudes toward sex; third, a well-developed, usable value system that provides input into sexual decisions; and, finally, some degree of emotional comfort and stability in relation to sexual activities in which the individual and others engage.

Phase–Etiology Grid

An overhead display or sheet is prepared that includes a blank 3×3 grid. Across the horizontal axis are the three phases of the sexual response cycle: desire, excitement, and orgasm. On the vertical axis on the left are three etiological explanations of dysfunction: situational, relational, and intrapsychic. Students are asked to think of dysfunctions that might be placed in each of the nine cells. For example, in the upper left-hand corner, a desire–situational problem may arise when, for example, a person does not feel sexual desire when sleeping with his or her partner at either partner's parents' home.

Practice in History Taking

Various models of sex history taking (already discussed to some extent; see also "Key Books, Chapters, and Articles") include at least the following major components: (1) questions that enable one to make a differential diagnosis between a dysfunction of organic etiology and one of psychogenic etiology; (2) questions about the duration and course of the dysfunction; and (3) questions about the current sexual behavior of the client. Since modeling and practice of a complete sexual history can often be too time-consuming, these components can be modeled/practiced in different class sessions.

Student Reports on Dysfunctions

Students may be asked to make oral presentations or write term papers on the most current information regarding the major dysfunctions. A suggested outline includes (1) definitions, (2) incidence, (3) etiology, (4) consequences of the dysfunction for the individual or couple, (5) treatment, and (6) prognosis and outcome, as suggested by research.

Multiple Conceptualization Exercise

The students should be familiar with various authors such as Kaplan, Schnarch, and Leiblum and Rosen, who afford the students the opportunity to conceptualize dysfunctions from a variety of viewpoints. In small groups, students can be assigned a specific sexual dysfunction and challenged to indicate how it would be conceptualized and treated by the various authors. Also, the students can be asked how their own conceptualizations and treatment programs would differ from those of these recognized experts.

Sensate Focus Instructions

Since sensate focus is a common element in many treatment plans, students need to learn to practice giving the rationale and specific instructions for this task. Examples of verbatim instructions are found in Kaplan (1974) and Munjack and Oziel (1980).

Exercise in Specific Treatment Strategies

Although treatment must, of course, be tailored to the individual client or couple, there is some advantage in knowing (perhaps even memorizing) a basic sequence one might typically follow for treating each of the major dysfunctions. Kaplan (1979, Chap. 3) offers a succinct outline of treatment steps for each dysfunction. The class is divided into triads. The instructor calls out the name of a particular dysfunction and asks person *A*, *B*, or *C*, to delineate the steps. The two individuals in each triad who are not being targeted help out if the first person gets stuck. The triads can then discuss the circumstances under which this treatment strategy might not be appropriate.

Ethics Exercise

The instructor prepares a handout containing a list of 12 behaviors actually engaged in by some sex therapists. All of these behaviors might be considered ethically objectionable by some therapists, whereas others might be quite comfortable with them. Individually, students are asked to rank-order the behaviors from 1 (least objectionable to them personally) to 12 (most objectionable to them personally). The results are then discussed in small groups. Examples of such therapist behaviors might include (1) using sexually explicit materials as part of therapy; (2) counseling a person who wants the therapist to facilitate a sexual activity that the therapist considers unethical for him- or herself, although not necessarily unethical for others (e.g., a client who wants help in working through jealousies related to "swinging," which the therapist does not personally endorse); or (3) having sexual relations with a client, sincerely believing that this will be helpful to him or her.

Training and Research Centers

Since training opportunities are continuously changing, people looking for training in sex therapy should contact the professional organizations listed in this chapter for current listings. Below are some examples of training opportunities.

- Institute for Advanced Study in Human Sexuality, 1523 Franklin Street, San Francisco, CA 94109 (offers master's and doctorate in Human Sexuality).
- Masters and Johnson Institute, One Campbell Plaza, 59th Street & Arsenal, St. Louis, MO 63139.
- New York University, Department of Health Studies, 35 West 4th Street, 12th Floor, New York, NY 10003 (offers master's and doctorate in Human Sexuality).
- Program in Human Sexuality, The Medical School, University of Minnesota, Department of Family Practice and Community Health, 1300 South 2nd Street, Minneapolis, MN 55454.

Producers of Films and Videotapes on Sex Therapy

- Multi-Focus, Incorporated, 1525 Franklin Street, San Francisco, CA 94109 (800-821-0514).
- Sinclair Institute, 1829 East Franklin Street, Suite 1014, Chapel Hill, NC 27514 (919-929-3797).

Journals Related to Sex Therapy

- *Archives of Sexual Behavior,* Plenum Publishing Corporation, 233 Spring Street, New York, NY 10013.
- *Journal of Homosexuality,* The Haworth Press, 10 Alice Street, Binghamton, NY 13904-1580.
- *Journal of Sex Education, Counseling, and Therapy,* American Association of Sex Educators, Counselors, and Therapists, 435 North Michigan Avenue, Suite 1717, Chicago, IL 60611.
- *Journal of Sex and Marital Therapy,* Brunner/Mazel, 19 Union Square West, New York NY 10003.
- *Journal of Sex Research,* Society for the Scientific Study of Sex, Inc., P.O. Box 208, Mount Vernon, IA 52314.
- *SIECUS Report,* Sex Information and Education Council of the United States, 130 West 42nd Street, New York, NY 10036.

National Organizations Concerned with Human Sexuality

- American Academy of Clinical Sexologists, 1929 18th Street, N.W., Suite 1166, Washington, DC 20009 (202-462-2122). This organization publishes the *Journal of Sex and Marital Therapy* and offers postgraduate training courses.
- American Association of Sex Educators, Counselors, and Therapists, 435 North Michigan Avenue, Suite 1717, Chicago, IL 60611. In addition to publishing a journal (listed), the organization conducts many national and regional workshops and certifies sex educators counselors, and therapists.
- American Board of Sexology, 1929 18th Street, N.W., Suite 1166, Washington, DC 20009 (800-533-3521). This organization provides board certification as a "clinical sexologist."
- Sex Information and Education Counsel of the United States (SIECUS), 130 West 42nd Street, New York, NY 10036. This organization publishes the *SIECUS Report,* an excellent bimonthly newsletter telling what is happening in the field and offering both book and audiovisual reviews. It also publishes excellent study guides and pamphlets such as an updated film resource guide. You may write them and ask for a list of publications.
- Society for the Scientific Study of Sex (SSSS), P.O. Box 208, Mount Vernon, IA 52314. SSSS is an international organization of professionals dedicated to the advancement of sexual knowledge. Besides publishing the *Journal of Sex Research,* SSSS also publishes the *Annual Review of Sex Research* and the society newsletter.

- Society for Sex Therapy and Research (SSTAR), c/o Dr. P. Schreiner-Engel, Mt. Sinai Medical Center, 1176 Fifth Avenue, Box 1170, New York, NY 10029. The Society for Sex Therapy and Research is a small organization with a newsletter and annual meeting. Its primary focus is on clinical and research issues of sexual dysfunctions.

RESEARCH ISSUES

Although a number of voices have called for better research in sex therapy, and the "Key Books, Chapters, and Articles" section contains some examples of good research, clinical folklore rather than a solid empirical base still dominates the field. Samples, with some exceptions, tend to be small. Most of the research studies, including Masters and Johnson's work, have been uncontrolled (Zilbergeld & Evans, 1980). A considerable amount of the "research" has been case studies. Much of what we "know" about the relationship of client variables to outcome is speculation. There is almost no research on therapist variables in sex therapy.

Concerning treatment variables, it is difficult to determine the curative value of various techniques, since therapy usually consists of a combined-technique approach. Two techniques do seem to be fairly robust; they are the "squeeze" or "stop–start" for premature ejaculation, and the "dilation" procedure for vaginismic women. In addition, the general therapeutic technique of anxiety reduction is clearly beneficial for the large number of clients whose sexual dysfunction is related to anxiety. However, since the treatment interventions reported are generally broad-spectrum combinations, there are few attempts to differentiate the "active ingredients" from the "inert fillers" in the total package (Heiman et al., 1981). There is, in summary, little evidence to support the differential effectiveness of various modalities of therapy.

The problem of dependent variables may be the most serious issue in the sex therapy research literature. There are clearly no well-operationalized and generally accepted standards as to what constitutes a "success" or a "failure," and measurement techniques are in their infancy. As in other areas of family therapy outcome literature (Gurman & Kniskern, 1981), it will be necessary to have multiple measures from multiple vantage points. One could utilize patient, partner, or therapist reports. Data could include questionnaires, physiological evidence, or behavioral indices. For a brief review of treatment outcome in sex therapy, see pages 10–12 in Rosen and Leiblum (1995).

In surveying sexologists, Apt, Hurlbert, and Clark (1994) found several areas that have been neglected and are in need of further research. These include "healthy" sexual behaviors and relationships, outcome studies of various therapies with diverse populations, and theoretical studies of possible causes of dysfunctions.

One area that has shown progressive research is in the medical aspects of sexual dysfunction and treatment (e.g., pharmacology or chronic illness). For example, several authors have described the use and effectiveness of injection treatments for impotence (Eid & Pearce, 1993; Levitt & Mulcahy, 1995; Wagner & Kaplan, 1993).

KEY BOOKS, CHAPTERS, AND ARTICLES

Araoz, D. L. (1982). *Hypnosis and sex therapy.* New York: Brunner/Mazel.

This relatively short book (178 pages) is a remarkably comprehensive and truly integrative treatise on these two disciplines. The result of this synthesis is a "hypnobehavioral model" that incorporates principles of cognitive therapy, imagery conditioning, and behavior modification within an interactional perspective.

Atwood, J. D., & Dershowitz, S. (1992). Constructing a sex and marital therapy frame: Ways to help couples deconstruct sexual problems. *Journal of Sex and Marital Therapy, 18,* 196–218.

Based on social constructionism, this article integrates the theoretical and therapeutic ideas from marital therapy into marital and sexual therapy. It offers a therapeutic stance that utilizes sexual meaning systems and sexual scripts in working with couples.

Barbach, L. (1980). *Women discover orgasm: A therapist guide to a new treatment approach.* New York: Free Press

This is an excellent book for therapists who are leading or want to lead sex therapy groups for preorgasmic women. It includes discussions of forming a group, therapy methods, homework assignments dealing with resistance, working with the client's partners, cotherapists' problems, and the limitations of the group method.

Eid, J. F., & Pearce, C. E. (1993). *Making love again: Regaining sexual potency through the new injection treatment.* New York: Brunner/Mazel.

This short book provides a complete explanation of injection therapy for impotence, covering the process of assessment and methods for treatment.

Genhard, P., & Johnson, A. (1979). *The Kinsey data: Marginal tabulations of the 1938–1963 interviews conducted by the Institute for Sex Research.* Philadelphia: Saunders.

This work is an important revision of and supplement to the previously published Kinsey data. It includes 45 pages of text, with 580 statistical tables, and thus offers a valuable opportunity for researchers to compare their current findings with Kinsey's figures from an earlier generation.

Heiman, J., LoPiccolo, L., & LoPiccolo, J. (1988). *Becoming orgasmic: A sexual growth program for women* (rev. ed.). Englewood Cliffs, NJ: Prentice-Hall.

This book outlines a detailed growth program for women who have problems in experiencing orgasm. The book also includes a section relating to male partners. The emphasis is on orgasm as a part of, rather than the only or primary goal of sexuality and sexual experience.

Kaplan, H. S. (1974). *The new sex therapy.* New York: Quadrangle Books.

This classic work is an interesting synthesis of psychoanalytic, behavioral, and systems approaches to sex therapy. The first 116 pages cover the physiology of sexual response. Then the author turns to general approaches to treatment, with six very detailed chapters on the six major dysfunctions. In addition, the book has sections on the results of sex therapy, sexual therapy with psychiatric patients, the relationship of sexual therapy and marital therapy, and so on.

Kaplan, H. S. (1979). *Disorders of sexual desire and other new concepts and techniques in sex therapy.* New York: Brunner/Mazel.

This is a groundbreaking work, in which the author articulates her triphasic model of sexual response that includes "desire." After reviewing the physiology, etiology, and treatment guidelines for the basic dysfunctions, Kaplan devotes four chapters specifically to desire-phase disorders of males and females. She posits that desire disorders are typically related to deeper, often unconscious causes, and are therefore less amenable to brief, behaviorally oriented sex therapy. She believes their treatment often requires longer, insight-oriented approaches. This book has been followed with Kaplan's (1995) *The Sexual Desire Disorders: Dysfunctional Regulation of Sexual Motivation* (see listed review).

Kaplan, H. S. (1983). *The evaluation of sexual disorders: Psychological and medical aspects.* New York: Brunner/Mazel.

This impressive book focuses on the diagnosis and evaluation of sexual disorders, with a special emphasis on the differential diagnosis of psychogenic and organic etiology. In the first section, Kaplan describes her general process of psychosexual evaluation of dysfunctional patients. In the second section, a group of colleagues detail the medical evaluation of the major dysfunctions. In the final section, Kaplan details her specific assessment criteria (both medical and social–psychological) for gender identity disorders, the major psychosexual dysfunctions, sexual phobias and avoidance, and unconsummated marriage. The volume is an excellent resource on information concerning differential diagnosis.

Kaplan, H. S. (1995). *The sexual desire disorders: Dysfunctional regulation of sexual motivation.* New York: Brunner/Mazel.

In her second book on sexual desire disorders, Kaplan integrates theory, research and clinical skills to provide an excellent resource for evaluating and treating desire disorders. Kaplan also incorporates many case studies and includes specific chapters focusing on psychiatric disorders and medical conditions.

Leiblum, S. R., & Rosen, R. C. (Eds.). (1989). *Principles and practice of sex therapy* (2nd ed.): *Update for the 1990s*. New York: Guilford Press.

The second edition of this excellent book offers many updates, as well as several new chapters. This book is more useful than the typical edited work, in that the authors have been asked to describe treatment failures as well as successes. The volume attempts to identify some of the factors leading to varying degrees of success with different clients and problems. The book demonstrates the enormous diversity of both conceptualization and treatment in sex therapy. Valuable introductory chapters by the editors describe the development of the field and critical issues facing it.

Leiblum, S. R., & Rosen, R. C. (Eds.). (1988). *Sexual desire disorders*. New York: Guilford Press.

This book focuses on the theory, research, and treatment of sexual desire disorders. It offers conceptual frameworks from several major theories, such as psychodynamic, object relations, cognitive, and behavioral systems, and biomedical approaches.

Mason, M. J. (1991). Family therapy as the emerging context for sex therapy. In A. S. Gurman & D. P. Kniskern (Eds.), *Handbook of family therapy* (Vol. 2). New York: Brunner/Mazel.

This chapter is an excellent overview of sex therapy and its relation to family therapy. Mason discusses how familial issues impact sexual functioning, as well as reviewing the literature for the major areas of sexual dysfunctions. The chapter also covers clinically relevant tools and issues in sex therapy.

Masters, W. H., & Johnson, V. E. (1970). *Human sexual inadequacy*. Boston: Little, Brown.

On the basis of 11 years of careful clinical research, Masters and Johnson present findings for the treatment of impotency, ejaculatory disorders, inadequate female response, vaginismus, dyspareunia, and sexual problems of aging. The book is a basic and essential resource for all therapists and counselors, as well as for others seriously interested in human sexuality. The publication of this book was perhaps the single most important milestone in the history of sex therapy.

Reinisch, J. M., Beasley, R., & Kent, D. (1990). *The Kinsey Institute new report on sex: What you must know to be sexually literate*. New York: St. Martin's Press.

This book reports the results of a new national survey on sexual literacy by the Kinsey Institute. The book states that Americans are sexually illiterate and offers answers to the most frequently asked questions about sexuality.

Rosen, R. C., & Leiblum, S. R. (Eds.). (1992). *Erectile disorders: Assessment and treatment*. New York: Guilford Press.

This book provides the reader with a complete overview of current methods for assessment, conceptualization, and therapy for erectile disorders. This edited work provides different perspectives and methods, ranging from intrapsychic concepts to the use of vacuum devices and injection treatments.

Rosen, R. C., & Leiblum, S. R. (Eds.). (1995). *Case studies in sex therapy.* New York: Guilford Press.

Through a comprehensive collection of case studies, this book offers an overview of the current state of sex therapy. With chapters written by experts in each area, this practice-oriented book provides readers with up-to-date information and theory in an applied clinical format. The book is divided into three main sections: sexual desire disorders, sexual performance problems, and sexual addiction and compulsion.

Rosen, R. C., Leiblum, S. R., & Spector, I. P. (1994). Psychologically based treatment for male erectile disorder: A cognitive-interpersonal model. *Journal of Sex and Marital Therapy, 20,* 67–85.

This article provides a five-part cognitive-interpersonal treatment method for impotence, including both theoretical conceptualization and case examples.

Schnarch, D. M. (1991). *Constructing the sexual crucible: An integration of sexual and marital therapy.* New York: Norton.

This book offers an alternative view to current sex therapy practices that focus primarily on sexual functioning and symptom removal. Schnarch focuses on the role of intimacy and personal differentiation in sexual relationships. He offers a theoretical framework that combines behavioral, object relations, and systems theory in order to "construct the sexual crucible." This framework also integrates emotional and biological functioning.

Schover, L. R., & Jensen, S. B. (1988). *Sexuality and chronic illness: A comprehensive approach.* New York: Guilford Press.

This book is a comprehensive source for sex therapists with clients who have chronic illnesses. It provides an explanation of the effects of chronic illness on sexuality, as well as covering the assessment and treatment (including examples) of several specific illnesses. This book emphasizes the need for a balance between psychological and biological assessment and treatment.

Wagner, G., & Kaplan, H. S. (1993). *The new injection treatment for impotence: Medical and psychological aspects.* New York: Brunner/Mazel.

This in-depth book provides clinicians with information regarding injection treatment for impotence. It covers assessment and treatment procedures, as well as the psychological and relational aspects of this form of treatment.

Weeks, G. R., & Hof, L. (Eds.). (1987). *Integrating sex and marital therapy: A clinical guide.* New York: Brunner/Mazel.

This edited book offers an integration of sex therapy with marital therapy. It focuses on the conceptualization and assessment of sexual issues from a relational or systemic framework and offers several clinical applications.

REFERENCES

Althof, S. E., & Kingsberg, S. A. (1992). Books helpful to patients with sexual and marital problems: A bibliography. *Journal of Sex and Marital Therapy, 18,* 70–79.

American Psychiatric Association. (1994). *Diagnostic and statistical manual of mental disorders* (4th ed.). Washington, DC: Author.

Annon, J. (1975). *The behavioral treatment of sexual problems: Intensive therapy.* Honolulu: Enabling Systems.

Annon, J. (1976). *The behavioral treatment of sexual problems: Brief therapy.* New York: Harper & Row.

Apt, C., Hurlbert, D. F., & Clark, K. J. (1994). Neglected subjects in sex research: A survey of sexologists. *Journal of Sex and Marital Therapy, 20,* 237–243.

Atwood, J. D., & Dershowitz, S. (1992). Constructing a sex and marital therapy frame: Ways to help couples deconstruct sexual problems. *Journal of Sex and Marital Therapy, 18,* 196–218.

Carl, D. (1990). *Counseling same-sex couples.* New York: Norton.

Coleman, E. (1995). Treatment of compulsive sexual behavior. In R. C. Rosen & S. B. Leiblum (Eds.), *Case studies in sex therapy.* New York: Guilford Press.

Comfort, A. (1972). *The joy of sex.* New York: Crown.

Derogatis, L., & Melisaratos, N. (1979). The DSFI: A multidimensional measure of sexual functioning. *Journal of Sex and Marital Therapy, 5,* 244–281.

Eid, J. F., & Pearce, C. E. (1993). *Making love again: Regaining sexual potency through the new injection treatment.* New York: Brunner/Mazel.

Eichel, E. D., Eichel, J. D., & Kule, S. (1988). The technique of coital alignment and its relations to female orgasmic response and simultaneous orgasm. *Journal of Sex and Marital Therapy, 14,* 129–141.

Eichel, E. W., & Nobile, P. (1992). *The perfect fit: How to achieve mutual fulfillment and monogamous passion throughout the new intercourse.* New York: Fine.

Ellis, A. (1962). *Reason and emotion in psychotherapy.* New York: Lyle Stuart.

Ellis, A. (1980). Treatment of erectile dysfunction. In S. B. Leiblum & L. A. Pervin (Eds.), *Principles and practice of sex therapy.* New York: Guilford Press.

Fischer, N., & Corcoran, K. (1994). *Measures of clinical practice* (Vols. 1 & 2, 2nd ed.). New York: Free Press.

Fish, L., Fish, R., & Sprenkle, D. (1984). Treating inhibited sexual desire: A marital therapy approach. *American Journal of Family Therapy, 12,* 3–12.

Fisher, J., & Gochros, H. (1977). *A handbook of behavior therapy with sexual problems* (Vols. 1 & 2). New York: Pergamon Press.

Goldstein, I., & Rothstein, L. (1990). *The potent male: Facts, fiction, future.* Los Angeles: Body.

Gonsiorek, J. (Ed.). (1982). *Homosexuality in psychotherapy: A practitioner's handbook of affirmative models.* Binghamton, NY: Haworth.

Gurman, A., & Kniskern, D. (Eds.). (1981). *Handbook of family therapy.* New York: Brunner/Mazel.

Hartman, W., & Fithian, M. (1972). *Treatment of sexual dysfunction.* Long Beach, CA: Center for Marital and Sexual Studies.

Hastings, D. W. (1963). *Impotence and frigidity.* Boston: Little, Brown.

Heiman, J. R., & LoPiccolo, J. (1988). *Becoming orgasmic: A sexual growth program for women.* Englewood Cliffs, NJ: Prentice-Hall.

Heiman, J., LoPiccolo, L., & LoPiccolo, J. (1981). The treatment of sexual dysfunction. In A. Gurman & D. Kniskern (Eds.), *Handbook of family therapy.* New York: Brunner/Mazel.

Hurlbert, D. F., & Apt, C. (1995). The coital alignment technique and directed masturbation: A comparative study on female orgasm. *Journal of Sex and Marital Therapy, 21,* 21–29.

Jacobsen, F. M. (1992). Fluoxetine-induced sexual dysfunction and an open trial of yohimbine. *Journal of Clinical Psychiatry, 53,* 119–122.

Kaplan, H. S. (1974). *The new sex therapy.* New York: Quadrangle Books.

Kaplan, H. S. (1979). *Disorders of sexual desire.* New York: Brunner/Mazel.

Kaplan, H. S. (1983). *The evaluation of sexual disorders: Psychological and medical aspects.* New York: Brunner/Mazel.

Kaplan, H. S. (1989). *PE: How to overcome premature ejaculation.* New York: Brunner/Mazel.

Kaplan, H. S. (1995a). *The sexual desire disorders: Dysfunctional regulation of sexual motivation.* New York: Brunner/Mazel.

Kaplan, H. S. (1995b). Sexual aversion disorder: The case of the phobic virgin, or an abused child grows up. In R. C. Rosen & S. R. Leiblum (Eds.), *Case studies in sex therapy.* New York: Guilford Press.

Kaplan, H. S., & Staff (1992). Does the CAT technique enhance female orgasm? *Journal of Sex and Marital Therapy, 18,* 285–291.

Kaplan, H. S., Fyer, J., & Novick, A. (1982). The treatment of sexual phobias: The combined use of antipanic medication and sex therapy. *Journal of Sex and Marital Therapy, 8,* 3–28.

Kaplan, P. M. (1994). The use of serotonergic uptake inhibitors in the treatment of premature ejaculation. *Journal of Sex and Marital Therapy, 20,* 321–324.

Kinsey, A. C., Pomeroy, W. B., & Martin, C. E. (1948). *Sexual behavior in the human male.* Philadelphia: Saunders.

Kinsey, A. C., Pomeroy, W. B., Martin, C. E., & Gebhard, P. H. (1953). *Sexual behavior in the human female.* Philadelphia: Saunders.

Kolodny, R. C. (1981). Evaluating sex therapy: Process and outcome at the Masters and Johnson Institute. *Journal of Sex Research, 17,* 301–318.

Lazarus, A. (1965). The treatment of a sexually inadequate man. In L. P. Ullmann & L. Krasner (Eds.), *Case studies in behavior modification.* New York: Holt, Rinehart & Winston.

Lazarus, A. (1980). Psychological treatment of dyspareunia. In S. R. Leiblum & L. A. Pervin (Eds.), *Principles and practices of sex therapy.* New York: Guilford Press.

Leiblum, S. R., & Rosen, R. C. (Eds.). (1989). *Principles and practice of sex therapy* (2nd ed.): *Update for the 1990s.* New York: Guilford Press.

Levine, S. B. (1980). Conceptual suggestions for outcome research in sex therapy. *Journal of Sex and Marital Therapy, 6,* 102–108.

Levitt, E. E., & Mulcahy, J. J. (1995). The effect of intracavernosal injection of papaverine hydrochloride on orgasm latency. *Journal of Sex and Marital Therapy, 21,* 39–41.

LoPiccolo, J. (1978). Direct treatment of sexual dysfunction. In J. LoPiccolo & L. LoPiccolo (Eds.), *Handbook of sex therapy.* New York: Plenum Press.

LoPiccolo, J., & Steger, J. C. (1974). The Sexual Interaction Inventory: A new instrument for assessment of sexual dysfunctions. *Archives of Sexual Behavior, 3,* 585.

Maddock, J. W. (1976). Sexual health: An enrichment and treatment program. In D. H. Olson (Ed.), *Treating relationships.* Lake Mills, IA: Graphic.

Maddock, J. W., & Larson, N. R. (1995). *Incestuous families: An ecological approach to understanding and treatment.* New York: Norton.

Masters, W. H., & Johnson, V. E. (1966). *Human sexual response.* Boston: Little, Brown.

Masters, W. H., & Johnson, V. E. (1970). *Human sexual inadequacy.* Boston: Little, Brown.

Metz, M. E., & Weiss, K. E. (1992). A group therapy format for the simultaneous treatment of marital and sexual dysfunctions: A case illustration. *Journal of Sex and Marital Therapy, 18,* 173–195.

Munjack, D. J., & Oziel, L. J. (1980). *Sexual medicine and counseling in office practice.* Boston: Little, Brown.

Nichols, M. (1989). Sex therapy with lesbians, gay men, and bisexuals. In S. R. Leiblum & R. C. Rosen (Eds.), *Principles and practice of sex therapy* (2nd ed.): *Update for the 1990s.* New York: Guilford Press.

Nichols, M. (1995). Sexual desire disorder in a lesbian–feminist couple: The intersection of therapy and politics. In R. C. Rosen & S. R. Leiblum (Eds.), *Case studies in sex therapy.* New York: Guilford Press.

Olson, D. H. (1982). *Prepare–Enrich: Counselor's manual.* Minneapolis: Prepare–Enrich.

Patterson, W. M. (1993). Fluoxetine-induced sexual dysfunction. *Journal of Clinical Psychiatry, 54,* 71.

Regas, S., & Sprenkle, D. (1983). Functional family therapy and the treatment of inhibited sexual desire. *Journal of Marital and Family Therapy, 10,* 63–72.

Rosen, R. C., & Leiblum, S. R. (Eds.). (1995). *Case studies in sex therapy.* New York: Guilford Press.

Schiavi, R., Derogatis, L., Kuriansky, J., O'Connor, D., & Sharpe, L. (1979). The assessment of sexual function and marital interaction. *Journal of Sex and Marital Therapy, 5,* 169–224.

Schnarch, D. M. (1991). *Constructing the sexual crucible: An integration of sexual and marital therapy.* New York: Norton.

Schover, L. R., & Jensen, S. B. (1988). *Sexuality and chronic illness: A comprehensive approach.* New York: Guilford Press.

Semans, J. H. (1956). Premature ejaculation: A new approach. *Southern Medical Journal, 49,* 353–357.

Snyder, D. (1981). *Marital Satisfaction Inventory (MSI): Manual.* Los Angeles: Western Psychological Services.

Talmadge, L. D., & Talmadge, W. L. (1990). Sexuality assessment measures for clinical use: A review. *American Journal of Family Therapy, 18,* 80–105.

Tavris, C. (1992). *The Mismeasure of woman: Why women are not the better sex, the inferior sex, or the opposite sex.* New York: Touchstone.

Tiefer, L. (1995). *Sex is not a natural act and other essays.* Boulder, CO: Westview Press.

Trepper, T. S., & Barrett, M. J. (1989). *Systemic treatment of incest: A therapeutic handbook.* New York: Brunner/Mazel.

Wagner, G., & Kaplan, H. S. (1993). *The new injection treatment for impotence: Medical and psychological aspects.* New York: Brunner/Mazel.

Walen, S. (1980). Cognitive factors in sexual behavior. *Journal of Sex and Marital Therapy, 6,* 87–101.

Weeks, G. R., & Hof, L. (1987). *Integrating sex and marital therapy: A clinical guide.* New York: Brunner/Mazel.

Wolpe, J. (1958). *Psychotherapy by reciprocal inhibition.* Stanford, CA: Stanford University Press.

Zilbergeld, B. (1980). Alternatives to couples counseling for sex problems: Group and individual therapy. *Journal of Sex and Marital Therapy, 6,* 3–18.

Zilbergeld, B., & Ellison, C. (1980). Desire discrepancies and arousal problems in sex therapy. In S. R. Leiblum & L. A. Pervin (Eds.), *Principles and practice of sex therapy.* New York: Guilford Press.

Zilbergeld, B., & Evans, M. (1980, August). The inadequacy of Masters and Johnson. *Psychology Today,* pp. 29–43.

8

Divorce Therapy

DOUGLAS H. SPRENKLE
PILAR GONZALEZ-DOUPÉ

THE 1970s gave birth to a new form of family intervention—divorce therapy. It was necessitated not only by the large increase in the number of divorces, but also by an increased awareness that divorcing people need help uncoupling (Olson, Russell, & Sprenkle, 1980).

The family field, however, was somewhat reluctant to accept this new emphasis. As Emily Brown (1985), a pioneer in divorce intervention has written:

> Historically, the marriage centers wanted no part of divorce. Success meant keeping couples together, not helping them end their marriage. Those who saw a need for divorce counseling and tried to interest the established marriage and family agencies received a chilly response until very recently. Therefore, as with many new ideas, the innovative work in developing divorce services was done outside the mainstream, usually in small, private organizations which focused on one or more aspects of divorce. (p. 159)

Hence, the interventions described in this chapter have gained public as well as professional respectability only in the last 25 years. This might help us to understand why, although there is an enormous body of literature on divorce in general, attention to divorce therapy has been both late and underdeveloped. We may hope that the field has moved past the association of divorce with pathology and the belief that divorce therapy is "antifamily" or "antimarriage" (Sprenkle, 1985).

By 1986, there were only two published general texts on divorce therapy (Rice & Rice, 1986; Sprenkle, 1985). Books had been written about certain special topics such as mediation (Coogler, 1978; Haynes, 1981; Irving, 1980) and treating postdivorce families (Hansen, 1982; Sager et al., 1983; Visher & Visher, 1979). In addition, overview articles and book chapters on divorce therapy began appearing in the literature (Brown, 1976; Kaslow, 1981; Storm, Sprenkle, & Williamson, 1985).

By 1995, several new texts on divorce therapy appeared (Isaacs, Montalvo, & Abelsohn, 1986; Textor, 1989). Books on mediation flourished (Emery, 1994; Folberg & Milne, 1988; Marlow & Sauber, 1990), as did books in the self-help genre (Ahrons, 1994; Everett & Volgy Everett, 1994). Books also began considering the effects of divorce on special populations, such as adult children of divorce (Beal & Hochman, 1991; Berman, 1991), young children experiencing divorce and custody battles (Garrity & Baris, 1994; Warshak, 1992), men (Myers, 1989), and stepfamilies (Visher & Visher, 1988). The effects of divorce on minority populations were minimally considered (Chiriboga, Catron, & Associates, 1991). Other books also introduced the need to build new rituals for the divorced population (Ahrons, 1994; Imber-Black & Roberts, 1992; Isaacs et al., 1986).

DEFINING DIVORCE THERAPY

In its strictest sense, marital therapy can be defined as relationship treatment that focuses on maintaining, enhancing, and strengthening the marital bond. Conversely, divorce therapy can be defined as relationship treatment that focuses on decreasing the function of the marital bond, with the eventual goal of dissolving it.

Unfortunately, however, such a clear-cut dichotomy is not often found in clinical practice. Marital and divorce therapy are not so much distinct clinical entities as they are segments of a continuum that cannot be easily demarcated. One or both partners who present themselves for marital therapy frequently have desires and often behave in ways suggesting that they want out of their relationship. Conversely, divorce therapy clients are often ambiguous about uncoupling. Establishing and redefining therapeutic contracts are often major aspects of this work.

We favor a broad definition of the term "divorce therapy" and consider some definitions found in the literature to be too narrow. For example, Gurman and Kniskern (1978) have defined the goals of divorce therapy as limited to "aiding the divorced and separated partner to deal with his/her loss, resolving ambivalence, fostering autonomy, and self-esteem as a separate person" (p. 881). We conceptualize divorce therapy more broadly as helping couples and families through the stages of (1) predivorce decision making, (2) divorce restructuring, and (3) postdivorce recovery and remarriage.

In the first stage, therapists help couples to look at divorce as one alternative to relationship difficulties and appraise the consequences of such a major decision. The therapist also encourages nondestructive communication about the decision so that family members are better prepared for the major changes that will follow. In the second stage, the therapist helps family members make the legal, emotional, financial, social, and parental arrangements necessary for the transition from marriage to the postmarriage family. During the third stage, the therapist facilitates the growth of the divorced spouses as autonomous individuals with stable lifestyles and helps them to develop social relationships independent of the former love relationship (goals similar to Gurman and Kniskern's definition, as noted previously). Continuing difficulties related to parent–child relationships, sibling relationships, and custody–visitation issues often occupy the therapist during this postdivorce stage. Preparation for remarriage and facilitating the remarriage process can also be included here. Alternatively, remarriage can be considered a fourth stage, since the majority of divorcing families will experience remarriage of one or both spouses (Sprenkle, 1985).

It is important to note that these stages are more heuristic than literally descriptive of all divorces, since divorces vary widely and issues cycle and recycle among the various stages. Some individuals, for example, have no time or even the option to think about the decision to divorce, since they are abruptly abandoned (Sprenkle & Cyrus, 1983). Other persons, far into the second stage, reevaluate their decision and reconcile. Nonetheless, these stages are generally accurate and serve as useful benchmarks of the divorce process.

We describe in this chapter the types of interventions carried out in each of the stages.

THERAPY FOR PREDIVORCE DECISION MAKING (STAGE 1)

The first stage in our conceptualization is the least developed of the areas. Nathan Turner (1980, 1985) is one of the few scholars who has written specifically on the intricacies of predivorce decision making and ways in which therapists can facilitate the process. Turner has drawn upon the social–psychological decision-making theories of Janis and Mann (1977) to make some sense of the often puzzling decisional behavior of clients contemplating divorce—frequently marked by seeming irrationality, extraordinary ambivalence, regressive behavior, decisional reversals, and impulsive behavior (Turner, 1985). Turner delineates stages of predivorce decision making as well as typical coping patterns and common problems of people undergoing decisional stress. Turner recommends stress inocula-tion (Janis, 1983), emotional role playing (Janis, 1983), and the decisional balance sheet (Janis & Mann, 1977) as useful techniques for therapists during this stage of the divorce process.

Building on the work of Storm and Sprenkle (1982), who recommend that this stage calls for a high emphasis on conjoint therapy and a low emphasis on both individual and family therapy, Salts (1985) offers a variety of helpful suggestions for couple work. She demonstrates how techniques of circular questioning can be utilized to clarify the clients' commitment to the marriage. For couples with serious doubts about continuing the relationship, Salts recommends a decision-making contract that enables them to determine whether their needs can be met *within* the marriage (not necessarily *by* the marriage).

Everett and Volgy Everett (1994) delineate two types of separations: (1) an experimental separation to diffuse conflict and test the future of the relationship, and (2) a separation that represents an eventual transition into divorce. Experimental, or structured, separation is sometimes used with couples who do not appear to be benefiting from marriage counseling but who are doubtful that divorce is the best alternative. Different models of structured separation are reviewed by Granvold (1983). Most require a written contract that specifies the ground rules of the separation. Time limits are set (typically 4 weeks to a year), and interaction is structured in such a way as to maintain a balance between "absence makes the heart grow fonder" and "out of sight, out of mind" (Granvold, 1983, p. 407). All of the models require couples to attend therapy, usually once a week, and the therapist attempts to create a more rational environment for decision making. Everett and Volgy Everett (1994) prescribe a 7-point guide to planning a healthy physical separation for both the parents and the children.

Since the few follow-up studies of this method suggest a high rate of marital termination (Greene, Lee, & Lustig, 1973; Toomin, 1972), it is important to match the technique to the needs of the couple. Granvold (1983) offers some guidelines for assessing whether this technique is either premature or too late for a couple.

THERAPY FOR DIVORCE RESTRUCTURING (STAGE 2)

Ideally, if the couple's decision to divorce has been facilitated by a therapist who has created a mutually acceptable decision and hence has toned down the intensive emotions surrounding the divorce, then the couple is ready to explore alternative ways to carry out this decision (Salts, 1985). The decision to divorce entails the legal, emotional, financial, social, and parental arrangements necessary to make the shift from marriage to single status

(Storm & Sprenkle, 1982). This is the time of inordinate stress because of the multitude of changes that often occur—moving, lowering standards of living, shifting parental arrangements, changing social networks, and so on. The difficulty in this stage depends, in part, on the process used to arrive at the decision to divorce. If one spouse feels callously "dumped" and is desperately "holding on," restructuring will be more difficult. Ideally, conjoint couple therapy, with family therapy to deal with children's issues, is preferable here. Of course, people who have been "left" will often first seek help at the time of physical separation, and even the most engaging therapist will have difficulty getting the other spouse to participate (Salts, 1985).

Often, children are neglected emotionally during this period, because parents are overwhelmed by their own needs (Salts, 1985). Since there is research evidence that children's postdivorce adjustment is directly related to the parents' own adjustment (Wallerstein & Kelly, 1980), therapists may gain leverage to encourage partners to continue working on their own emotional issues by informing them of the benefits for the children (Kaslow, 1984; Salts, 1985). Fortunately, there are a variety of resources for the professional (Cantor & Drake, 1983; Gardner, 1976; Emery, 1994; Hetherington, Cox, & Cox, 1981; Kurdek, 1983; Nichols, 1984, 1985; Stuart & Abt, 1981; Wallerstein & Kelly, 1980) and for parents themselves (Francke, 1983; Newman, 1981; Oakland, 1984) to help with parenting and children's issues. There are also several excellent books written for children (Gardner, 1971, 1978, 1982; Rofes, 1982). In recent years, there has also been a push to involve fathers more in their children's lives after the divorce (Ahrons, 1994; Everett & Volgy Everett, 1994; Furstenberg & Cherlin, 1991).

The form of intervention most directly related to restructuring is divorce mediation. Although mediation has been widely accepted in other aspects of life (e.g., labor disputes), it has been only recently applied to divorce, as Cohen (1985) notes in his interesting history of divorce mediation. The movement arose as a reaction to the destructive dimensions of the adversary legal system and was made possible by a confluence of social, economic, and legal changes, including the widespread acceptance of no-fault divorce. Mediation does not replace the legal system but attempts to circumvent its more negative aspects. The mediation process is typically present centered and time limited, and focuses on the goal of reaching agreement on such crucial issues as custody, visitation, and finances. Typically, the end product is a nonlegal written agreement by the couple, which must then be formalized by the attorneys.

Early mediation services developed as an extension of ongoing services provided by professionally staffed counseling units, called "conciliation courts," that were attached administratively to a judicial jurisdiction. Originally, these services were designed to provide marriage counseling, focusing on the reconciliation of couples who had filed for divorce or were considering it (Cohen, 1985). As divorce rates began to climb, conciliation courts expanded their services to include the mediation of custody and visitation disputes. Non–court-related mediators are more likely to include financial mediation among their services. There are only a small number of full-time private practice mediators; more typically, mental health professionals provide divorce mediation in addition to other services. Lawyers also provide this service, but typically continue to practice more traditional law while offering mediation to selected clients (Cohen, 1985). An interdisciplinary team approach involving attorneys and therapists has also been advocated (Bernstein, 1977; Kaslow & Steinberg, 1981). The rationale is that therapists cannot keep up with the complex issues related to property, pensions, taxes, support, and the like, and attorneys are often not trained to deal with the complex emotional issues surrounding divorce. Fortunately, therapists desiring to learn more about mediation have a variety of books to consult (Coogler, 1978; Emery, 1994; Folberg & Milne, 1988; Haynes, 1981; Irving, 1980; Marlow & Sauber, 1990; Saposnek, 1983; Shapiro & Caplan, 1983).

The role of the mediator or therapist in facilitating custody decisions has received considerable attention in recent years. Typically, mediated divorces are much more likely to result in joint custody arrangements than nonmediated divorces, and valuable resources are now available for mediator/therapists who wish to learn more about such options. Howell and Toepke (1984) summarize the joint custody laws for the 50 states. Folberg (1991) offers the most recent comprehensive collection of papers on this theme. Marlow and Sauber (1990), in their comprehensive handbook on the theory and practice of mediation, address the issue of power imbalances in mediation, paying particular attention to the needs of women and children in mediation. Volgy and Everett (1985) offer five criteria that may be used to determine whether couples are adaptive enough to make joint custody work. These authors stress that joint custody, like mediation, is not to be viewed as a panacea, and therapists cannot be blind to contraindications to these approaches.

THERAPY FOR POSTDIVORCE RECOVERY AND REMARRIAGE (STAGE 3)

Following initial restructuring, the therapist can begin to focus more on individual issues, such as coping with loneliness, regaining self-confidence, and rebuilding social relationships (Storm & Sprenkle, 1982).

Unless there are continuing problems with parent–child relationships or custody–visitation issues, or unless remarriage issues are the focus, the individual is the unit of treatment during this stage (Storm & Sprenkle, 1982). The therapist's goals include helping the individual to develop an autonomous lifestyle, altering self-destructive cognitions about the divorce and the self, and mobilizing resources to achieve personal goals and ambitions. M. D. Brown (1985) demonstrates how a structural–strategic approach may be utilized with such individuals to help create "new realities" for the recently divorced.

More has been written about group and educational approaches than about techniques for therapists working with individuals. A variety of such programs and their goals are reviewed by Storm et al. (1985). Typically, a group format is used to normalize the divorce experience and to generate support and acceptance. Groups are also typically less expensive than individual therapy. Formats include short, didactic educational emphases, skills training, group therapy, or combinations of these.

Group leaders, as well as individual therapists, often suggest bibliotherapy for divorced persons at this time. Among the most popular self-help books are those by Ahrons (1994), Everett and Volgy Everett (1994), Kayser (1993), Vaughn (1986), Fisher (1981) and Bernard and Hackney (1983). Older but still well-received works are those by Johnson (1977), Krantzler (1974), Smoke (1976), and Weiss (1975).

Imber-Black and Roberts (1992) speak to the difficulty of life-cycle transitions such as divorce that often go unmarked. They encourage the creation of new life-cycle rituals, such as redecorating the house to suit the person's own tastes and inviting people to a party, or having an anniversary party to celebrate the divorce date as the first day of new singlehood. Other rituals, such as holiday celebrations, birthdays, mealtimes, and good-byes, which can be made difficult by divorce, are also addressed.

The single-parent phase following divorce is often problematic, and Weiss (1979) offers a text that is valuable for mental health professionals and the single parent. Both Weltner (1982) and Isaacs (1982) offer structural family therapy models for single-parent families. Eno (1985) addresses a greatly neglected area of divorce therapy literature: sibling relationships in families of divorce and ways in which these relationships can be affected therapeutically.

Perhaps the most impressive divorce intervention literature is in the area of the transition from divorce to remarriage. Crosbie-Burnett and Ahrons (1985) offer therapists a detailed guide for the issues and problems families face at this time. Ahrons (1979, 1994) has coined the term "binuclear family" to describe the context in which remarriage occurs. Therapists must frequently dispel courtship expectations and the myth that the remarried family will replace the nuclear family. One of Ahron's theoretical tenets is the boundary ambiguity inherent in remarried families and the greater need for boundary permeability than is the case for nuclear families. Such issues as movement between households, exchange of money, and shared decision making between "coparents" (ex-spouses) reflect this need for permeability and also underscore the potential for difficulty. Role ambiguity in remarried families is often the "twin" of boundary ambiguity. Therapists must help clients define roles, while encouraging them to be flexible (Sprenkle, 1985).

The classic text on treating the remarried family is that by Sager et al. (1983). These authors prefer the term "remarried (REM) family" and examine it on three levels: "family systems," "life cycle," and "intrapsychic." Other important recent texts include those by Hansen (1982) and Visher and Visher (1979, 1982, 1988). Visher and Visher (1988) delineate with text and charts the therapeutic needs of stepfamilies who come to therapy. The important area of the impact of divorce on the extended family is explored in a collection of articles by Fisher (1982).

DIVORCE THEORY

Kaslow (1981) has written that what therapists need is not simply a new technique for doing divorce therapy (as virtually any existing therapeutic modality may be applied), but a deeper understanding of the phenomenon of divorce. Similarly, Gurman and Kniskern (1981) have written that there is little that is strategically or technically unique to divorce therapy itself. This section briefly reviews the major theoretical approaches that have been taken to understand the phenomenon of divorce, in the hope that they will increasingly affect the work of practitioners.

Textor (1989) developed 10 goals for divorce therapy, including cognitive and emotional acceptance of the finality of divorce, taking personal responsibility, social networking, developing personal health, negotiating the legal process, and assisting children's adjustment.

The theory most widely used to explain the causes of divorce (on the individual as opposed to the societal level) has been social exchange theory. It has been used by Levinger (1976), Spanier and Lewis (1980), and other scholars to explain how individuals assess the costs and rewards associated with both staying in and terminating a relationship. In Levinger's (1976) highly influential formulation, people remain in a relationship on the basis of an unconscious accounting of three factors: (1) their attractions to the relationship, (2) barriers they perceive to divorce, and (3) comparisons they make between their current relationship and the alternatives they perceive are available to them. If internal attractions to the marriage and barrier forces to divorce become distinctly weaker than alternative attractions, the consequence is marital breakup.

The sociological version of crisis theory, originally developed by Hill (1949) and others, has been used by family stress researchers to describe, predict, and explain when a stressor event will cause a crisis or disorganization in a family and also to predict the extent of the crisis (Raschke, 1982). Hill's (1949) "ABCX" theory posits that A, the stressor or event, is mediated by B, the crisis meeting resources of the family, and C, the definition of the situation by the family, to produce X, the crisis (Raschke, 1982). Sprenkle and Cyrus (1983), for example, have utilized this basic scheme to predict the relative level of stress experienced by persons abruptly abandoned by their spouses.

Other forms of crisis theory were developed during the 1970s by clinically oriented researchers to describe the developmental process of adjustment to divorce. These writers generally view divorce as a series of overlapping stages based on the psychological–emotional consequences of separation and divorce (Raschke, 1982). For example, several writers (Froiland & Hozeman, 1977; Weisman, 1975) describe the divorce process as analogous to the grief process articulated by Kübler-Ross (1969). Smart (1977) has used Erikson's (1963) "eight stages of man" typology as a model for the divorce process. Other frequently cited stage theories are those of Bohannan (1970), Kessler (1975), Weiss (1975), and Brown (1976). Everett and Volgy (1994) describe a 14-stage model of the divorce process, which is the most comprehensive to date.

Theses crisis theories that conceive of divorce in stages must be envisaged more as theoretical models than as full-fledged theories with interrelated propositions. Nonetheless, they do have considerable descriptive and explanatory power for the process of adjustment (Raschke, 1982). Several useful tables that compare the various models are found in Price-Bonham and Balswick (1980) and Salts (1979).

KEY CONCEPTS

Adjustment. Basically, the process of adapting to the difficulties and challenges both of ending a marriage and of beginning a new lifestyle (Spanier & Casto, 1979). Beginning with Goode (1956, p. 19) and Waller (1967, p. xxi), and continuing to Kitson and Raschke (1981, p. 16), there have been a variety of influential definitions of divorce adjustment. Divorce adjustment is considered constructive when a divorced person is able to develop a lifestyle and identity independent of the previous marriage and the ex-spouse, and to function satisfactorily in the new identity and lifestyle (Ahrons, 1994; Isaacs et al., 1986; Kitson & Raschke, 1981). Sutton and Sprenkle (1985) have postulated 10 criteria for long-term constructive adjustment to divorce and have developed a scale that is being used to measure the perceptions of therapists (Sutton, 1983), divorced people (Cantrell, 1985), attorneys (Sprenkle & Cantrell, 1986), and clergypersons (Wong, 1986) about constructive divorce. Holley (1980) has prepared an analysis of existing divorce adjustment measures. Isaacs et al. (1986) consider longitudinal aspects of postdivorce adjustment, specifically for the custodial parent and children. Ahrons (1994, p. 77) speaks to the five transitions inherent in the divorce process: the decision, the announcement, the separation, the formal divorce, and the aftermath.

Attachment. The bond that frequently persists between partners following separation and divorce, even after the "erosion of love" (Weiss, 1975). Kitson (1982) believes that attachment is the primary cause of emotional distress experienced by those divorcing and that the failure to "let go" can hinder adjustment. Ahrons (1980) indicates, however, that one needs to differentiate between "normal" attachment, based on realistic caring and friendship, and "pathological" holding on. Thompson and Spanier (1983) have developed an 11-item scale for attachment (Acceptance of Marital Termination, or AMT), developed on the basis of previous work by Kitson (1982).

Binuclear family. A term coined by Ahrons (1979, 1994) to describe the organization of the nuclear family after divorce into two interrelated households or two nuclei. Ahrons argues that although there are two households, there is one family system, and the term holds whether or not the households have equal importance in the child's life experience. The term is more inclusive than "remarried (REM) family" or "stepfamily" but less inclusive than "REM suprasystem" (see listed entries for these terms).

Blended family. A synonym, along with "reconstituted family," for the postdivorce family. These terms are less widely used today, because they do not make sufficiently clear the distinction between the postdivorce and the nuclear family. The connotation that parts of two previous nuclear families can be "blended" or "reconstituted" into something approximating the nuclear family is misleading. See also Binuclear family; Remarried (REM) family; Stepfamily.

Custody. A term used by the courts to describe a variety of arrangements for the raising and rearing of children after divorce. The most common custody arrangement has been and continues to be "sole custody," which typically means that the children live with a "custodial" parent, and the other ("noncustodial") parent has "visitation" time. With this arrangement, the custodial parent has full authority and full responsibility to make medical, educational, and religious decisions, as well as to give consent for a minor child to marry or enter the armed forces (Association of Family and Conciliation Courts, 1982). Until the 1980s, most other arrangements were called "divided custody" or "alternating custody." In such arrangements, each parent has physical custody and legal authority for a specified period of time (e.g., alternate years, or school year vs. summer). "Divided custody" (or, more commonly, "split custody") is also used to describe the arrangement whereby one parent has custody of some of the children, and the other parent has custody of the remaining children. Although the term "joint custody" is sometimes used to describe a divided custody arrangement, the term typically goes beyond it. The typical hallmark of joint custody is that both partners have *shared decision-making authority* regarding all important matters concerning the children, such as educational, medical, and religious decisions. The terms also implies that both parents have the *responsibility* for raising the children and carrying out such tasks as guiding and disciplining them. The mother and father are often referred to as "coparents" and the process as "coparenting" (Galper, 1978). The granting of joint custody does *not* imply a fixed arrangement for physical custody. Typically, it allows parents to plan creatively for the residential arrangements that they think make the most sense. Sometimes the court will determine physical custody arrangements, and joint custody may de facto not be that much different from sole custody with visitation. This is sometimes called "joint legal" to distinguish it from "joint physical" custody. Nonetheless, the nonresidential parent in a joint custody arrangement, even of this nature, typically feels less demeaned and more "involved." The term "shared custody" has been offered to describe the arrangement whereby parents share major decisions, but the residential parent makes day-to-day decisions.

Divorce rates. A number of different methods are used to report on the incidence of divorce. One can, of course, simply count the number of couples divorcing each year. For example, this figure, in 1994, was 1,191,000 (Singh, Mathews, Clarke, Yannicos, & Smith, 1995). Because the population is increasing, however, this figure alone does not give one a "rate" that can be compared with previous years. The least satisfactory divorce "rate" is that frequently offered by the popular press, which gives a ratio of divorces decreed in a particular year to marriages performed in that year. For example, in 1994, there were about 1.2 million divorces and 2.4 million marriages, and hence the marriage–divorce ratio was 50%. This is a misleading "rate," because few of those divorces came from the marriages contracted in 1994. The vast majority came from marriages started in earlier years (Reiss, 1980). The "crude" divorce rate is a better alternative. It is the number of divorces occurring each year for each 1,000 persons in the population. The crude divorce rate for 1994 was 4.6, which means that 4.6 out of every 1,000 men, women, and children in the United States divorced in 1994. The "refined" divorce rate was 20.5. This means that if a random sample were taken of any 1,000 marriages in the United States in 1994, approximately 20.5 (21) of them would have ended in divorce.

The difficulty with both the crude and refined divorce rates is that they do not make any assumptions about future years. For this reason, demographers have also devised a "cohort" approach that tracks the percentage of marriages that have actually ended in divorce for marriages that began each year (e.g., for marriages beginning in 1964, 29.7% of these marriages had resulted in divorce by 1980). Using the technique called "demographic projection," the cohort approach also predicts the percentage of these marriages that will eventually end in divorce. For example, 42.2% of marriages commencing in 1964 are projected to eventually end in divorce (Weed, 1980). Utilizing these techniques, Glick (1984) projects that 49% of those born between 1946 and 1955 will dissolve their first marriage.

Leaver and left. The perceptions individuals have of themselves concerning whether they are the initiators or noninitiators of the divorce. In his popular text, Fisher (1981) uses the terms "dumper" and "dumpee." These terms are described here as "perceptions," since the individual who thinks he or she is being left at the time of the divorce may have been involved in subtle or not-so-subtle "leaving" behavior for many years. Nonetheless, typically, the experience at the time of divorce is more painful for the one "left," since he or she feels out of control or emotionally abandoned. Utilizing his Divorce Adjustment Scale, Fisher (1976) found that after 1 year, "left" spouses attained a level of adjustment equal to that of "leavers" at the time of the overt break in their relationships. Typically, however, a "leaver" experiences more pain during a marriage, or at least during the period prior to the decision to terminate the relationship (Sprenkle & Cyrus, 1983).

Mediation. A specific type of intervention by a trained therapist designed to help divorcing couples in conflict over custody, visitation, spouse and child support, and issues related to the economic settlement. It also can be utilized to address postdivorce disputes related to remarriage, visitation, and child support issues (Cohen, 1985; Folberg & Milne, 1988; Marlow & Sauber, 1990). Described in more detail elsewhere in this chapter, mediation can be viewed as an alternative to self-help, on the one hand, and litigation on the other. Rather than being an advocate for a particular point of view, the mediator(s) is a neutral facilitator who helps the couple reach a consensual agreement around disputed issues. The process does not circumvent the legal system, since mediated agreements are usually subsequently written up in legal language by lawyers. Nonetheless, it is envisaged as a constructive alternative to the adversarial nature of the legal process.

No-fault divorce laws. Basically, laws that obviate the necessity for establishing a "guilty" and "innocent" party in a divorce and allow divorce on the basis of "irreconcilable differences" or following a separation for a specified period of time. Beginning with California's groundbreaking legislation in 1970, some form of no-fault divorce legislation has been adopted by all the states. No-fault divorce has not eliminated the adversarial process, since custody and property settlements can still be contested. Nonetheless, no-fault laws have resulted in a savings of time and legal expense, as well as eliminating a degree of shame from the courtroom.

Remarried (REM) family. The term of choice in the classic work *Treating the Remarried Family* (Sager et al., 1983). It is defined as a family created by the marriage (or living together in one domicile) of two partners, one or both of whom have been previously married, then divorced or widowed. There may or may not be children from prior marriages who visit or reside with them. The adult couple and the children comprise the REM family system (Sager et al., 1983, p. 3). Since children are not *required,* the REM family presumably need not be a stepfamily, even if one or both of its members are stepparents. As defined, the REM family could be a part of a binuclear family. See also Binuclear family; Stepfamily.

REM suprasystem. Another term used by Sager et al. (1983) to describe the network of people and relationships created through a prior divorce and remarriage. It includes the former spouses of one or both the REM adults (alive or dead), the families of origin of all of the adults, the REM couple themselves, and the children of each of these adults. Hence, grandparents, aunts, uncles, cousins, and stepgrandparents are included. Bohannan (1971) has used the term "divorce chains" to describe this entourage (Sager et al., 1983, p. 3).

Separation. A term that is used in a variety of ways. In its most informal sense, a couple is considered to be "separated" when they are not living together due to conflict or dissatisfaction. The term is typically not applied to couples living apart because of vocational choice (as in commuter marriages) or because of hospitalization, military service, or the like. The term "legal separation" applies to a formalized legal agreement that regulates such matters as custody, visitation, finances, and residential access. Most legal separations are preliminaries to divorce, although a small minority are entered into in lieu of divorce by persons for whom divorce is not a viable alternative. The extent of informal separations is not known, although they are more frequent than divorces. Weiss (1975) has written that "almost certainly not more than half of all separations go on to divorce" (p. 11).

The term "structured separation" refers to a therapeutic technique used for couples who are undecided about divorce. It has been described previously in this chapter.

Single-parent family. Once a popular term for the postdivorce family prior to remarriage; however, it is now being criticized, because it connotes noninvolvement of the nonresidential, generally noncustodial parent (Ahrons, 1979, 1994; Bernard & Hackney, 1983). Ahrons believes that although the terms "single parent" is appropriate, the "family" of the children following a divorce should be conceptualized as a "binuclear family" (listed).

Stages of divorce. A number of authors have postulated that divorce is typically experienced as the unfolding of certain stages. A number of major theories have been noted previously in this chapter (see section "Divorce Theory"). Although stages underlying these theories have considerable descriptive appeal and are heuristic for the therapist, stage categories have not been empirically confirmed.

Stepfamily. According to Visher and Visher (1979, p. 4), a family in which at least one partner of a couple is a stepparent. The only difference between a stepfamily and an REM family is that the former requires at least one partner to have previously had children. Like that REM family, the stepfamily could be a part of a binuclear family. Visher and Visher (1979, p. 19) emphasize that the stepfamily has five structural characteristics distinguishing it from the nuclear family: (1) There is a biological parent elsewhere; (2) virtually all members have recently sustained a primary relationship loss; (3) the relationship between one adult (parent) and a child predates the marriage; (4) a child is a member of more than one household; and (5) one adult (stepparent) is not legally related to a child (stepchild). See also Binuclear family and Remarried family.

TEACHING TOOLS AND TECHNIQUES

Values Clarification Exercises

Divorce is a topic that is replete with value implications for both the instructor and the students. There are a variety of values clarification exercises that also serve as excellent "warm-up" tasks for classes or groups. On an overhead projector or in a handout, an instructor can do a sentence-completion exercise with the following sentence stems: "Divorce means . . . "; "The best thing about divorce is . . . "; "The worst thing about divorce is . . . "; "My children will react to my divorce by . . . "; "My parents, other relatives, church, friends, employer, and colleagues will react to my divorce by . . . "; and so on.

Another exercise is to say a series of statements about divorce and ask class members to go to one of four corners in the room designated "strongly agree," "agree," "disagree," and "strongly disagree." The statements might include such opinions as "I believe that divorce is a sensible solution to many unhappy marriages," or "Divorce is harder on children than on the divorcing parents." Once the group is divided into these categories, the instructor can also stimulate debates by asking people in the opposite corners to give rationales for their "strongly agreeing" or "strongly disagreeing."

Still another exercise is to draw an imaginary line across the room that represents a continuum of opinions about divorce. Class members are then asked to position themselves on the line between two opposites, such as "acceptable–sinful," "selfish–caring," "failure–success," "relief–trauma." Once class members have positioned themselves on the continuum, they are asked to discuss with another person why they placed themselves at the point they did. They may then be asked to move to the point on the continuum where they would "like to be." This move may be debriefed by asking them to discuss what would have to happen to make this change possible.

Grid Balance Sheet

The grid balance sheet is one of the techniques described by Turner (1985) in his discussion of divorce decision making and is adapted from the work of Janis (1983, p. 171). Students are asked to imagine that they themselves are anticipating divorce. Either on an overhead projector or through a handout, they are asked to consider two columns called "positive anticipations" and "negative anticipations." A grid is formed utilizing the following "rows": "tangible gains and losses for self"; "tangible gains and losses for others"; "self-approval or disapproval"; and "social approval or disapproval." A separate sheet is made out for each major alternative, such as "remaining married" or "trial separation." The procedure requires the decision maker to investigate carefully all alternatives and systematically consider the major gains and risks that might be otherwise overlooked (Turner, 1985).

Outcome Psychodrama

The instructor can model the psychodrama procedure for the class through either the use of a videotape or a role-play simulation with class volunteers. A person simulating decisional conflict concerning divorce is asked to assume one side of the ambivalence, for example, "Let us say you have decided to get a divorce." Turner (1985) describes the procedure:

> The therapist leads the person through all of the consequences of that decision. "You are now telling your husband/children. What are you saying? How does that feel?" The client is led further. "You are now in the court. What are you feeling as you look over at your partner across the room/as you leave the courtroom as a newly single person?" The sequence progresses. "It is now six months after the divorce. What are you doing? What do you feel? How much support are you receiving?"
>
> The process is then repeated taking the other polarity. You have decided to stay in your marriage. You are telling your husband of that decision. "What are you saying? How does that feel?"
>
> By giving the client the freedom to fantasize about the consequences of both outcomes, there is the opportunity to clarify thoughts and feelings and to assess the emotional readiness for a given decision. (pp. 35–36)

Following the second drama, the instructor can debrief the experience with the volunteers and then with the class itself.

We have also adapted this exercise for use in divorce therapy. Ambivalent clients are asked to "picture" (fantasize) themselves acting out each decision, being aware of their feelings as they do so. Through this focused fantasy, clients are encouraged to get in touch with their affect related both to choosing divorce and to staying married.

Model of the Divorce Process

Class members are presented with various models of the divorce process, such as those by Kitson (1992), E. M. Brown (1976), Kessler (1975), and

Salts (1979). Class members are then challenged to develop a diagram of their conceptualization of the process and to produce a written commentary explaining it. They are free to draw upon the models developed by others but are also encouraged to add something that is original. Although this task is challenging, many report it to be the highlight of their course in divorce therapy. Class members also are asked to explicate their therapeutic implications of the various components of the model.

B. Fisher's Building Blocks

In his popular and highly readable self-help book for persons going through divorce, *Rebuilding: When Your Relationship Ends,* B. Fisher (1981) presents a series of building blocks that one must "assemble" on the "ascent" to divorce recovery. Each of these blocks constitutes a chapter in his book. Each chapter ends with a quiz that a divorcing person can use to assess his or her own progress. Although this is not a book for therapists, each of these chapters has many therapeutic implications. Class members can be asked to make a presentation that describes a particular building block and explicate the therapeutic implication of the topic under consideration (e.g., dealing with anger, friendships, sexuality, one's self-concept).

Divorce Interviews

Class members are assigned to interview one or more persons who have experienced divorce. Prior to the interview, they are warned that sometimes such interviews elicit powerful emotions, and they are given steps to take should this occur. If two interviews are possible, students can be encouraged to interview one person who was the "leaver" in the marriage and another who perceives him- or herself as the "left." In the case of the former, questions can be asked about the decision to divorce, utilizing the Levinger (1976) model described earlier (see the "Divorce Therapy" section). If students have developed their own model of the divorce process (see teaching strategy on "Model of the Divorce Process"), the interview can be structured around the model. It is important for the interviewer to ask whether the interviewee was engaged in divorce therapy and what was useful or not useful about the experience. If the interviewee did not seek therapy, what was his or her rationale, and what kinds of help (if any) facilitated his or her adjustment?

Visits to and from Representatives of the Legal System

Following an orientation, students can be asked to visit divorce court, preferably during a contested custody hearing. If possible, interviewing a divorce judge can be instructive. Inviting a divorce lawyer and/or a divorce mediator to class is often helpful and can be stimulating if they appear simultaneously on a panel.

"Ripple Effects" Exercise

Another exercise is designed to show the number of people who are affected by each divorce. A series of concentric circles is drawn on a blackboard or presented on an overhead projector or handout. The inner-most circle contains the word "individual," and in progressive concentric circles are the terms (one in each circle) "marital couple," "nuclear family," "extended family," "friends," "work associates," and "professional helpers."

Members of the class are to list the numbers of people affected by each "typical" divorce as its "ripple effect" is felt. The exercise demonstrates that although there are approximately 1.2 million divorces each year, the number of people affected directly or indirectly by these divorces constitutes a fairly large percentage of the population of the United States.

RESEARCH ISSUES

There has been much more research on divorce in general than on interventions related to divorce. In her decade review, White (1990) found that the research on divorce done in the 1980s used bigger and better data sets, used more appropriate analytic techniques, and garnered a growing body of conclusive empirical findings in the areas of demographic and life-course factors. However, there are still areas that are seen as needing more rigorous research: (1) family processes that contribute to high rates of divorce; (2) the dynamics of marriage, including mate selection, and benefits to marriage; (3) sex differences in the divorce process; (4) theoretical development; and (5) cross-cultural and historical research. Kitson and Morgan (1990), in their decade review, note several marked changes in the divorce literature, among them, (1) the growing recognition that divorce adjustment is a process, and (2) improved methodology. However, they, too, indicate new directions for future research: (1) better understanding of the causal relationship between divorce and its outcomes; (2) more representative sampling besides the standard white, middle-class, female population; (3) more longitudinal or panel studies on divorce outcome; (4) better quality of research instruments; (5) more sophisticated statistical analysis; (6) cross-cultural research on adjustment; and (7) a more multidimensional view of the consequences of divorce.

Prior to 1980, there were few available studies on remarriage and stepfamilies. Coleman and Ganong (1990), in their decade review, assert that the 1980s saw an incredible increase in empirical research done on remarriage and stepfamilies. However, there are still areas that remain understudied: (1) demographic characteristics of stepfamilies; (2) relationships within stepfamilies; (3) research on stepchildren; and (4) financial aspects of stepfamilies. In addition, they called for greater research and theory developments in the 1990s, including (1) more varied research methods and study designs, including descriptive, qualitative designs and longitudinal, single-case designs; (2) greater multidisciplinary collaboration between stepfamily clinicians and researchers; (3) more explicit use of frameworks and theoretical assumptions; and (4) greater theory-building efforts.

Turning to intervention research, in 1983, Sprenkle and Storm reviewed 22 empirical investigations of divorce intervention. They reported studies in the areas of mediation (n = 6), conciliation courts counseling (n = 4), consumer evaluation studies (n = 2), divorce groups (n = 6), structured separation techniques (n = 2), and marriage counseling with divorce as an unintended outcome (n = 2). Only the first two groups of studies utilized sound methodological procedures. Hence, results outside the areas of mediation and conciliation courts counseling were considered quite tentative. Fortunately, 13 studies did use replicable standardized treatments.

Sprenkle and Storm (1983) noted that the mediation studies used the most impressive designs and had equally impressive results. Until 1986, divorce mediation research did not include examinations of the mediation of property settlement and child support, although private mediators, in particular, were frequently facilitating agreements on such matters. In the last decade, several comprehensive guidebooks have addressed the issue of mediating property, taxes, and child support (Folberg & Milne, 1988; Marlow & Sauber, 1990). The field still awaits research on this type of mediation.

In Sprenkle and Storm's (1983) review, in all but one of the mediation studies (Irving, Benjamin, Bohm, & MacDonald, 1981), mediation was compared with the traditional adversary method of resolving disputes. In these direct comparisons, mediation produced the following results: (1) a considerably higher rate of pretrial stipulations or agreements; (2) a significantly higher level of satisfaction with the agreements reached; (3) a dramatic reduction in the amount of litigation following the final order; (4) an increase in joint custody arrangements; and (5) a decrease in public expenses, such as custody studies and court costs. However, one study (Pearson & Thoennes, 1982) suggests that attorney's fees may not be reduced by mediation (Sprenkle & Storm, 1983, p. 140).

The studies of conciliation court counseling utilized reconciliation as the major dependent variable. They showed a significantly greater number of reconciliations in experimental groups than in no-treatment control groups, but the follow-ups were completed at only 3, 4, and 9 weeks posttreatment. Hence, although these studies were otherwise generally well designed, only short-term results were reported.

The two studies of consumers of court-related counseling centers (P. Brown & Manela, 1977; Lee, 1979) indicated global satisfaction rates roughly similar to those in other uncontrolled studies of marital and family therapy.

Furthermore, two studies (Greene et al., 1973; Toomin, 1972) investigated structured separation techniques. Of the couples in these investigations, 44% and 67%, respectively, went on to divorce following structured separation. However, severe methodological problems in the two studies and the fact that there is no "base divorce rate" for those who are participating in conjoint marital therapy (Gurman, Kniskern, & Pinsof, 1986) make meaningful interpretation of these results difficult.

The studies of divorce education–adjustment groups indicated that such groups appeared to be helpful in aiding divorcing individuals to feel greater mastery of their environment and to gain more self-confidence (Sprenkle & Storm, 1983). In addition, at least short-term gains in measures of self-esteem and divorce adjustment were common outcomes. Typically ranging from 4 to 10 sessions, these group approaches included didactic and experiential components.

Since the publication of the Sprenkle and Storm's decade review (1983), there have been many more articles written on divorce interventions, including case reports, presentation of models, and empirical evaluations (Lee, Picard, & Blain, 1994). In their review article, Lee et al. (1994) critique published studies on interventions for divorce adjustment on the basis of their findings, methodological sophistication, and psychometric adequacy. The authors also delineate three major foci of interventions: (1) adult-focused treatment, (2) child-focused treatment, and (3) family-focused treatment. Overall, these writers conclude that there has only been modest improvement in the methodology of divorce intervention research since the Sprenkle and Storm (1983) review.

By 1986, none of the studies of divorce therapy had investigated the effects of treatment on the children of divorce, nor had a single study included children as participants in the therapy experience. Since then, investigations including children's responses to divorce have been considered crucial for public policy as well as clinical reasons (Gurman et al., 1986). In their methodological review, Lee et al. (1994) report more intervention studies in which children are included, but much more research is needed. Almost all of the studies they reported were on groups for children rather than children in family therapy.

To the best of our knowledge, there is still very little outcome research on interventions related to remarriage or single-parent families, in spite of the excellent books on theory and technique in this area (Sager et al., 1983; Visher & Visher, 1979, 1982, 1988). One notable exception is the Stepfamily Association of America sponsored study on consumer satisfaction with counseling around stepfamily issues reported by Pasley, Rhoden, Visher, and Visher (in press).

The field of divorce intervention is still empirically underdeveloped (Lee et al., 1994). Aside from the firm conclusion that the mediation of custody and visitation disputes are preferable to the traditional adversary process, there is no strong database on which to conclude that any other form of divorce intervention except for group treatments is superior to receiving no treatment at all. There is no controlled research about what is probably the most widely practice form of divorce therapy, namely, individuals or couples going to therapists for help in getting through the trauma of divorce. In short, basic controlled research on the process and outcome of divorce therapy has yet to be done (Sprenkle & Storm, 1983, p. 255).

Finally, there is a need to control for client variables that theoretically may have relationships with divorce outcome. Specifically, the stages of the dissolution process should be controlled in future research, because it is unwise to lump together persons in crises immediately following separation with subjects who are many months into the single life. It is also conceivable that there will be significant differences in the nature of adjustment experience between those who perceive themselves as the "leaver" and those who see themselves as the "left" in the divorce (Sprenkle & Storm, 1983). Bray and Jouriles (1995) review the small amount of literature there is on the long-term efficacy of marital therapy in preventing marital separation and divorce. It will behoove investigators to compare various forms of treatment. For example, no one has examined the results of individual versus conjoint versus family treatment for persons going through divorce. On theoretical grounds, Storm and Sprenkle (1982) have argued that specific units of treatment (individual, conjoint, family, and group) are most appropriate for persons in certain stages of the dissolution process, but research is urgently needed to verify such speculation.

KEY BOOKS, CHAPTERS, AND ARTICLES[1]

Adjustment for the Divorced Person

Everett, C., & Volgy Everett, S. (1994). *Healthy divorce.* San Franciso, CA: Jossey–Bass.

This book offers an alternative way of viewing divorce: that it *is* possible for both parents and children to maintain emotional stability and a sense of security—if the process has been conducted as a *healthy* divorce. With this encouraging note, they outline 14 stages of divorce and address such tough issues as how to tell your children you're getting a divorce, how to plan a separation, and how to cope with

[1]This section is an expanded version of (1) "Divorce and Divorce Therapy: An Annotated Bibliography" by R. G. Cantrell (1985), in D. H. Sprenkle (Ed.), *Divorce Therapy*, Binghamton, NY: Haworth, and (2) "Divorce Therapy" by D. H. Sprenkle (1986), in F. P. Piercy and D. H. Sprenkle (Eds.), *Family Therapy Sourcebook*, New York: Guilford Press. Used by permission.

your feelings of anger, grief, and abandonment. The authors offer practical advice on using mediation to reduce conflict, coparenting to maintain stability, and organizing to form a happy, blended family. This book is a wonderful, hands-on guide to navigating the difficult channels of divorce; its pages are filled with helpful checklists and various examples.

Fisher, B. (1981). *Rebuilding: When your relationship ends.* San Luis Obispo, CA: Impact.

This is an excellent handbook for those going through the divorce process. Using the metaphor of climbing a mountain, Fisher divides the process into 16 rebuilding blocks. This most readable book normalizes what divorced people go through and gives suggestions on how to deal with each rebuilding block.

Kayser, K. (1993). *When love dies: The process of marital disaffection.* New York: Guilford Press.

Kayser coins the new term "marital disaffection" to define the gradual loss of emotional attachment between partners in marriage. She first analyzes in-depth interviews with 49 spouses on their feelings, thoughts, and actions as they fell out of love with their partners. Then, Kayser incorporates data from a random sample survey, comparing troubled spouses with nondisaffected spouses, thereby exploring the relationships between marital disaffection, psychological well-being, commitment, attribution, and gender. She presents a new theoretical model on the process of marital disaffection and its key stages of disillusionment, hurt, anger, ambivalence, and disaffection. This is a good resource for therapists, researchers, and for newly divorced persons who want to make sense of what went wrong in their marriage.

Weiss, R. S. (1975). *Marital separation.* New York: Basic Books.

Here is a book both for those going through a divorce and for the professional. Weiss describes the process of divorce and separation. He includes many accounts of those who are in the process, to give the flavor of what it is like. Areas covered include why separation takes place, the emotional impact of separation, various aspects of relationships between the separating spouses and with friends and relatives of each, difficulties that are likely to come up with children, and how to establish a new life. Weiss does a good job of explaining and demonstrating the attachment felt between separating spouses.

Children's Books

Gardner, R. A. (1971). *The boys' and girls' book about divorce.* New York: Bantam Books.

Gardner, R. A. (1978). *The boys' and girls' book about one-parent families.* New York: Bantam Books.

Gardner, R. A. (1982). *The boys' and girls' book about stepfamilies.* New York: Bantam Books.

Each of these books is written for both children and parents to read. Each is written at the third- to fourth-grade level, although younger children can understand as parents read. Each book includes an introduction for parents and one for children. An excellent description of each situation is given, including feelings that a child may expect and suggestions for how to deal with individual situations. It is highly recommended for parents and children to discuss issues covered in the books.

Krasny Brown, L., & Brown, M. (1986). *Dinosaurs divorce.* Boston: Little, Brown.

This is a delightfully illustrated book geared toward children whose parents are going through a divorce. Key divorce words are defined in easy-to-understand language, children's feelings and reactions are normalized, and different scenarios are provided to explain the various outcomes of parents' divorce. The book addresses what can happen after a divorce, including living with one parent, having two homes, celebrating holidays and special occasions, dealing with parents dating other people, living with stepparents, and living with stepbrothers and stepsisters. The authors sensitively portray how children can react to their parents' divorce and make suggestions as to how children can best adapt to different situations, making this a good read for both parents and children.

Rofes, E. (Ed.). (1982). *The kids' book of divorce: By, for, and about kids.* New York: Vintage Books.

This book is written by 20 youngsters, aged 11 to 14, who have either experienced divorce personally or through a friend or relative. (Professionals are also interviewed.) The contributors explain what happens during the divorce process and give many suggestions on how to deal with divorce. Some topics included are how parents should tell kids, legal issues, counseling, "weekend Santa", stepparents, and gay parents. This book is appropriate for both parents and children.

Custody

Bricklin, B. (1995). *The custody evaluation handbook: Research-based solutions and applications.* New York: Brunner/Mazel.

This book advocates a test-based approach to be used during custody evaluations to determine the degree of success parents have parenting their children. The book describes several tests and tools for accessing valuable information from children and parents, but especially from children. Brickling further provides us with a specific system of nonadversarial communication strategies that can be used in all interactions with clients. This book is recommended for all mental health professionals who work closely with families as a custody evaluator.

Folberg, J. (Ed.). (1991). *Joint custody and shared parenting* (2nd ed.). New York: Guilford Press.

Like its predecessor published in 1984, this second edition is a comprehensive, well-organized collection of articles dealing with joint custody. Part I provides a historical perspective, definitions, different living arrangements, and review of the literature. Chapters in Part II examine factors that may influence the decision to implement joint custody and the success of shared parenting. Research findings are discussed in Part III, including what we know and what we have yet to learn. Finally, Part IV deals with issues and trends in the law in different geographical locations. Appendices include an excellent chart of state-by-state custody statutes and judicial interpretations, and a sample joint custody agreement, with alternative provisions.

Leupnitz, D. A. (1982). *Child custody.* Lexington, MA: Lexington Books.

The study reported in this book indicates better overall results for joint custody than for sole custody. Specifically, parents with joint custody were more likely to maintain contact with each other; the fathers were more likely to support the children financially, and parents were less likely to feel overwhelmed by child-care responsibilities. The major disadvantages of joint custody found in this investigation were that the parents felt too tied to each other and that some complained of lack of geographical mobility.

Warshak, R. A. (1992). *The custody revolution: The father factor and the motherhood mystique.* New York: Poseidon Press.

This book attributes many of the problems of divorce to custody practices. Based on scientific research, Warshak questions the routine practice of awarding custody to mothers and shows why children often adjust better to living with the same-sex parent. Warshak explores the potential benefits, especially for boys, of involving fathers in single parenting. The book makes a strong argument for balance in custody decisions, strongly emphasizing the needs of children.

Extended Family

Fisher, E. O. (Ed.). (1982). *Impact of divorce on the extended family.* Binghamton, NY: Haworth.

The impact of divorce on the extended family is explored in this collection of articles. Some of the topics examined include the dynamics of relationships within the extended family after divorce and remarriage, the role of extended kin in the adjustment to divorce/separation, effects of those in the role of grandparents and parents of an adult son or daughter, visitation rights of grandparents, the beneficial impact of divorce on the extended family, and services and interventions for this population.

Mediation

Emery, R. E. (1994). *Renegotiating family relationships: Divorce, child custody, and mediation.* New York: Guilford Press.

This book provides a good overview of divorce, child custody, and mediation in light of the latest psychological research and contemporary divorce law. Describing concrete techniques and detailed case examples, Emery shows how he helps estranged couples renegotiate their relationship by defining new boundaries of intimacy and power between the different members of the family. The role of children in the divorced family system is also explored, and strategies are offered for setting up visitation schedules, disciplinary tactics, joint physical custody, and other parenting arrangements. Mediation is shown to be an effective tool in increasing out-of-court settlements, encouraging parents' involvement with the children, and replacing the "win–lose" mentality with a "win–win" attitude. This is a good resource guide for the mental health and legal professional.

Folberg, J., & Milne, A. (Eds.). (1988). *Divorce mediation: Theory and practice.* New York: Guilford Press.

This is a state-of-the-art resource on divorce resolution, compiling the work of leading practitioners who define the theory of divorce mediation and outline (1) techniques and strategies, (2) ethical considerations and constraints, (3) standards of practice, and (4) policy issues. Mediation's role in important and controversial matters such as domestic violence disputes is also addressed. The book concludes with a discussion on the research results in the field, a longitudinal comparison of mediated versus adversarial divorce, and an in-depth descriptive analysis of common divorce-mediation behaviors. This comprehensive guidebook considers both the legal and psychological dimensions of divorce and is written in a style that is accessible to mediators, therapists, lawyers, social workers, and any other dispute-resolution professionals.

Marlow, L., & Sauber, S. R. (1990). *The handbook of divorce mediation.* New York: Plenum Press.

This detailed guidebook to mediation is written for the mental health professional who has little or no previous experience in mediation. It can also be an excellent resource guide for practiced mediators. The book has two sections: The first, entitled "Theory," defines and examines assumptions implicit in the authors' view of divorce mediation; the second section, entitled "Practice," takes the practitioner through a complete mediation, discussing the key subjects that a mediator is expected to address (i.e., debts, real and personal property, custody (parenting), support, medical and life insurance, college education). An appendix compiles the forms and letters that are useful for communication between the mediator and clients.

Parenting and Children

Ahrons, C. R. (1994). *The good divorce.* New York: HarperCollins.

This book provides divorcing and divorced parents with some hope that divorce does not automatically result in damaged children, broken homes, and a dysfunctional family. Based on her two decades of research and clinical practice with families of divorce, Ahrons clearly delineates the different stages of divorce, indicating what works and what does not at each stage. Ahrons coins the term "binuclear" family to describe the divorced family in more inclusive terms than "single-parent" family. She insists on looking at the realities of divorce and equally insists that we consider the possibilities of a "good divorce" by (1) removing the stigma of divorce; (2) helping parents and children establish new roles, rules, and rituals in keeping with their new family structure; and (3) applying divorce strategies and parenting solutions that help healthy development. This is an excellent resource for mental health professionals and divorcing parents alike.

Francke, L. B. (1983). *Growing up divorced.* New York: Linden Press.

Through interviews with children and experts in the field, the author describes the effects of divorce on children according to their age level: babies and toddlers, preschoolers, 6- to 8-year-olds, 9- to 12-year-olds, and teenagers. At the end of each chapter is a section on what parents can do to help. The latter part of the book looks at the roles that the institution (e.g., schools, courts, government) can and cannot fill.

Furstenberg, F. F., Jr., & Cherlin, A. J. (1991). *Divided families: What happens to children when parents part.* Cambridge, MA: Harvard University Press.

To illustrate the difficulties of divorce, the authors present us with the case of a typical middle-class couple as they struggle through separation, divorce, and remarriage. The authors claim that most children can adapt successfully after a divorce if two conditions are met: (1) the custodial parent (usually the mother) is able to provide love, a predictable routine, and consistent, moderate discipline, and (2) conflict between the parents is minimal. An added benefit is if the children can maintain an ongoing relationship with their father; however, more often than not, the relationship between fathers and their children deteriorates, because fathers lose touch with their children after they move out of the home. The authors also consider what economic and legal aspects must be in place to allow for more positive outcomes of divorce.

Garrity, C. B., & Baris, M. A. (1994). *Caught in the middle: Protecting the children of high-conflict divorce.* New York: Lexington Books.

This book provides mental health professionals with a guide to helping divorcing parents resolve their relentless conflict. Ongoing disputes between parents present a serious obstacle to children's adjustment in childhood as well as later in life. The first chapters of the book offer clues to detecting the origins of parental conflict and outline how divorce affects children of different ages. The remainder of the book is dedicated to discussing mediation by a parenting coordinator and creating a parenting plan that involves both parents. In the appendices, the Parenting Plan, the Parenting Checklist, and written agreements are included for handy reference.

Hetherington, E. M., Cox, M., & Cox, R. (1981). The aftermath of divorce. In E. M. Hetherington & R. D. Parke (Eds.), *Contemporary readings in child psychology.* New York: McGraw-Hill.

This chapter describes one of the best-designed studies on the effects of divorce on mothers, fathers, and children. In this study, continued involvement of the noncustodial father proved to be most important. The study demonstrates that a conflict-ridden, intact home is more detrimental to all members of the family than a stable home in which the parents are divorced.

Kurdek, L. A. (Ed.). (1983). *New directions for child development: Children and divorce.* San Francisco: Jossey-Bass.

The unifying theme of this collection of articles is the child's view of divorce. Each author has addressed some aspect of the question "What is the child's view of the divorce?" Rather than relying on parent reports, these authors have gone directly to the children themselves. Areas covered are children's understanding of their parents' divorces, young adolescents' responses, exploration of father-custody and mother-custody homes, correlates of children's adjustment, and a divorce adjustment project.

Oakland, T. (1984). *Divorced fathers: Reconstructing a quality life.* New York: Human Sciences Press.

This book is written as a primer to help divorced fathers to understand what they are going through, how their children are affected, and how to reconstruct their lives. Topics covered include psychological and social changes faced by fathers, understanding children and the effects of divorce, how to anticipate children's problems and deal with them, legal issues, and managing a household.

Wallerstein, J. S., & Kelly, J. B. (1980). *Surviving the breakup: How children and parents cope with divorce.* New York: Basic Books.

The California Children of Divorce Project is described in this book. Findings at the time of initial separation, 1 year later, and 5 years later are discussed in detail. The authors look at the reactions of parents, children, and school personnel at all three time periods. The chapter on how children respond to their parents' divorces is an exceptionally good one. Using developmental theory, Wallerstein and Kelly describe the reactions of the children in their study according to their developmental stage. Another excellent chapter on understanding the process of divorce and its ramifications presents the implications of their findings.

Adult Children of Divorce

Beal, E. W., & Hochman, G. (1991). *Adult children of divorce: Breaking the cycle and finding fulfillment in love, marriage, and family.* New York: Delacorte Press.

This book focuses on the experiences of adults who grew up as children of divorce. Since 1972, more than a million children have been involved in divorce every year. The authors review the short-term effects of divorce but concentrate on the lasting effects of divorce for children of divorce who grow up and form relationships of their own. Based on years of research and more than 300 case studies, the authors posit that the lasting effects of divorce depend on every family's unique style of coping with problems *before, during,* and *after* the divorce. This is an invaluable resource for those who have seen parents and loved ones go through the trauma of divorce and want to recover a sense of connectedness and wholeness.

Berman, C. (1991). *Adult children of divorce speak out.* New York: Simon & Schuster.

Berman shares her findings after conducting extensive, in-depth interviews with adult men and women on their experiences as children of divorce. Certain patterns make themselves apparent: problems with self-esteem; concerns with sexuality; a strong need to control; difficulty committing to relationships; and repeating parents' behavior, including divorce. Ways of moving through the painful experience of divorce also emerge: confronting and letting go of anger; seeking support from significant others; learning to manage conflict; demystifying the past; and forgiving and reconnecting with parents. This book validates the difficulties experienced by children of divorce and is recommended not only to adult children, but also to concerned parents who are contemplating divorce and want to help their children overcome the hardships of divorce.

Economic Consequences

Everett, C. A. (Ed.). (1994). *The economics of divorce: The effects on parents and children.* Binghamton, NY: Haworth.

This book offers a collection of studies on the economic consequences of divorce on postdivorce families . The articles focus on the mother's financial situation after a divorce and effects of maternal employment on economic well-being and attitudes toward divorce. Methods, results, and discussion are elaborated upon in each article. This is a concise text that is a handy reference for mental health professionals and students.

Postdivorce Families

Hansen, J. C. (Ed.). (1982). *Therapy with remarriage families.* Rockville, MD: Aspen Systems Corporation.

Information and techniques are provided for the therapist who is working with family members going through the remarriage cycle. Articles have been arranged according to the temporal sequence of this process. Several articles look at the concerns and needs of children and adults in dealing with the losses they encounter in the separation process. Others explore concepts and techniques to assist the remarried family in resolving problems.

Sager, C. J., Brown, H. S., Crohn, H., Engel, T., Rodstein, E., & Walker, L. (1983). *Treating the remarried family.* New York: Brunner/Mazel.

This comprehensive book is a must for the mental health professional who is working with remarried (REM) families. The authors examine the REM family on three levels: family systems, life cycle, and intrapsychic. This well-organized volume discusses in great detail the theory, structure, treatment, special issues, and prevention in dealing with this population. Case examples are well utilized. An appendix of forms and checklists for clinician use is included.

Visher, E. B., & Visher, J. S. (1979). *Stepfamilies: A guide to working with stepparents and stepchildren.* New York: Brunner/Mazel.

The Vishers help those in the mental health field realize the uniqueness of stepfamilies and how to help them. The first three chapters discuss the cultural and structural characteristics of stepfamilies and the research done on them. The rest of the book looks at different constellations of family members in stepfamilies. The authors explore what difficulties to expect and how to deal with them as a therapist.

Visher, E. B., & Visher, J. S. (1982). *How to win as a stepfamily.* New York: Dembner Books.

In this book, the Vishers cover mainly the same material as in *Stepfamilies: A Guide to Working with Stepparents and Stepchildren.* The difference lies in the audience for which the book has been written—stepfamilies themselves. The authors do an excellent job of explaining stepfamilies and the difficulties they face. Included in these difficulties are dealing with former spouses, grandparents of remarriage, legal issues, and helping children adjust. The Vishers have succeeded in normalizing stepfamily interactions. Information and suggestions are given on how to make a stepfamily work. References for stepparents and children are included at the end of the book.

Visher, E. B., & Visher, J. S. (1988). *Old loyalties, new ties: Therapeutic strategies with stepfamilies.* New York: Brunner/Mazel.

In this new book, the authors again make the argument that stepfamilies are viable family structures that are not imperfect replicas of nuclear families, but healthy family systems created from the integration of old loyalties and new ties. The Vishers underscore the importance of the therapist's role in validating stepfamilies' uniqueness by reducing their sense of helplessness, enhancing their self-esteem, teaching negotiation skills, and encouraging dyadic relationships. This is an extremely helpful guidebook for therapists helping stepfamilies resolve such difficulties as change and losses, unrealistic beliefs, life-cycle discrepancies, loyalty conflicts, boundary problems, power struggles, and juggling closeness and distance.

Schools

Allers, R. D. (1982). *Divorce, children, and the school.* Princeton, NJ: Princeton Books.

If the therapist plans on involving the school as part of the therapeutic program, this book will prove to be most helpful. The first half of the book describes both the child's and parents' experience of divorce. The role of the school is described in the last half. The role of the teacher is explored in relation to what would be helpful and what would not. Allers also describes a program to be led by mental health professionals to help children of divorce in the school. A bibliography for children and adults is included.

Theory, Therapy, and Research

Cherlin, A. J. (1981). *Marriage, divorce, remarriage.* Cambridge, MA: Harvard University Press.

The author examines overall trends in the United States over the last several decades in relation to marriage, divorce, and remarriage. He first examines the demographic data and then outlines the trends. Cherlin continues with explanations for these trends for each decade, from the 1950s to the 1980s. Consequences of these trends for spouses, parents, and children are then explored. In his last chapter, Cherlin looks at differences in family patterns of Black families and White families.

Chiriboga, D. A., Catron, L. S., & Associates. (1991). *Divorce: Crisis, challenge or relief?* New York: New York University Press.

This book is written by an interdisciplinary team of social and behavioral scientists on their life-span study of divorced adults. The authors base their findings on hundreds of face-to-face interviews with adults ranging in age from 20 to 79, and of different ethnic background and sexual orientation. The major contribution of this research is that subjects were randomly selected from county courthouse records, rather than relying on specific divorce recovery groups or clinical samples. The authors address such key topics as demographic issues, life before separation, divorce as a transitional process, childhood stress as a shaper of adult adaptation, divorce stress and coping, the role of social supports, locus of control, mental health, and emotional well-being. The authors use clear, descriptive language and case examples to highlight their findings.

Everett, C., & Volgy, S. S. (1991). Treating divorce in family-therapy practice. In A. S. Gurman & D. P. Kniskern (Eds.), *Handbook of family therapy* (Vol. 2). New York: Brunner/Mazel.

In this chapter, the authors provide an organized and coherent framework for therapists to clarify assessment and evaluation during the divorce process. The authors' major contribution is in offering a descriptive systemic and developmental model of the family dissolution process. Using this 14-step model, clinicians can understand the salient aspects of the divorce process and thus develop appropriate treatment goals and strategies for families seeking their assistance.

Guttman, J. (1993). *Divorce in psychosocial perspective: Theory and research.* Hillsdale, NJ: Erlbaum.

This book offers a comprehensive perspective on the process of divorce and its effects on children, adults, and the family. Guttman integrates and analyzes current research, theory, and clinical practice in the divorce domain, and introduces a new psychosocial lens to studying the phenomenon of divorce. This is a great reference book for students, clinicians, and family theorists.

Isaacs, M. B., Montalvo, B., & Abelsohn, D. (1986). *The difficult divorce: Therapy for children and families.* New York: Basic Books.

Drawing on their longitudinal study, Families of Divorce Project, the authors present a new method of face-to-face problem solving with families in the therapy room that helps parents control their anger and focus on their children's welfare. Using several case examples and concise language, the authors define the different goals for therapy, including managing preseparation crises, mediating between lawyers and clients, reducing hostility, strengthening sibling ties, and conducting custody evaluations. This is a practical guide for therapists and lawyers who work with families undergoing the difficult process of divorce.

Jacobson, G. F. (1983). *The multiple crisis of material separation and divorce.* New York: Grune & Stratton.

Following a review of the literature, the author describes a study of 159 females and 79 males subdivided into three groups: (1) married/discussing separation, (2) separated and divorced within the previous 14 months, and (3) separated and divorced more than 14 months. Subjects had all sought professional help. Data are reported on the relationship of gender, time, age, the presence of children, relationships with ex-spouses, and social relationships, to the mental health of the subjects.

Kaslow, F. W. (1981). Divorce and divorce therapy. In A. S. Gurman & D. P. Kniskern (Eds.), *Handbook of family therapy.* New York: Brunner/Mazel.

In this chapter, Kaslow gives an overview of divorce. Topics covered include divorce statistics, factors that lead to divorce, various models of stages of the divorce process, the impact of divorce on children, intervention strategies, research on divorce therapy, and training of the divorce therapist.

Kaslow, F. W. (1984). Divorce: An evolutionary process of change in the family system. *Journal of Divorce,* 7(3), 21–39.

Kaslow explores divorce from a combination of perspectives: family systems, the individual life cycle, and stage theories of development. The choice of treatment varies according to where one is in the divorce process, one's ego strength, one's cognitive functioning, and available social and resource networks. Kaslow includes an excellent chart of stages, feelings, actions and tasks, and the most appropriate therapeutic interventions. Case vignettes are also presented to elaborate further Kaslow's thinking.

Kitson, G. C., & Holmes, W. M. (1992). *Portrait of divorce: Adjustment to marital dissolution.* New York: Guilford Press.

This is a welcome addition to the current research on divorce. The authors integrate 50 years of prior research with original data and introduce a new model of divorce adjustment. The book considers the process of adjustment, beginning in the period of estrangement, through the divorce process, and on to 4 years after the couple has separated. The authors also consider various causes of divorce, impact of divorce on children, economic factors, social support systems, and life after divorce. One of the book's unique contributions to the field is contrasting divorcing people with a comparable sample of people who remain in intact marriages, thereby allowing the detection of factors that facilitate or hinder divorce adjustment for Blacks and Whites, and men and women, both cross-sectionally and longitudinally.

Kitson, G. C., & Raschke, H. J. (1981). Divorce research: What we know; what we need to know. *Journal of Divorce,* 4(3), 1–37.

Kitson and Raschke explore the divorce process through an extensive review of the literature. The main focus is on antecedents and consequences of divorce. They examine the sociological and psychological factors, the causes, and various theoretical perspectives of divorce. Much information is shared in this clearly written review, with an excellent bibliography at the end.

Rice, J. K., & Rice, D. G. (1986). *Living through divorce: A developmental approach to divorce therapy.* New York: Guilford Press.

Although written by practicing therapists, this book stresses theory as well as technique. The authors believe that divorce needs to be integrated theoretically in the individual, marital, and family life cycles. They also stress that "a therapist [who] thoroughly understands the processes of narcissistic injury and role disorientation accompanying divorce . . . is in a better position to help the client accomplish the related therapeutic and developmental tasks: ego reparation and role restructuring" (p. xi). This is one of the most comprehensive texts on divorce therapy.

Sprenkle, D. H. (Ed.). (1985). *Divorce therapy.* Binghamton, NY: Haworth.

This collection of articles is organized around therapeutic interventions related to the following stages of divorce: (1) divorce decision making; (2) restructuring therapy for children, mediation, and custody; and (3) postdivorce recovery and remarriage. This book also contains a helpful overview article on criteria for a constructive divorce and a comprehensive, annotated bibliography. It is one of the first general texts on divorce therapy.

Sprenkle, D. H., & Cyrus, C. L. (1983). Abandonment: The stress of sudden divorce. In C. R. Figley & M. I. McCubbin (Eds.), *Stress and the family: Coping with catastrophe.* New York: Brunner/Mazel.

As illustrated in this chapter, the sudden divorce has its own unique circumstances with which one must deal. The authors examine, both theoretically and practically, one specific type of divorce—abandonment. Areas covered include (1) the meaning of emotional abandonment, (2) why this stressor is so painful for all involved, (3) factors determining the level of stress experienced, (4) constructive and destructive coping methods, (5) useful interventions, (6) the constructive potential for the survivor, and (7) gaps in our knowledge and recommendations for future research.

Sprenkle, D. H., & Storm, C. L. (1983). Divorce therapy outcome research: A substantive and methodological review. *Journal of Marital and Family Therapy, 9,* 239–258.

The authors provide a substantive and methodological review of 22 empirical studies related to divorce therapy. The studies are divided into the following six areas: (1) mediation, (2) conciliation courts counseling, (3) consumer evaluation, (4) divorce groups, (5) separation techniques, and (6) marriage counseling with divorce as an unintended outcome. An excellent chart comparing the studies is included. There is strong evidence for the superiority of mediation to traditional adversary methods in custody and visitation disputes. There appears to be an increase in the number of reconciliations in the short term for those using conciliation counseling. Due to the weakness of the methodologies of many of the studies, other conclusions remain tentative.

Storm, C. L., & Sprenkle, D. H. (1982). Individual treatment in divorce therapy: A critique of an assumption. *Journal of Divorce, 6,* 87–97.

The authors critically examine the commonly held maxim that the treatment of choice in divorce is working with the individual. Conjoint and family treatment are explored as alternatives. A model of divorce therapy using all three modes of treatment is offered. Storm and Sprenkle propose conjoint and/or family treatment as most effective in the decision-making and restructuring stages. Individual treatment is the most appropriate mode for the recovery phase.

Textor, M. (1989). *The divorce and divorce therapy handbook.* Northvale, NJ: Jason Aronson.

This book presents important findings on divorce, as well as various therapeutic interventions developed by clinicians. Part I, entitled "Therapy," deals with the special problems of divorce: pragmatic issue, interpersonal and social issues, and family-related issues. Part II, entitled "Divorce Therapy," illustrates the various approaches to divorce and postdivorce recovery: marital and family therapy; crisis intervention treatment; grief and bereavement counseling; and, educational–supportive counseling, including school interventions and group work. Part III, entitled "New Family Systems," addresses the practical realities of divorce, including economic hardship and new family configurations. Textor compiles the writings of several well-known practitioners in the field of divorce, making this a very comprehensive handbook for all mental health professionals.

Walsh, F. (1991). Promoting healthy functioning in divorced and remarried families. In A. S. Gurman & D. P. Kniskern (Eds.), *Handbook of family therapy* (Vol. 2). New York: Brunner/Mazel.

This chapter speaks to the process of reorganization and adaptation in divorced and remarried families. In addition, Walsh offers clinical guidelines to depathologize family distress that is associated with complications in various transitions and promote optimal functioning in each family arrangement. The author makes note of factors that affect vulnerability and resiliency to distress, as well as short- and long-term tasks and challenges facing these families on the road to functional postdivorce adjustment.

Women's Issues

Colleta, S. D. (1983). Stressful lives: The situation of divorced mothers and their children. *Journal of Divorce, 6*(3), 19–31.

In this study, 72 divorced and married mothers were interviewed. The results suggest that the negative situations of divorced mothers and children are largely due to the low income of divorced mothers, rather than the fathers' absence.

Langelier, R., & Deckert, P. (1980). Divorce counseling guidelines for the late divorced female. *Journal of Divorce, 3*(4), 403–411.

Based on research, this article offers divorce counseling guidelines for females who divorce after being married a minimum of 20 years. Guidelines are given in the six following areas: emotions, divorce grounds, finances and budgeting, children, lifestyle changes, and independence.

Robertson, C. (1980). *Divorce and decision making: A woman's guide.* Chicago: Follett.

This is an excellent how-to book for women going through the divorce process. It is full of information, activities, and questions that a woman needs to ask as she goes through a divorce. Part I deals with emotional supports, values, plans for the future, and decision-making ability. Part II deals with specific decisions that need to be made in the following areas: legal help, the divorce settlement, children, money, career, and social life. The last chapter discusses the use of assertiveness in implementing decisions. An excellent bibliography and list of resources are included at the end of the book.

Men's Issues

Myers, M. F. (1989). *Men and divorce.* New York: Guilford Press.

This book focuses specifically on men and their reactions to divorce in a wide array of circumstances. Using many clinical examples, Myers illustrates the unique dynamics and symptomatology of separations that are husband-initiated, wife-initiated, and mutually initiated. There is also a chapter on divorcing men who come out as gay, with consideration given to the impact on both the men and their families. Myers, a physician, adopts a biopsychosocial perspective to look at such emotions as anger, dependency, intimacy, control, grief, male inexpressiveness, loneliness, and isolation. This is an invaluable resource for any mental health professional working with individuals and couples.

REFERENCES

Ahrons, C. R. (1979). The binuclear family: Two households, one family. *Alternative Lifestyles, 2,* 499–515.

Ahrons, C. R. (1980). Divorce: A crisis of family transition and change. *Family Relations, 4,* 533–540.

Ahrons, C. R. (1994). *The good divorce.* New York: HarperCollins.

Association of Family and Conciliation Courts (1982). *Joint custody: A new way of being related.* (Available from Association of Family and Conciliation Courts, c/o Nova University Law Center, 3100 S.W. Ninth Avenue, Fort Lauderdale, FL, 33315.)

Beal, E. W., & Hochman, G. (1991). *Adult children of divorce: Breaking the cycle and finding fulfillment in love, marriage, and family.* New York: Delacorte Press.

Berman, C. (1991). *Adult children of divorce speak out.* New York: Simon & Schuster.

Bernard, J. M., & Hackney, H. (1983). *Untying the knot: A guide to civilized divorce.* Minneapolis: Winston Press.

Bernstein, B. (1977). Lawyer and counselor as an interdisciplinary team: Preparing the father for custody. *Journal of Marriage and Family Counseling, 3,* 29–40.

Bohannan, P. (1970). The six stations of divorce. In P. Bohannan (Ed.), *Divorce and after.* Garden City, NY: Doubleday.

Bohannan, P. (1971). Divorce chains, households of remarriage, and multiple divorces. In P. Bohannan (Ed.)., *Divorce and after: An analysis of the emotional and social problems of divorce.* New York: Anchor Books.

Bray, J. H., & Jouriles, E. N. (1995). Treatment of marital conflict and prevention of divorce. *Journal of Marital and Family Therapy, 21*(4), 461–473.

Brown, E. M. (1976). Divorce counseling. In D. H. Olson (Ed.), *Treating relationships.* Lake Mills, IA: Graphic.

Brown, E. M. (1985). The comprehensive divorce treatment center: The divorce and marital stress clinic model. In D. H. Sprenkle (Ed.), *Divorce therapy.* Binghamton, NY: Haworth.

Brown, M. D. (1985). Creating new realities for the newly divorced: A structural strategic approach for divorce therapy with an individual. In D. H. Sprenkle (Ed.), *Divorce therapy.* Binghamton, NY: Haworth.

Brown, P., & Manela, R. (1977). Client satisfaction with marital and divorce counseling. *Family Coordinator, 26,* 294–303.

Cantor, D. W., & Drake, E. A. (1983). *Divorced parents and their children: A guide for mental health professionals.* New York: Springer.

Cantrell, R. (1985). *Defining constructive adjustment to divorce: I. Comparison between groups of divorcées; II. Comparison of therapists and divorcées.* Unpublished doctoral dissertation, Purdue University, West Lafayette, IN.

Chiriboga, D. A., Catron, L. S., & Associates. (1991). *Divorce: Crisis, challenge or relief?* New York: New York University Press.

Cohen, S. N. (1985). Divorce mediation: An introduction. In D. H. Sprenkle (Ed.), *Divorce therapy.* Binghamton, NY: Haworth.

Coleman, M., & Ganong, L. H. (1990). Remarriage and stepfamily research in the 1980s: Increased interest in an old family form. *Journal of Marriage and the Family, 52*(4), 925–940.

Coogler, O. J. (1978). *Structural mediation in divorce settlement.* Lexington, MA: Lexington Books.

Crosbie-Burnett, M., & Ahrons, C. R. (1985). From divorce to remarriage: Implications for therapy with families in transition. In D. H. Sprenkle (Ed.), *Divorce therapy.* Binghamton, NY: Haworth.

Emery, R. E. (1994). *Renegotiating family relationships: Divorce, child custody, and mediation.* New York: Guilford Press.

Eno, M. M. (1985). Sibling relationships in families of divorce. In D. H. Sprenkle (Ed.), *Divorce therapy.* Binghamton, NY: Haworth.

Erikson, E. K. (1963). *Childhood and society* (2nd ed.). New York: Norton.

Everett, C. A. (Ed.). (1994). *The economics of divorce: The effects on parents and children.* Binghamton, NY: Haworth.

Everett, C. A., & Volgy Everett, S. (1994). *Healthy divorce.* San Franciso, CA: Jossey-Bass.

Fisher, B. (1976). *Identifying and meeting needs of formerly married people through a divorce adjustment seminar.* (Available from Family Relations Learning Center, 450 Ord Drive, Boulder, CO 80303.)

Fisher, B. (1981). *Rebuilding: When your relationship ends.* San Luis Obispo, CA: Impact.

Fisher, E. O. (Ed.). (1982). *Impact of divorce on the extended family.* Binghamton, NY: Haworth.

Folberg, J. (Ed.). (1991). *Joint custody and shared parenting* (2nd ed.). New York: Guilford Press.

Folberg, J., & Milne, A. (Eds.). (1988). *Divorce mediation: Theory and practice.* New York: Guilford Press.

Francke, L. B. (1983). *Growing up divorced.* New York: Linden Press.

Froiland, D. J., & Hozeman, T. L. (1977). Counseling for constructive divorce. *Personnel and Guidance Journal, 55,* 525–529.

Furstenberg, F. F., Jr., & Cherlin, A. J. (1991). *Divided families: What happens to children when parents part.* Cambridge, MA: Harvard University Press.

Galper, M. (1978). *Co-parenting: Sharing your child equally.* Philadelphia: Running Press.

Gardner, R. A. (1971). *The boys' and girls' book about divorce.* New York: Bantam Books.

Gardner, R. A. (1976). *Psychotherapy with children of divorce.* New York: Jason Aronson.

Gardner, R. A. (1978). *The boys' and girls' book about one-parent families.* New York: Bantam Books.

Gardner, R. A. (1982). *The boys' and girls' book about stepfamilies.* New York: Bantam Books.

Garrity, C. B., & Baris, M. A. (1994). *Caught in the middle: Protecting the children of high-conflict divorce.* New York: Lexington Books.

Glick, P. (1984). Marriage, divorce, and living arrangements: Prospective changes. *Journal of Family Issues, 5,* 7–26.

Goode, W. J. (1956). *After divorce.* Glencoe, IL: Free Press.

Granvold, D. K. (1983). Structured separation for marital treatment and decision-making. *Journal of Marital and Family Therapy, 9,* 403–412.

Greene, B. L., Lee, R. R., & Lustig, N. (1973). Transient structured distance as a maneuver in marital therapy. *Family Coordinator, 20,* 15–22.

Gurman, A. S., & Kniskern, D. P. (1978). Research on marital and family therapy: Progress, perspective and prospect. In S. Garfield & A. Bergin (Eds.), *Handbook of psychotherapy and behavior change* (2nd ed.). New York: Wiley.

Gurman, A. S., & Kniskern, D. P. (1981). Editor's note to "Divorce and divorce therapy." In A. S. Gurman & D. P. Kniskern (Eds.), *Handbook of family therapy.* New York: Brunner/Mazel.

Gurman, A., Kniskern, D., & Pinsof, W. (1986). Research on the process and outcome of marital and family therapy. In S. Garfield & A. Bergin (Eds.), *Handbook of psychotherapy and behavior change* (3rd ed.). New York: Wiley.

Hansen, J. M. (1982). *Therapy with remarriage families.* Rockville, MD: Aspen Systems.

Haynes, J. M. (1981). *Divorce mediation: A practical guide for therapists and counselors.* New York: Springer.

Hetherington, E. M., Cox, M., & Cox, R. (1981). The aftermath of divorce. In E. M. Hetherington & R. D. Parke (Eds.), *Contemporary readings in child psychology.* New York: McGraw-Hill.

Hill, R. (1949). *Families under stress.* New York: Harper Press.

Holley, P. (1980). *An analysis of divorce adjustment measures.* (Available from Department of Social Sciences, Southwestern Oklahoma State University, Weatherford, OK 73096.)

Howell, R. J., & Toepke, K. E. (1984). Summary of the child custody laws for the fifty states. *American Journal of Family Therapy, 12,* 56–60.

Imber-Black, E., & Roberts, J. (1992). *Rituals for our times: Celebrating, healing, and changing our lives and our relationships.* New York: HarperCollins.

Irving, H. H. (1980). *Divorce mediation.* New York: Universe Books.

Irving, H. H., Benjamin, M., Bohm, P., & MacDonald, G. (1981). *A study of conciliation counseling in the Family Court of Toronto: Implications for socio-legal practice.* Toronto: Department of National Health and Welfare and the Ontario Ministry of the Attorney General.

Isaacs, M. B. (1982). Helping mom fail: A case of a stalemated divorcing process. *Family Process, 21,* 225–234.

Isaacs, M. B., Montalvo, B., & Abelsohn, D. (1986). *The difficult divorce: Therapy for children and families.* New York: Basic Books.

Janis, I. L. (1983). *Short-term counseling: Guidelines based on recent research.* New Haven, CT: Yale University Press.

Janis, I. L., & Mann, L. (1977). *Decision making: A psychological analysis of conflict, choice, and commitment.* New York: Free Press.

Johnson, S. M. (1977). *First person singular.* Philadelphia: Lippincott.

Kaslow, F. W. (1981). Divorce and divorce therapy. In A. S. Gurman & D. P. Kniskern (Eds.), *Handbook of family therapy.* New York: Brunner/Mazel.

Kaslow, F. W., & Steinberg, J. (1981). Ethical divorce therapy and divorce proceedings: A psycho-legal perspective. In L. L'Abate (Ed.), *Values, ethics, legalities, and the family therapist.* Rockville, MD: Aspen Systems.

Kayser, K. (1993). *When love dies: The process of marital disaffection.* New York: Guilford Press.

Kessler, S. (1975). *The American way of divorce: Prescriptions for change.* Chicago: Nelson-Hall.

Kitson, G. C. (1982). Attachment to the spouse in divorce: A scale and its applications. *Journal of Marriage and the Family, 44,* 379–393.

Kitson, G. C., & Raschke, H. J. (1981). Divorce research: What we know; what we need to know. *Journal of Divorce, 4*(3), 1–37.

Kitson, G. C., & Morgan, L. A. (1990). The multiple consequences of divorce: A decade review. *Journal of Marriage and the Family, 52*(4), 913–924.

Krantzler, M. (1974). *Creative divorce.* New York: Signet.

Kübler-Ross, E. (1969). *On death and dying.* New York: Macmillan.

Kurdek, L. A. (Ed.). (1983). *New directions for child development: Children and divorce.* San Francisco: Jossey-Bass.

Lee, B. E. (1979). Consumer evaluation of a family court service. *Conciliation Courts Review, 17,* 49–54.

Lee, C. M., Picard, M., Blain, M. D. (1994). A methodological and substantive review of intervention outcome studies for families undergoing divorce. *Journal of Family Psychology, 8*(1), 3–15.

Levinger, G. (1976). A social psychological perspective on divorce. *Journal of Social Issues, 32,* 21–47.

Marlow, L., & Sauber, S. R. (1990). *The handbook of divorce mediation.* New York: Plenum Press.

Myers, M. F. (1989). *Men and divorce.* New York: Guilford Press.

Newman, G. (1981). *101 ways to be a long distance super-dad.* Mountain View, CA: Blossom Valley Press.

Nichols, W. C. (1984). Therapeutic needs of children in family system reorganization. *Journal of Divorce, 7,* 23–44.

Nichols, W. C. (1985). Family therapy with children of divorce. In D. H. Sprenkle (Ed.), *Divorce therapy.* Binghamton, NY: Haworth.

Oakland, T. (1984). *Divorced fathers: Reconstructing a quality life.* New York: Human Sciences Press.

Olson, D. H., Russell, C. S., & Sprenkle, D. H. (1980). Marital and family therapy: A decade review. *Journal of Marriage and the Family, 42,* 973–993.

Pasley, K., Rhoden, L., Visher, E. B., & Visher, J. S. (in press). Successful stepfamily therapy: Client's perspectives. *Journal of Marital and Family Therapy.*

Pearson, J., & Thoennes, N. (1982). The benefits outweigh the costs. *Family Advocate, 4,* 26–32.

Price-Bonham, S., & Balswick, J. O. (1980). The noninstitutions: Divorce, desertion, and remarriage. *Journal of Marriage and the Family, 42,* 959–972.

Raschke, H. J. (1982). *Divorce and marital separation.* Unpublished manuscript, Department of Psychology and Sociology, Austin College, Sherman, TX.

Reiss, I. L. (1980). *Family systems in America.* New York: Holt, Rinehart & Winston.

Rice, J. K., & Rice, D. G. (1986). *Living through divorce: A developmental approach to divorce therapy.* New York: Guilford Press.

Rofes, E. (Ed.). (1982). *The kid's book of divorce: By, for and about kids.* New York: Vintage Books.

Sager, C. J., Brown, H. S., Crohn, H., Engel, T., Rodstein, E., & Walker, L. (1983). *Treating the remarried family.* New York: Brunner/Mazel.

Salts, C. J. (1979). Divorce process: Integration of theory. *Journal of Divorce, 2,* 233–240.

Salts, C. J. (1985). Divorce stage theory and therapy: Therapeutic implications throughout the divorcing process. In D. H. Sprenkle (Ed.), *Divorce therapy.* Binghamton, NY: Haworth.

Saposnek, D. T. (1983). *Mediating child custody disputes.* San Francisco: Jossey-Bass.

Shapiro, T. J., & Caplan, M. S. (1983). *Parting sense: A couple's guide to divorce mediation.* Lutherville, MD: Greenspring.

Singh, G. K., Mathews, T. J., Clarke, S. C., Yannicos, T., & Smith, B. L. (1995). Annual summary of births, marriages, divorces, and deaths: United States, 1994. *Monthly Vital Statistics Report, 43*(13), 1–44.

Smart, L. S. (1977). An application of Erikson's theory to the recovery-from-divorce process. *Journal of Divorce, 1,* 67–79.

Smoke, J. (1976). *Growing through divorce.* Irving, CA: Harvest House.

Spanier, G. B., & Casto, R. F. (1979). Adjustment to separation and divorce: An analysis of 50 case studies. *Journal of Divorce, 2,* 241–253.

Spanier, G. B., & Lewis, R. A. (1980). Marital quality: A review of the seventies. *Journal of Marriage and the Family, 42,* 825–839.

Sprenkle, D. H. (Ed.). (1985). *Divorce therapy.* Binghamton, NY: Haworth.

Sprenkle, D. H., & Cantrell, R. G. (1986). *Attorney conceptions of constructive divorce.* Unpublished manuscript, Purdue University, West Lafayette, IN.

Sprenkle, D. H., & Cyrus, C. (1983). Abandonment: The sudden stress of divorce. In C. R. Figley & H. I. McCubbin (Eds.), *Stress and the family* (Vol. 2). New York: Brunner/Mazel.

Sprenkle, D. H., & Storm, C. L. (1983). Divorce therapy outcome research: A substantive and methodological review. *Journal of Marital and Family Therapy, 9,* 239–258.

Storm, C. L., & Sprenkle, D. H. (1982). Individual treatment in divorce therapy: A critique of an assumption. *Journal of Divorce, 5,* 87–97.

Storm, C. L., Sprenkle, D. H., & Williamson, W. (1985). Innovative divorce approaches developed by counselors, conciliators, mediators, and educators. In R. Levant (Ed.), *Psychoeducational approaches to family therapy.* New York: Springer.

Stuart, I. R., & Abt, L. E. (Eds.). (1981). *Children of separation and divorce: Management and treatment.* New York: Van Nostrand Reinhold.

Sutton, P. (1983). *Defining divorce adjustment: A study of marriage and family therapists' criteria for constructive long-term adjustment to divorce.* Unpublished doctoral dissertation, Purdue University, West Lafayette, IN.

Sutton, P., & Sprenkle, D. H. (1985). Criteria for a constructive divorce: Theory and research to guide the practitioner. In D. H. Sprenkle (Ed.), *Divorce therapy.* Binghamton, NY: Haworth.

Textor, M. (1989). *The divorce and divorce therapy handbook.* Northvale, NJ: Jason Aronson.

Thompson, L., & Spanier, G. (1983). The end of marriage and acceptance of marital termination. *Journal of Marriage and the Family, 45,* 103–113.

Toomin, M. K. (1972). Structured separation with counseling: A therapeutic approach for couples in conflict. *Family Process, 11,* 299–310.

Turner, N. W. (1980). Divorce in mid-life: Clinical implications and applications. In W. Norman & T. J. Scaramella (Eds.), *Mid-life: Developmental and clinical issues.* New York: Brunner/Mazel.

Turner, N. W. (1985). Divorce: Dynamics of decision therapy. In D. H. Sprenkle (Ed.), *Divorce therapy.* Binghamton, NY: Haworth.

Vaughn, S. (1986). *Uncoupling.* New York: Oxford University Press.

Visher, E. B., & Visher, J. S. (1979). *Stepfamilies: A guide to working with stepparents and stepchildren.* New York: Brunner/Mazel.

Visher, E. B., & Visher, J. S. (1982). *How to win as a stepfamily.* New York: Dembner Books.

Visher, E. B., & Visher, J. S. (1988). *Old loyalties, new ties: Therapeutic strategies with stepfamilies.* New York: Brunner/Mazel.

Volgy, S. S., & Everett, C. A. (1985). Systemic assessment criteria for joint custody. In D. H. Sprenkle (Ed.), *Divorce therapy.* Binghamton, NY: Haworth.

Waller, W. W. (1967). *The old and the new: Divorce and adjustment* (3rd ed.). Carbondale, IL: Southern Illinois University Press.

Wallerstein, J. S., & Kelly, J. B. (1980). *Surviving the breakup: How children and parents cope with divorce.* New York: Basic Books.

Warshak, R. A. (1992). *The custody revolution: The father factor and the motherhood mystique.* New York: Poseidon Press.

Weed, J. A. (1980). *National estimates of marriage dissolution and survivorship: United States* (Vital and Health Statistics: Series 3, Analytical Studies, No. 19; Department of Health and Human Services, Pub. No. 81-1403). Hyattsville, MD: National Center for Health Statistics.

Weisman, R. S. (1975). Crisis theory and the process of divorce. *Social Casework, 56,* 205–212.

Weiss, R. S. (1975). *Marital separation.* New York: Basic Books.

Weiss, R. S. (1979). *Doing it alone: The family life and social situation of the single parent.* New York: Basic Books.

Weltner, J. S. (1982). A structural approach to the single-parent family. *Family Process, 21,* 203–210.

White, L. K. (1990). Determinants of divorce: A review of research in the eighties. *Journal of Marriage and the Family, 52*(4), 904–912.

Wong, R. (1986). *Defining constructive adjustment to divorce: Comparison of Protestant, Catholic and Jewish clergy.* Unpublished doctoral dissertation, University of Washington.

9

Deconstructing Gender in Family Therapy[1]

JUDITH MYERS AVIS

ATTENTION TO gender has evolved significantly in the field of family therapy over the past 17 years. In examining this evolution, I locate myself as a feminist who increasingly uses social constructionist and narrative ideas in conjunction with feminist ones to illuminate my understanding of gender. As a feminist, I understand gender as a fundamental organizing principle of human experience and social relations, usually involving domination and unequal power, and interacting with other categories of oppression, such as race and class. As a social constructionist, I understand gender and gender relations as socially constructed and therefore capable of being deconstructed, reconstructed, and transformed. I also realize that my understanding of gender is necessarily shaped by my own engendered experience, and I can never completely free myself from distortions resulting from that experience. The ideas I discuss in this chapter, then, represent only one possible perspective on the subject of gender, rather than any attempt to distill "truth." They are a work in progress, a statement of my evolving thinking at this particular point in time.

[1]Portions of this chapter have been presented in different form in "Deepening Awareness: A Private Study Guide to Feminism and Family Therapy" by J. M. Avis (1986), in L. Braverman (Ed.), *Women, Feminism, and Family Therapy*, Binghamton, NY: Haworth.

220

THE HISTORY OF GENDER CONSCIOUSNESS
IN FAMILY THERAPY

An awareness of gender as a fundamental dimension of personal and social organization—of personal identity, family relationships, therapeutic relationships, sociocultural privilege and oppression—has grown from virtual nonexistence in the field of family therapy prior to 1978 to one of general recognition in 1995. However, although there is, today, general agreement that gender is important, there is no matching agreement on why or how it is important, on how to think about it, or on how to attend to it in practice.

Attention was first drawn to issues of gender in the field by a handful of feminist or feminist-informed family therapists in the late 1970s and early 1980s (Avis, 1985; Bograd, 1984; Goldner, 1985a, 1985b; Hare-Mustin, 1978, 1979, 1980; Jacobson, 1983; James, 1984; James & McIntyre, 1983; Libow, Raskin, & Caust, 1982), who began examining dominant family therapy models and critiquing them in terms of their failure to recognize gender and power in intimate relationships. In the early 1980s there was no "feminist family therapy" and only a few feminist critiques of family therapy as it was usually practiced. These early writings were often seen as radical and controversial, challenging as they did the dominant systems views of neutrality and circular causality, and suggesting that family therapists often did therapy "on the backs of women," reinforced traditional gender roles, and held women responsible for family relationships.

In the second half of the 1980s, feminist voices in family therapy grew stronger and more audible with a mushrooming of conference presentations, articles, and the appearance of the first feminist books in the field (Ault-Riche, 1986; Braverman, 1988; Goodrich, Rampage, Ellman, & Halstead, 1988; Luepnitz, 1988; McGoldrick, Anderson, & Walsh, 1988; Walters, Carter, Papp, & Silverstein, 1988). These books marked the beginning of more concentrated efforts to define what feminist approaches to family therapy might look like, rather than simply critiquing existing models. With the advent of the *Journal of Feminist Family Therapy* in 1989 and other literature articulating more gender-conscious approaches to training and supervision (Ault-Riche, 1988; Avis, 1989a; Wheeler, Avis, Miller, & Chaney, 1988), as well as to therapy (Goodrich, 1991), feminist theorizing evolved from being predominantly critique into the generation of new ideas about working with gender and power in therapy and in training.

Up to this time, feminist writings had taken as their point of departure the perspective of women as both clients and therapists. Gender was written about in terms of how gender stereotypes and imbalances affected and oppressed women, and of ways to practice therapy in nonoppressive and empowering ways. Little was written from the perspective of how gender affected the lives and experience of men, or of working with men in gender-conscious ways. In the 1990s, this gap has begun to be addressed by the efforts of both feminists and nonfeminists to examine the experiences of men in families and in family therapy (Bograd, 1990; Dienhart & Avis, 1994; Jenkins, 1990; Meth & Pasick, 1990; White, 1992).

In the 1990s, there is also beginning to emerge a greater sensitivity to women's diversity and to the interaction of multiple sources of oppression, such as gender, class, race, culture, and sexual orientation (Greene, 1994; Kliman, 1994; Laird, 1994; Mirkin, 1994; Nichols, 1994; Pressman, 1994; Tamasese & Waldegrave, 1993). Earlier feminist writings tended to speak from the perspective of White, middle-class North American women and to ignore the differing perspectives and experiences of poor women, immigrant women, women of color, and lesbian and bisexual women. Some more recent writings emphasize the contribution of each source of oppression to the experience and definition of the others. Kliman (1994), for example, points out that "people of color are generally more oppressed on the basis of race than of gender. Race therefore tends to be more salient to family members than gender, even when there is tension or even hatred between the sexes" (p. 34).

Finally, in the mid-1990s there is emerging a postmodern or social constructionist feminist perspective in the field, with emphasis on how gender relations are constructed and co-constructed in families and in therapy (Avis & Turner, 1996; Hare-Mustin, 1994; Weingarten, 1991, 1992). This perspective examines the construction and consequences of dominant gender discourses and practices, takes a self-reflexive stance in examining the oppressive potential of feminist theories themselves, deemphasizes any attempt to reach "truth," and values diversity and multiplicity in feminist perspectives.

FEMINIST FAMILY THERAPY

Is there such an entity as "feminist family therapy," possible to define in the same way we might, for example, structural family therapy? There has been a great deal of debate among feminists and nonfeminists on this question. Some fear that using the word "feminist" appears to exclude men, both as clients and therapists, whereas others argue that it is important to use the word "feminist" because of the particular political stance it communicates about recognizing and addressing women's oppression. Some have wanted to call what they do "feminist-informed" therapy, whereas a few have used the designation "gender-sensitive." Many feminists regard this latter designation as inadequate in its neutrality. By not naming the relationship between gender and power, it appears to disguise or ignore this link and to imply that women and men are equally disadvantaged by the politics of gender:

Until recently, family therapy has been profoundly mute on the subject of power and its unequal distribution either in the family or in the society. Even now, the depth and breadth of women's inequality seem glossed over, for scarcely had we begun to examine the implications for therapy when we glided into "gender sensitivity" and "gender bias" instead. By creating the safe harbor of studying a seemingly two-sided phenomenon, we have been rescued from noticing how one-sided has been the damage of our traditional work. (Goodrich, 1991, p. 17)

Whatever designation is used, it has become increasingly evident that there is no single entity that can be called "feminist family therapy," just as there is no single feminism. There are, rather, multiple feminisms and multiple feminist *approaches* to family therapy. Many therapists, both women and men, consider themselves feminist and bring to their practice an awareness of gender and power relations. Yet, these therapists may practice in widely differing ways, depending on the particular family therapy models that guide their work. Thus, therapists practicing from such diverse methods as Bowen Family Systems, narrative, psychodynamic, solution-focused and behavioral models may all regard themselves as feminist or feminist-informed family therapists. Feminist family therapy, then, is best thought of as a *perspective* on gender relations, as a lens through which a therapist views his or her clients and work. This lens differs depending on the particular feminist theories the therapist embraces while these theories are, themselves, rapidly developing and evolving. With so much variation, can we say anything definitive about feminist perspectives on family therapy? Despite their differences, I believe most feminist therapists would agree with Flax (1990) that "one of the distinguishing features of feminist theories is the claim that gender relations, at least as they have been organized so far, are (variable) forms of domination. Feminist theorists are motivated in part by an active concern with justice and a desire to contribute to the overcoming of women's subordinations" (p. 139).

Where feminists in family therapy differ is in their thinking about how the dynamics of gender-based oppression actually work, and how best to address gender and power imbalances in their clients' lives. Thus, in the later section on key clinical skills, the skills reported will be a sampling of those most discussed in the field. They are not, however, skills that all family therapists practicing from feminist perspectives would necessarily utilize. From a social constructionist or postmodern feminist perspective, such diversity is welcomed and promoted, with multiplicity of ideas and approaches regarded as enriching and no single perspective regarded as embodying "truth."

The central focus of concern in relation to gender consciousness in family therapy has been the relationship between gender and power in intimate relationships. This concern relates both to power relations in

families and to those between therapist and family, with a growing awareness
that the gender-*un*aware therapist will almost certainly act in ways that
maintain and reinforce oppressive dynamics in the family. Despite this
growing awareness and the existence of a strong feminist critique, "traditional work still holds sway in many quarters" (Goodrich, 1991, p. 17). There
follows a brief review of the feminist critique in family therapy as it has
evolved over the past 18 years. A reference guide to books and articles
written during the first 10 years of the critique has been compiled by Avis
(1989b).

THE FEMINIST CRITIQUE OF FAMILY THERAPY

The Inadequacy of the Family Systems Metaphor

The primary focus of the feminist critique has been on the field's use of
family systems theory, devoid of any analysis of gender and power, as the
dominant framework for understanding family difficulties. Expressed in the
abstract, neutral language of cybernetics, the family systems metaphor likens
families to machines, functioning according to specific systemic rules and
divorced from their historical, social, economic, and political contexts. When
family therapists view families in isolation from these contexts, they tend
to see family difficulties as arising entirely within interpersonal relationships
in specific families and ignore the repetitive patterns of difficulty occurring
across families. By overlooking the relationship between sociopolitical
contexts and family functioning, they miss seeing how gender and power
relations in the wider culture are mirrored in families (James & McIntyre,
1983; Lerner, 1988). When family functioning is further conceptualized
outside its historical context, understanding of the impact of social change
on such things as family structure and the gendered division of labor is lost.

The systemic concepts of circularity, neutrality, and complementary
have been singled out as particularly problematic for developing adequate
accounts of gender-based inequalities in families.

Circularity. This concept, often referred to as "circular causality," implies
that family members engage in a never-ending, repetitive pattern of
mutually reinforcing behaviors, without regard for differences in power or
agency. When applied to problems such as battering, rape, and incest, the
concept of circular causality subtly removes responsibility from the aggressor
(most often male) and transfers it to the victim of the aggression (most
often female) by implying that she is a coresponsible participant in the
interactional pattern that ends in violence or abuse (Bograd, 1984). The
consequences of this way of thinking led Goldner (1985a) to suggest that
the concept of circularity looks "suspiciously like a hypersophisticated
version of blaming the victim and rationalizing the status quo" (p. 33). By

implying that all interactional behavior originates within the interaction itself, circular "causality" makes it impossible to conceptualize causes external to the interaction, such as cultural beliefs about appropriate gender behavior, a preexisting propensity to use violent behavior, or differences in power with which each partner entered the relationship. Circular "causality" is, then, a misnomer. It is actually a theory of problem maintenance posing as one of etiology (James & McIntyre, 1983), and, as such, renders it difficult for therapists to even raise questions about the causes of family problems (Taggart, 1985).

Neutrality. Similarly, the systemic concept of neutrality suggests that all parts of the system contribute *equally* to the production and maintenance of problems and thus render invisible the differences between family members in power and influence. As Taggart (1995) points out, within a systemic framework, questions of individual rights and responsibilities tend to disappear. An explanation is constructed in which the buck never stops and no one is ultimately responsible for anything.

Complementarity. The concept of complementarity is similarly problematic in its suggestion that men and women take complementary gender roles that are equal although different. By "obscur[ing] aspects of power and domination by appealing to the prettier, democratic construct of 'separate but equal' " (Goldner, 1985a, p. 37), the concept of complementarity may be seen as increasing family therapists' vulnerability to gender blindness.

Attempts to Integrate Feminist and Systems Ideas

Another theme in the feminist critique has been debate over whether feminist and family systems ideas are, in fact, incompatible with each other. Some early writers spoke of their struggles and dilemmas in trying to integrate these two perspectives (Libow et al., 1982). Some have argued that feminist theory can, by challenging traditional family systems theory to include broader social contexts, enable it to become more truly systemic (Lerner, 1988; Taggart, 1985).

Others argue that feminism is "dangerous" to family therapy (Goldner, 1985b; Hare-Mustin, 1980), and any genuine encounter between the two must involve a fundamental rethinking of many basic family therapy axioms and assumptions, as well as the introduction of new categories of analysis. These categories include gender, individual functioning, and "the material and social bases of interpersonal power . . . money, power, access to power, fairness, the ability to leave" (Goldner, 1985b, p. 23).

Gender as a Fundamental Category

A further theme in feminist theorizing is an understanding of gender as a fundamental and "irreducible category of clinical observation and theorizing" (Goldner, 1985b, p. 22), similar to other categories of oppression, such as race and class. Reducing this category to constructs such as "gender issues" and "gender roles" is seen as potentially trivializing of gender and obscuring of power differences between men and women (Goldner, 1985b; James, 1984; Thorne, 1982, 1985). The construct of sex roles, for example, implies that, similar to work or social roles, one can choose to "play" them or not, and men and women are equally disadvantaged by this "common enemy" (Goldner, 1985b). Feminist writers argue for the importance of understanding the whole of human experience as being gendered, including society, the family, and individual identity. They hold as equally necessary an understanding of the symbolic dimensions by which patriarchy is embedded in language, culture, and experience, and is thus subtly communicated and internalized from the moment of birth (Goldner, 1985b; James, 1984; Taggart, 1985).

Ignoring Gender Scholarship in Other Disciplines

Feminists have puzzled over the surprising lack of attention in family therapy to the voluminous theory and research on gender developed in the social sciences over the past 20 years. Until recently, this knowledge was largely ignored and only rarely integrated into clinical theorizing (Avis, 1985; Goldner, 1985a; James & McIntyre, 1983; Lerner, 1988). Knowledge about wife abuse, sexual abuse, and gender-related power and control are notable examples of such traditional gaps in knowledge in the field (Avis, 1992; Bograd, 1984, 1992; James & MacKinnon, 1990; Lamb, 1991). Feminists argue that it is family therapy's single-minded commitment to systemic ideas, especially those of neutrality and circularity, that has been largely responsible for its lack of receptivity to scholarship from other disciplines. Additional but less central reasons for the field's ignoring gender knowledge include the early predominance of male leaders and family therapists' faith that systemic thinking protects them from sexist or blaming practice (James & McIntyre, 1983).

Reinforcement of Traditional Gender Roles

The unquestioned reinforcement of stereotypical gender roles is a further area of gender blindness in the field (Hare-Mustin, 1978). A family therapist who has not developed her or his own gender consciousness is at high risk for having stereotypical expectations of men and women and for seeing traditional relationship arrangements as most desirable or most functional. They are also unlikely to comprehend the impact of gender socialization and cultural gender prescriptions on men's and women's lives and relationships. Without gender awareness, family therapists literally practice unconsciously, unable to prevent themselves from unintentionally reinforcing these prescriptions. These dominant cultural discourses on gender are embedded in the androcentric theories of development, behavior, and relationships that have been central to North American professional education for the past 40 years. Without a reexamination of these theories, therapists will continue to view their clients through the distorted lens of male-defined reality and theories that view women's socialized behaviors as signs of inherent weakness, passivity, or masochism (Weiner & Boss, 1985).

In 1975, the American Psychological Association (APA) Task Force on Sex Bias and Sex-Role Stereotyping in Psychotherapeutic Practice found the following biases particularly prevalent among family therapists: (1) assuming that remaining in a marriage would result in better adjustment for women; (2) demonstrating less interest in and sensitivity to a woman's career than a man's; (3) perpetuating the belief that a child's problems and child rearing are primarily women's responsibilities; (4) exhibiting a double standard regarding a wife's versus a husband's extramarital affair; and (5) deferring to a husband's needs over a wife's. Although 20 years have passed since the Task Force identified these biases, they continue to be dominant in the culture and affect the practice of gender-*un*conscious family therapists.

Tendency to Blame Mothers for Family Difficulties

The belief that a child's problems and child rearing are primarily women's responsibilities has been the focus of significant feminist critique (Bograd, 1984; Caplan & Hall-McCorquodale, 1985; Haig, 1988; Layton, 1984; Wheeler, 1985). The assumption of women's primary responsibility for child-rearing frequently results in a parallel assumption of their primary responsibility for causing problems in their children. Although mother-blaming is pervasive in all areas of psychotherapeutic theory and practice (Caplan, 1985; Caplan & Hall-McCorquodale, 1985; Ehrenreich & English, 1978; Penfold & Walker, 1983), several studies have found it to be particularly prevalent in family therapy.

Caplan and Hall-McCorquodale's (1985) study of nine major clinical journals (in psychiatry, psychoanalysis, psychology, and family therapy), found 72 different types of child problems attributed to mothers by therapists. Although extensive mother-blaming was found throughout all of the journals examined, it was most extreme in the psychoanalytic and family therapy journals. In another study, Haig (1988) examined clinical examples in four family therapy journals in two target years, and found mother-blaming to be a serious and pervasive problem that had increased slightly between 1978 and 1988. She found 17 areas in which there was a significant difference in the way fathers and mothers were treated by family therapists. These included such areas as being described negatively, being seen as the source of children's problems, and being the focus of treatment.

The gender blindness promoted by family systems concepts has led to a failure in the field to recognize the central dilemma of many women's lives: The cultural prescription for motherhood requires women to devote themselves to their families and to assume primary (and often sole) responsibility for raising their children, even at the cost of their own needs, even when they are employed full time, and even when they lack the power or resources to do so. When children develop problems, it is their mothers who are then seen as having failed in their responsibility. There is no parallel prescription for fathers. Their absence from the home is regarded as expected and "normal," and these studies found that they are rarely seen as the source of their children's difficulties.

As a result of this cultural prescription for women and the underlying beliefs about women's responsibility, family therapists are at risk of behaving in ways that hold women more responsible than men for family well-being. Goldner (1985a) suggests that family therapists often exploit women's sense of responsibility for their families by pushing them harder than they do their partners to effect family change. When a structural family therapist attempts to engage a peripheral father by asking him temporarily to take charge of some aspect of parenting, the implicit message is that the mother has failed in some way, and the father will show her how to do it properly. The other message is that the responsibility for the family is actually the mother's, and the father is either teaching her more effective parenting skills or temporarily helping her out, or giving her a holiday. As Taggart (1985) points out, practices such as these "project onto the woman as her pathology, what are consequences of the cultural bias in the first place" (p. 4).

The other side of mother-blaming is father-idealizing (Caplan & Hall-McCorquodale, 1985). Unlike mothers, fathers are often described in the clinical literature in only positive or neutral terms, appreciated simply for coming to therapy, given credit for family change, and placed in teaching and supervisory roles in relation to their wives (Haig, 1988).

These practices can result in very different experiences for women and men in family therapy, with men being underchallenged to assume their share of responsibility, and women being asked to assume more than theirs. Such practices are disrespectful of both men and women, and simply perpetuate in the therapy room the dominant cultural narratives about gender.

Blindness to the Political Dimensions of Therapy

Another way in which family therapists may remain gender blind is by failing to recognize the political dimensions of their work. Many therapists attempt to maintain a neutral stance with regard to gender and power arrangements in their client families, believing that such a stance shows maximum respect for a family's own values. Many models encourage therapist neutrality in the name of multipartiality or, in the case of some social constructionist approaches, of therapist curiosity and "not-knowing" (Anderson & Goolishian, 1988, 1992). However, such a position ignores the power inherent in the therapeutic relationship, the reality that therapists cannot, in fact, *not* express values, and the realization that therapeutic neutrality is an impossible and often dangerous myth (Avis, 1985; Jacobson, 1983; White, 1994). Feminists raise concerns that therapists who attempt to maintain neutrality will, without realizing it, adopt political positions by what they choose to focus on, respond to, challenge, or ignore. In so doing, they may well reinforce traditional values, ideas, or arrangements oppressive to women. Such reinforcement occurs primarily by default: The therapist's failure to challenge traditional arrangements, for example, or to raise questions about indications of violence, may then be perceived by clients as tacit approval. Avoiding this situation requires therapists to develop an awareness of their own values and beliefs, and to consciously choose what values they wish to reinforce (Avis, 1985; Gurman & Klein, 1984; Jacobson, 1983; White, 1994).

Failure to Recognize or Address Abuse, Violence, and Control

In recent years, feminists have strongly criticized family therapy for its failure to adequately address violence and sexual abuse in either theory or practice. Despite growing documentation of the extensive dimensions of physical and sexual violence committed by husbands and fathers against wives and children, family therapists have been ill prepared by their training or theory to attend to these issues in their clients' lives (Avis, 1992; Bograd, 1984, 1992; James & MacKinnon, 1990; Lamb, 1991). Family therapy journals, compared with those in other disciplines, have published relatively few articles on the subject, while Lamb (1991) found a high incidence of linguistic avoidance of male responsibility for wife battering in family therapy journal articles. She found that, of four disciplines examined, family therapy journal articles were highest in the area of diffusion of responsibility, that is, in causing the agent to disappear by referring to the battering of women by men as "spouse abuse," "marital aggression," "couples' violence," or "married couples experiencing violence." Lamb explains these findings as follows:

> Many family theorists [are] still rooted in the belief that systems are essentially "cooperative," apparently unaware that the superficial cooperation visible in a system may actually be the product of coercion. . . . For family systems theorists, a battering man's violence can be perceived as a result of an interaction, such as the joint escalation of an argument, thus obviating the need to assign an agent to the act itself. (p. 255)

Similar criticisms have been leveled against family therapy accounts of incest and sexual abuse. James and MacKinnon (1990) find these clinical accounts embedded with pervasive myths that serve both to blame the victim and to obscure the dimensions of gender and power.

Critique of Specific Models

In addition to the generalized issues outlined previously, specific models of family therapy have been individually critiqued for their embedded gender assumptions and blind spots. The most extensive critique of individual models is found in Luepnitz (1988). She examines the work of Nathan Ackerman, Murray Bowen, Virginia Satir, Salvador Minuchin, Ivan Boszormenyi-Nagy, and Carl Whitaker, as well as strategic family therapy and Milan systemic therapy. The politics of James Alexander's Functional Family Therapy is critiqued by Avis (1985).

It can safely be said that *all* models of family therapy involve some degree of inherent gender bias, since their developers were a product of their time and culture, and themselves lacked gender consciousness. Without such consciousness, they could not avoid replicating in their theories and models the dominant cultural discourses on gender. This does not mean that no traditional models can be useful to a feminist or gender-conscious family therapist. Most models have some, even many, useful ideas and concepts. What it *does* mean is that, before it can be safely used, any model must first be carefully deconstructed to reveal its gender assumptions and biases and then reconstructed to incorporate the dimensions of gender and power.

CONCEPTUAL AFFIRMATIVE ACTION

The work of feminist theorists from other disciplines has been drawn on by feminist family therapists to provide "conceptual affirmative action" (Weiner & Boss, 1985), that is, theoretical assistance in reconceptualizing women's development over the life cycle and challenging traditional assumptions regarding women's behavior and development. The following three examples illustrate this theoretical assistance. Chodorow's (1978) theory of the social construction of mothering has been widely cited for its linking of the sexual division of labor to the economic dictates of Western capitalism, and women's primary responsibility for child care to the development of different relational capacities in boys and girls.

Dinnerstein's (1976) work has been helpful in expanding thinking about the distinctly different ways in which male and female power are experienced. She hypothesizes that the domination of infant care by women results in exaggerated images and deep-seated fears of women's power, in a perception of women's power as irrational and engulfing, and a tendency to displace rage at adult powerlessness onto women.

Another example is the utilization of Jean Baker Miller's (1976) model of adulthood, which is based not on the traditional male model of separation, but on a female model of connectedness (i.e., of valuing enlarging and deepening human relationships). Miller's model values and validates women's traditional capacities for nurturing and cultivating relationships and suggests that, as capacities essential to the human community, they must be valued and shared by men as well as by women.

THERAPY WITH MEN

Since the advent of the 1990s, a slowly developing body of literature has begun to examine issues related to working with men in family therapy. This literature reflects a growing recognition, among both feminist and nonfeminist family therapists, of the high cost to men of their privilege; of the failure of dominant psychological, family systems, and psychotherapeutic theories to reflect the subjectively lived experience of men as well as of women (Bograd, 1990); and of the reality that family therapy committed to liberating women's lives from gender oppression must necessarily be committed to liberating men's. As Bograd (1990) points out:

> A feminist perspective is characterized by binocular vision that combines awareness of the pain and struggles of individual men with that of their adaptation and unquestioning compliance to cultural dictates that give them power at the cost of a certain humanity. . . . The challenges then become how to translate a feminist awareness into caring, effective clinical practice with men; how to extend feminist insights about women to encompass human systems; and how to bring men and women together from their divergent experiences and positions that so conspire against mutual understanding and collaboration. (pp. xiv–xv)

Although still sparse, literature on working with men emphasizes deconstructing traditional masculinity and male socialization (Allen & Laird, 1990; Meth & Pasick, 1990; White, 1992); exploring feminist and politically aware alternatives for therapy with men (Bograd, 1990; Dienhart & Avis, 1990; Ganley, 1990); and approaches to working with violent and sexually abusive men (Almeida & Bograd, 1990; Jenkins, 1990; Wheeler, 1989). In the Dienhart and Avis (1994) Delphi study of gender-sensitive ways to work with men in family therapy, 36 family therapists (23 women and 13 men) endorsed 131 interventions as appropriate and effective for working with male clients. This group of therapists emphasized the importance of therapists developing an understanding of their own gender socialization, values, and biases, including their stereotypical ideas about men, as essential to developing an awareness of gender issues in working with men. They also emphasized interventions that assess the distribution of responsibility in families and promote shared responsibility between men and women for family life and for resolving family difficulties. Similar to Meth and Pasick's (1990) contention that challenging socialized attitudes and behaviors is a major focus of therapy with men, the Dienhart and Avis (1994) participants endorsed many interventions designed to challenge men's socialization, including psychoeducation, cognitive restructuring, role reversals, examining family-of-origin issues, and direct challenge. They also supported interventions for assessing and challenging the balance of power in families. However, surprisingly few interventions (only four of 46 suggested) were endorsed relative to encouraging men's affective expression. In contrast, Meth and Pasick (1990) consider it critically important that therapists explore men's feelings in therapy, at the same time, understanding the enormous consequences of men's socialization to repress feeling.

Feminist and nonfeminist literature about family therapy with men tends to differ in its conceptualization and degree of emphasis on issues of power, control, and violence. Although feminists emphasize the negative consequences of male power and control, and personal accountability for abuse of this power, nonfeminists attend more to gender roles and socialization, affect, and cognitive change. Bograd (1990), for example, argues that "a feminist approach to the therapy of men keeps power at the center of personal and clinical concern" (p. 145), whereas Meth and Pasick (1990) suggest that male power is more burden than privilege and cite Farrell's (1986) conclusion that "men actually have very little power, if power is redefined as autonomy over one's own life" (p. 13). They argue that gender hierarchy has resulted from traditional expectations of men to be powerful and successful, and from the lack of socially acceptable alternatives to traditional male behaviors.

Our thinking about how to work most effectively in family therapy with men, and with gender as it is played out in men's lives, is clearly in an early stage. Much more theoretical and clinical development needs to be done in this area as we struggle to find more effective ways of inviting men to conscious and choiceful awareness, and to full partnership in their couple and family relationships.

KEY CONCEPTS

Agency. The ability to take action in one's own life and on one's own behalf is called agency. It is the freedom to make choices and to act on them. The ability to say "no," to assert, to do, by choice and without socialized guilt. Increasing women's sense of agency is an important focus of feminist therapy.

Collaboration. This is a therapeutic stance that emphasizes the client's expertise in her or his own life and the nonexpert position of the therapist. Therapy is seen as a cooperative and co-constructed endeavor between equals.

Constructed knowledge. Feminists view knowledge as socially constructed. Reality is not regarded as represented by science, but rather as *created* by theory builders and researchers. Power is the ability to have one's own construction of reality accepted as legitimate "knowledge." The critical question becomes "Whose interests are served by this particular construction of reality?" Commonly accepted "knowledge" about women is understood as having been largely constructed by men and as serving men's, not women's, interests. Therapy involves helping both women and men to deconstruct the impact of oppressive, dominant knowledges on their lives and construct new, liberating knowledge about themselves.

Deconstruction. The process of examining and challenging the assumptions about women and their roles embedded in dominant cultural beliefs, "knowledge," and practices is called deconstruction. As what is accepted as "the way things are" is deconstructed, the external sources of personal beliefs are illuminated and personal choice, free from cultural gender prescriptions, becomes possible.

Feminism. This is variously defined as (1) a *doctrine* recognizing asymmetric power in gender relations and espousing equal social, political, and economic rights for women with men; (2) an organized social *movement* for attaining those rights; (3) an *analysis* of the forces that maintain women's subordination and assertion of women's ideas, voice, experience, and construction of knowledge; and (4) a *commitment to broad social change* in order to achieve equal power between men and women (Lerner, 1986). Although most feminists incorporate the first three, there is disagreement on the necessity of the fourth.

Gender. A person's learned or cultural status as feminine or masculine, as distinct from his or her biological status as female or male, gender is "the cultural definition of behavior defined as appropriate to the sexes in a given society at a given time. [It] is a set of cultural roles. It is a costume, a mask, a straitjacket in which men and women dance their unequal dance" (Lerner, 1986, p. 238). Feminists emphasize the fundamental nature of gender as a basic category of social organization and discrimination, similar in nature to the categories of race and class (Flax, 1990; Goldner, 1985b; James, 1984).

Gender role. The culturally prescribed and learned behaviors, attitudes, and characteristics associated with being masculine or feminine are called the gender role (Greenglass, 1982). This concept has been criticized for depicting gender differences in sociopsychological rather than structural terms. Critics suggest that the concept of gender roles obscures the differences in power between the genders by implying both that one can choose whether to play one's gender role, and that men and women are equally disadvantaged by them (Goldner, 1985b; James, 1984).

Gender-sensitive. This is an awareness of the impact of gender socialization on an individual's psychological, emotional, and interpersonal functioning, as well as on his or her power, status, position, and privilege in social–cultural–political systems.

Liberal feminism. In this feminist framework emphasizing equality in terms of equal rights and equal opportunity for women, women's subordination is seen as caused by legal constraints and social policies that discriminate against women, resulting in inequality in civil rights and in educational and employment opportunities. Liberal feminists do not attempt a historical analysis of the causes of this discrimination but focus on removing sexist discrimination and economic and legal barriers to women's equal participation in the public sphere (Jaggar & Rothenberg, 1984).

Nonsexist. Nondiscrimination on the basis of sex (i.e., equal treatment of women and men) is called nonsexist behavior. This is distinct from feminist approaches that emphasize existing asymmetries in power and privilege between women and men, and deliberately works to redress them. This distinction is crucial. In marital therapy, for example, a nonsexist approach, by being evenhanded, may result in the perpetuation of preexisting inequities, whereas a feminist approach may give greater weight to a woman's requests for change than to a man's, in order to address the power imbalance between them (Jacobson, 1983).

Oppression. This term, meaning forceful subordination, "has been used to describe the subject condition of individuals and of groups, as in 'class oppression' or 'racial oppression'" (Lerner, 1986, p. 233). It is commonly used by feminists to describe the domination of women. Some feminist theorists, such as historian Gerda Lerner (1986), find the term problematic in its implication that women are primarily victims, and in its obscuring of the complexities of patriarchal dominance, including women's internalization of that dominance and their resulting unconscious participation in their own oppression.

Patriarchy. In its broad definition, patriarchy means "the manifestation and institutionalization of male dominance over women and children in the family and the extension of male dominance over women in society in general" (Lerner, 1986, p. 239). This concept recognizes men's power, and women's lack of access to it, in all important institutions in society. It does *not* imply, however, that women are totally powerless, that they do not protest their subordinate position, or that they have no rights, influence, or resources (Lerner, 1986).

"The personal is political." This concept emphasizes that what happens in the private sphere, in women's personal lives, is an expression of their experience of oppression in the wider public sphere. As Harriet Lerner

(1985) states, "There is a circular connection between the patterns of our intimate relationships and the degree to which women are represented, valued, and empowered in every aspect of society and culture. The patterns that keep us stuck in our close relationships derive their shape and form from the patterns of a stuck society" (p. 223). "The personal is political" emphasizes oppression as a process whereby dominant oppressive ideas from the culture are internalized and then acted upon (i.e., the oppressed begin to oppress themselves).

Power. There are a wide variety of definitions and distinctions about kinds of power, including the broad distinction between "power-over" (coercion, control, dominance) and "power-to" (the ability to act, to name, to influence, to comment, to say no, to define oneself, to act on one's own behalf, to have choice). Goodrich (1991) points out some of the contradictions and complexities in this simple delineation—that men's power, under patriarchy, to name and define reality (power-to), has been used to increase and justify their domination of women (power-over). Goodrich (1991) offers the following definition: "Power is the capacity to gain whatever resources are necessary to remove oneself from a condition of oppression, to guarantee one's ability to perform, and to affect not only one's own circumstances, but also more general circumstances outside one's intimate surroundings" (p. 10).

Radical feminism. This is a feminist framework that takes a number of different forms. However, all forms are based on the assumption that the oppression of women is the fundamental oppression: It has operated across time, culture, and class, is embedded in every aspect of life, and is therefore the hardest form of oppression to eradicate (Jaggar & Rothenberg, 1984). Radical feminists emphasize the personal as political and patriarchy as a social structure through which men of all classes and cultures dominate and exploit women. Women's problems and unhappiness are seen as a response to their oppression by the patriarchal system.

Sexism. Discrimination on the basis of sex, especially the denigration and oppression of women by, and in favor of, men is called sexism. "The ideology of male supremacy, of male superiority and of beliefs that support and sustain it" (Lerner, 1986, p. 240).

Socialist feminism. This feminist framework draws on Marxist traditions to analyze women's oppression. Like traditional Marxists, socialist feminists believe that human nature is created by the type of society and form of social organization in which people live. They also agree that equal opportunity is impossible in a class society. They do not, however, view women's oppression as simply a result of the class oppression embodied in capitalism; rather, they believe that in order to understand the oppression of women across classes, Marxist theory must be expanded from an analysis of the means of production to an analysis of the social organization of the means of reproduction, including sexuality, nurturing, and raising children

(Jaggar & Rothenberg, 1984). Socialist feminists argue that such an expanded analysis is necessary to explain why women in every class are subordinate to men, both within and outside the family. Some socialist feminists view patriarchy and capitalism as reciprocal and mutually reinforcing systems that allow men to control women's labor, and they suggest that both must be abolished before women can be liberated (Hartman, 1984).

Subordination. Meaning the position of being "of a lesser order or importance," "under the authority or control of another," and of being "put in a lower position or rank" (*Collins English Dictionary,* 1986, p. 1518), this term is used by feminists to describe women's historical position in society. Historian Gerda Lerner (1986) suggests that it is preferable to "oppression," because it does not imply that the dominant have evil intent and "it includes the possibility of voluntary acceptance of subordinate status in exchange for protection and privilege" (p. 234).

KEY CLINICAL SKILLS

A number of the skills discussed here are not unique to feminist therapy; what is unique is their intended purpose to address gender and rebalance power. Although different feminist therapists may emphasize different interventions, these skills appear repeatedly in the literature and form the core of feminist work. They have been organized under conceptual and intervention categories to emphasize the need for therapists to develop a conceptualization of gender and power before being able to intervene effectively in these areas. See Avis (1991), Libow (1986), and Wheeler et al. (1988) for further discussion.

Conceptual Skills

Understanding women in context. An in-depth understanding of the sociopolitical, economic, and biological forces that shape and constrain women's lives. These include the feminization of poverty, minimum wage, inadequate day care, sole-support parenting, violence, sexual abuse, cultural biases against women, gender socialization, guilt, the impact of women's biology on their lives and relationships, and the interaction of gender oppression with the oppressions of race, class, and sexual orientation.

Holding positive and empowering beliefs about women. A conceptual skill that first requires a conscious reexamination of the therapist's own beliefs and ideas about women and an honest confrontation with biases about women absorbed from the culture. It also involves deliberately cultivating a recognition of women's strengths and competencies, reconceptualizing many symptoms as survival mechanisms and appreciating women's essential reproductive, nurturing, and physical work in families.

Holding a positive, nonblaming attitude toward men. A skill that involves a recognition that men, as well as women, are victimized by their gender socialization, and developing a nonblaming attitude toward their socialized behaviors. This awareness in no way negates holding abusive or controlling men accountable for their misuse of power or use of coercion; rather, it means understanding these behaviors, and men, in their sociocultural and political contexts, and appreciating that it is these contexts, rather than innate male characteristics, that have taught and promoted male dominance and misuse of power. Such an understanding enables therapists to believe in men's ability to change, to engage with them in nonblaming ways, and to work with their strengths while challenging their socialized behaviors. This conceptual skill is perhaps best illustrated by the work of Alan Jenkins (1990).

Recognizing gender-based power inequities as a major factor in couple and family difficulties. Conceptualizing relationship functioning in terms of gender-based power and recognizing the impact of power inequities on individual, couple, and family well-being. This understanding helps family therapists avoid the pitfalls of such systemic notions as neutrality, circularity, and "the power of powerlessness."

Recognizing power issues as power issues. A conceptual skill that requires clarity about the difference between power issues and communication issues (Avis, 1991). Therapists are most likely to confuse one with the other in situations in which a man is ignoring or refusing his partner's requests that he take a more equitable share of responsibility for the relationship or the family. The unaware therapist may encourage the woman to communicate her needs and desires more effectively, failing to realize that the problem is not the woman's poor communication skills, but rather, the man's power to refuse and the woman's lack of power to persuade. Conceptual clarity in this area enables the therapist to focus intervention at the appropriate level (i.e., at the level of power, control, and responsibility, not of communication).

Intervention Skills

Empowerment. All approaches to family therapy endeavor to empower and strengthen family members. What is unique about a feminist approach is its recognition that women most often enter relationships, and therapy, with less power than their male partners in terms of economic and physical resources, agency, voice, and influence, while paradoxically having more responsibility for family maintenance and well-being. Feminist therapists believe that where such a power imbalance exists, working to empower men and women equally would simply maintain the same imbalance with which the couple entered therapy (Avis, 1985; Jacobson, 1983). They are, therefore, interested in shifting this imbalance by working with men to give up some of their power and privilege, and with women to assume more; however, feminist therapists recognize that the work of "empowerment" always takes place within an overarching sociocultural–political context of disempowerment. They distinguish between *feeling* more powerful and actually *having* power and emphasize that "empowering" work within the therapy room should not be mistaken as helping women to actually have power in the outside world or as a substitute for social action to change the oppressive social context.

All of the following specific interventions are designed to empower both women and men by challenging traditional gender prescriptions and promoting liberating relationships based on equality.

Regarding each woman as the best expert on herself. Perhaps the most important and empowering belief that a therapist can have is that the client is both competent and the best expert on herself. This attitude cannot be assumed as a therapeutic technique. To be effective, it must be deeply held and communicated to the client in a wide variety of ways. It involves really listening to women, validating their experience, ideas, and expertise; and helping them to listen to their own inner wisdom. Women often enter therapy disconnected to this inner voice, which they have been socialized to ignore in favor of dominant cultural voices that tell them how they should be as women. The first task of therapy, then, may be to help a woman begin to tune in to her own self-knowledge, to validate its authenticity, and to follow its guidance. Various interventions may be used to help this process, including visualization of her "inner guide," quietly listening to what is emerging within, journalizing, drawing, meditating, and listening to her symptoms as powerful messages from her inner self (Avis, 1991).

Encouraging women's agency, voice, and visibility. Having learned to listen to their own wisdom, the next step for many women is learning to take action in their own lives: to actually engage their strengths and competencies in working for their own best interests. Feminist therapists emphasize the importance of helping women to develop a sense of agency by such means as taking responsibility for that over which they do have control; claiming and expressing their anger directly; exercising direct forms of personal power such as saying "No"; finding their voice; asserting their ideas, needs, and wants; taking space; becoming visible to themselves and others; and taking action (Avis, 1991).

Challenging the client's internalized beliefs. Sometimes called "social analysis," this area of intervention is central to feminist therapy. It connects the personal and the political by challenging the oppressive beliefs about gender and about women that both women and men have internalized from the dominant culture—beliefs that lead them to unconscious participation in either their own oppression or that of their partner. Skills such as cognitive

restructuring and narrative questioning can be used to explore the relationship between the position of women and men in society and the client's
beliefs about her- or himself, about relationships, about what it is to be a
"good" woman, man, partner, mother, or father. Providing new information
further challenges oppressive beliefs.

Building respectful, collaborative therapeutic relationships. For feminist therapists, the therapeutic relationship is the most important element of therapy,
a template of the mutual, respectful, and balanced gender relationships that
the therapist seeks to foster. Emphasis is placed on developing relationships
which are nonhierarchical, highly respectful, and collaborative. Every effort
is made to equalize power in the therapeutic relationship, with the therapist
deliberately acting to decrease her or his expert power in the interests of
helping clients to increase theirs.

Demystifying therapy. Feminist therapists are committed to making the
processes of therapy as transparent as possible in the interests of maximizing
clients' power, agency, and choice. Therapists therefore openly share their
thinking, observations, goals, assumptions, beliefs, values, questions, approach
to therapy, and possible therapeutic options and choices, in an effort to
enable clients to participate from a position of maximum knowledge and
personal power and make informed choices about therapy.

Depathologizing women and their difficulties. This is the skill of redefining
as strengths, competence, and health those things the client may regard as
deficits, deviance, or pathology. It involves a therapeutic stance that understands the client in context and recognizes as healthy and adaptive a client's
responses to unhealthy circumstances. Depression may thus be seen as a
healthy reaction to a depressing relationship — as a message from the client's
inner self that something is wrong.

Making gender and power issues visible. A major focus of feminist work is
making gender and power dynamics visible to clients so that they may begin
to reexamine their gendered beliefs and assumptions. Typical interventions
are (1) including power and gender dimensions in problem definitions; (2)
exploring beliefs about such issues as money, leisure options, parenting
responsibilities, housekeeping, and child care; (3) making connections
between gender issues in the couple or family and those in the wider
culture; (4) questioning gender-stereotypical behaviors, attitudes, and expectations; and (5) exploring gender messages and assumptions in families
of origin.

Working to rebalance power in couple relationships. Interventions in this area
are based on the assumption that imbalances in power and privilege underlie
many couple conflicts. Feminist therapists usually address such imbalances
directly, seeking to resolve difficulties by redistributing power in the couple
system rather than by further disempowering the woman. They explicitly
discuss the distribution of power in such areas as the division of child care
and housekeeping responsibilities, money, spending, sex, decision making,

and differences in partners' economic power. They assess forms of control such as access to money and freedom to pursue one's own interests without partner approval. Furthermore, they assess for the existence of any form of intimidation, including physical, emotional, verbal, and sexual abuse. When a major power differential is uncovered, it is linked to the couple's presenting difficulties. The therapist then explores the couple's reasons for choosing this particular arrangement, challenges the beliefs underlying it, and encourages both partners to move toward a redistribution of power. An elaboration of this process can be found in Avis (1991) and in Dienhart and Avis (1994).

Skills training. This is a useful intervention for assisting women and men to develop skills neglected by their gender socialization. It may focus on such skills as (1) helping women learn how to express their ideas, needs and feelings, including anger, assertively and effectively; (2) using role play to enable clients to practice non-gender-normative behaviors; (3) helping women learn to assess and meet their own needs; (4) teaching men to ask for help; (5) helping men learn to recognize and express their feelings; (6) teaching men to listen to their partners' problems without taking or suggesting action; and (7) teaching men how to respond effectively to their families' emotional and nurturing needs; (8) helping both women and men to anticipate and deal with "change back" reactions from their families and others following change (Avis, 1991; Chaney, 1986; Dienhart & Avis, 1994).

TEACHING TOOLS AND TECHNIQUES

An in-depth discussion of ways to integrate gender into the family therapy curriculum can be found in Avis (1989). A summary of major teaching techniques from this discussion is presented here.

Course Content on Gender

Specific course content is necessary to promote shifts in trainees' thinking regarding gender. There are two methods for doing this. The first is through mainstreaming, whereby gender issues are raised in every course and in supervision, emphasizing the centrality of gender issues in all aspects of therapy. The second is through offering a separate course on gender, allowing a more in-depth examination of the issues and of the history behind the issues, which can be accomplished through mainstreaming. Ideally, both are needed for effective training in gender consciousness.

Actual course content includes a combination of theory and research on gender, including its interaction with other forms of discrimination, from the social sciences as well as from family therapy.

Required Readings

A broad spectrum of background reading is essential to developing gender consciousness. Students may be asked to read articles, research reports, autobiographies, and books that sensitize them to gender issues and feminist perspectives in general, and to the feminist critique of family therapy in particular.

Annotated Bibliographies

This is an assignment in which students write 30–35 annotations of course-related readings in lieu of a major paper. Each annotation consists of a brief summary of content, as well as of students' reactions and comments about how it relates to other readings. The assignment encourages students to read widely and to synthesize their thinking.

Open, Nondefensive Discussion

Group discussion is an important tool for allowing trainees to process their reactions to readings and lectures, to hear others' perspectives, and to resolve constructively strong feelings that may be aroused. This material touches participants deeply and often elicits intense reactions. To be effective, therefore, discussions must be made safe for all participants through setting group rules and discussion guidelines and helping participants learn how to listen to each other and deal with disagreement respectfully.

Making Gender and Power Issues Explicit

Trainers and supervisors can make gender and power issues, including those of class, race, and sexual orientation, explicit during training in a wide variety of ways. They can be raised as part of every topic and case discussion in both the classroom and in supervision. They can also be raised by asking questions that challenge trainees' gender assumptions and beliefs (such as questioning their assumptions about "normal" families, lesbian relationships, or single mothers); commenting on woman-blaming, father-ignoring, and sexist language whenever such biases occur in therapy or in training; and pointing out abuses of women in traditional therapies.

Use of Interpersonal Process in the Training Context

Interpersonal processes in the training context can be usefully identified and discussed as live illustrations of gender dynamics. Examples might be the tendency for men to interrupt women and to take up more airtime, and for women to hold back from expressing their views, to accommodate, and to let men interrupt them. When men comprise a small minority in a training group, the reverse may occur, with men feeling uncomfortable and marginalized. These feelings can be fruitfully explored and parallels drawn with the usual experience of women and racial minorities in a White male world. The key here is gentle, nonblaming, and supportive discussion.

Teaching What the Gender Issues Are

Through lectures and formal presentations, instructors can provide explicit information on gender and its interaction with other forms of oppression, including conceptual frameworks, statistics, historical perspectives, and the biases and limitations of traditional theory. Such presentations help trainees organize the large amounts of information acquired through their readings. Information is usually most effective when presented directly, openly, and nonapologetically.

Sharing One's Own Beliefs and Values; Changing Understanding, Learning, and Mistakes

By sharing with trainees her or his own journey in developing gender and sociopolitical awareness, an instructor can provide an invitation for open discussion and at the same time communicate that everyone is somewhere on the journey of developing consciousness.

Journal Writing

Journal writing can be an excellent tool for helping trainees to process their personal reactions, both cognitive and affective, aroused by readings, lectures, discussions, and class experiences. If journals are handed in to the instructor at regular intervals during a course, they can provide information about the issues a trainee is struggling with, as well as a wonderful opportunity for ongoing dialogue.

Gender Narratives

Trainees can be asked to interview each other using narrative questions to explore the gender narratives, rules, and expectations in their families of origin. Working in pairs, with about an hour in each role, trainees have an opportunity to experience the power of responding to gender narrative questions, as well as to practice asking them. A sampling of such questions includes the following: What were the dominant stories (both positive and negative) about women and about men in your family of origin? As you were growing up, what story did you have about what your life would be like as an adult woman or man? How was this idea formed? In what ways has your life benefited from these stories? In what ways has your life suffered from them? Which stories continue to have an impact on your life in the present?

Following this exercise, trainees may be asked to write a paper on their own gender narratives and values, and those in their families of origin.

Applying a Gender Analysis to Clinical Work

Require trainees always to (1) include an analysis of power and gender in conceptualizing relationship dynamics and presenting problems in their clinical work; (2) discuss sociopolitical and cultural forces and their impact upon presenting problems; (3) set treatment goals that are gender balanced; and (4) design interventions that address power and gender.

Case Analysis

Trainees may be presented with a case history, asked to develop various analyses of it, and then asked to discuss how some of these analyses may be subtly biased against women. Alternatively, trainees may present their current cases during group supervision, following which the group analyzes and discusses the gender dynamics in the family and the presenting problem.

Video Analysis and Role Play

Video analysis can be a particularly helpful tool for heightening trainees' awareness of gender issues in therapy. One method is to have therapists view tapes of themselves, watching for subtle signs in their own behavior that suggest that they respond differently to men than to women (e.g., being protective of the man, or talking to the woman about child care and to the man about finances). Role plays of therapy, videotapes, and training tapes may be used to analyze gender assumptions and blindness, as well as to develop gender hypotheses and interventions. Finally, exaggerated "how not to do therapy" role plays and videotapes may provide playful, memorable learning experiences.

Use of Media

Commercial, educational, and documentary films, as well as clips from television shows and commercials, can be extremely useful for demonstrating gendered behavior, gender relations, power dynamics, violence, abuse, and sexist attitudes. Used either in their entirety or as brief clips, films and videos are effective catalysts for raising issues, eliciting attitudes and values, and promoting discussion.

RESEARCH ISSUES

Research on gender is still scant in family therapy. Although there has been a growing feminist presence in the field for almost 20 years, there has been comparatively little feminist research, and few nonfeminists have been concerned with gender. In fact, there is a fundamental lack of attention to gender in family therapy research: Many studies fail to include even the most basic information regarding gender, and few explicitly study some dimension of gender relations. Feminist concerns regarding research generally fall into two main areas: (1) challenging family therapy research to attend more adequately to gender; and (2) doing feminist-informed research on aspects of gender and power relations in family therapy.

The first of these concerns is demonstrated by Woodard's (1991) study of 82 research studies published in four major family therapy journals in 1979 and 1989. She found that 30 relevant gender variables were not included in the majority of these studies. Some of the variables she looked for were very basic, including failure in the following areas: to report the sex of participants or research assistants; to discuss the possible impact of sex of research assistants on the findings; to analyze for sex differences; to note the relevance of gender to the findings; to state the researcher's own gender assumptions; to discuss gender concepts in the literature review; to state the reason for doing a single-sex study; and to discuss the gender bias of the instruments used. We see in these findings the gender blindness of the field expressed in its research.

Addressing this blindness requires attention to the areas identified by Woodard, as well as sensitivity to the ways family therapy research may reflect dominant cultural constructions of marriage and family. In research on marital change, for example, it is important to use outcome criteria that recognize increased conflict resulting from a wife's growing assertiveness as an indicator of positive, rather than negative, change, and to discriminate between positive and negative continuation of marriage outcomes.

The second feminist research concern (that of doing feminist research) is examined in depth in Avis and Turner (1996). A few of the most important issues are briefly summarized here.

Feminism provides a perspective on methods already used within the field, rather than being a distinct research method in itself (Reinharz, 1992). Thus, we can see feminist perspectives brought to such commonly used methods as survey, Delphi Technique, qualitative interviews, program evaluation, and content analysis. Furthermore, feminists use a multiplicity of research methods, recognizing that "there is no single 'feminist way' to do research" (p. 243). There is no attempt to define methodological "correctness"; rather, multiplicity, diversity, and expansion of methods are all valued and emphasized, including integrating methods and ideas from other disciplines. A central theme in feminist research is the explicit goal to create social change: to not only expand knowledge, but also to do so in a way that promotes greater gender equality and the transformation of gender relations (Reinharz, 1992).

Feminist research questions in family therapy are also varied and diverse, although all are concerned with some aspect of gender relations (Avis & Turner, 1996):

- How are gender-linked power imbalances expressed and maintained in relationships between family members, therapists and clients, trainers and trainees, researchers and participants, writers and journal editors?
- What approaches to therapy and to training are most effective in addressing gender–power imbalances?
- What therapeutic methods increase voice, visibility, and agency?
- How do oppressive gender relations interact with other relations of domination, such as race, class, and sexual orientation?

Some representative questions that have been examined by feminist researchers in family therapy include the fundamentals of a feminist approach to family therapy (Wheeler, 1985); the distinguishing characteristics of feminist approaches to supervision and training (Avis, 1986); feminist-informed approaches to working with men in family therapy (Dienhart & Avis, 1994); differences in the degree to which family therapists hold mothers and fathers accountable for their children's difficulties (Haig, 1988); the treatment of gender as a social category in family therapy research (Woodard, 1991); the adequacy of therapist training and preparation for responding to clients affected by child sexual abuse (Avis, Lero, & Guldner, 1992); and the linguistic ways in which family therapy clinical accounts minimize responsibility for violence perpetrated against women by men (Lamb, 1991). Two feminist instruments have been developed: the Feminist Family Therapist Behavior Checklist (Chaney & Piercy, 1988), which identifies the distinguishing behaviors of feminist therapists; and the Feminist Family Therapy Scale (Black & Piercy, 1991), designed to assess family therapists' gender sensitivity.

KEY BOOKS, CHAPTERS, AND ARTICLES

Avis, J. M. (1989). Reference guide to feminism and family therapy. *Journal of Feminist Family Therapy, 1,* 94–100.

A reference list of all family therapy literature related specifically to feminist, gender, and political issues up to the time of publication. A useful source for early feminist publications.

Avis, J. M. (1989). Integrating gender into the family therapy curriculum. *Journal of Feminist Family Therapy, 1,* 3–24.

An in-depth examination of key issues related to integrating gender into family therapy training, including approaches to integrating, course formats, training processes, teaching methods, and the impact of gender training on students.

Avis, J. M. (1991). Power politics in therapy with women. In T. J. Goodrich (Ed.). *Women and power.* New York: Norton.

An extensive discussion and elaboration of conceptual and intervention skills for empowering women in family therapy.

Avis, J. M., & Turner, J. (1996). Feminist lenses in family therapy research: Gender, politics, and science. In S. M. Moon & D. H. Sprenkle (Eds.), *Research methods in family therapy.* New York: Guilford Press.

An in-depth discussion of feminist research in family therapy. The authors examine the philosophical assumptions, methodologies, and themes of feminist research in the social sciences in general, and in family therapy in particular.

Bograd, M. (1984). Family systems approaches to wife battering: A feminist critique. *American Journal of Orthopsychiatry, 54,* 558–568.

An incisive analysis and critique of how subtle biases implicit in systems formulations are translated into practice, rendering systems theory an inadequate conceptual framework for intervening in situations of violence and abuse.

Bograd, M. (Ed.). (1990). *Feminist approaches for men in family therapy.* New York: Harrington Park Press.

Published simultaneously as a book and as a special issue of the *Journal of Feminist Family Therapy (2,* 3–4), this volume represents the first feminist work on family therapy with men. Its authors present many perspectives and ideas for working with men and examine some of the inherent challenges and dilemmas.

Bograd, M. (1992). Values in conflict: Challenges to family therapists' thinking. *Journal of Marital and Family Therapy, 3,* 245–256.

A powerful and challenging discussion of clinical and moral dilemmas posed by family therapy theory and practice related to men's violence toward their partners.

Braverman, L. (Ed.). (1988). *Women, feminism and family therapy.* Binghamton, NY: Haworth.

An excellent collection of articles by leading feminist family therapists that examine a wide range of issues related to women and to therapy.

Caplan, P. J., & Hall-McCorquodale, I. (1985). Mother-blaming in major clinical journals. *American Journal of Orthopsychiatry, 55,* 345–353.

This eye-opening study reports vivid examples of mother blaming and father idealizing in major clinical journals, with family therapy and psychoanalytic journals reported as most culpable. It is a great consciousness raiser regarding subtle biases in the literature.

Dienhart, A., & Avis, J. M. (1994). Working with men in family therapy: An exploratory study. *Journal of Marital and Family Therapy, 20,* 397–417.

A fascinating report of a Delphi study, in which a panel of family therapists endorsed 131 interventions as appropriate and effective for working with men. The interventions provide a thought-provoking summary of innovative ways to work with men, particularly around issues of gender and power.

Ehrenreich, B., & English, D. (1978). *For her own good: 150 years of the experts' advice to women.* Garden City, NY: Anchor Books.

This fascinating book recounts a history of women's experience at the hands of professional "experts," especially doctors, from the witch-hunts to the contemporary single woman. It is well-researched, witty, and highly illuminating.

Eisenstein, H. (1983). *Contemporary feminist thought.* Boston: Hall.

This is an excellent introduction and guide to contemporary feminist thought in America. Written for readers unfamiliar with feminism, it traces the progress of feminist thought since 1970 and helps make sense of changing ideas. It is highly recommended.

Goldner, V. (1985a). Feminism and family therapy. *Family Process, 24,* 31–47.

An eloquent and scholarly early feminist analysis of family therapy ideology and the complexities and dilemmas of sexual politics in family therapy practice.

Goldner, V. (1985b). Warning: Family therapy may be dangerous to your health. *Family Therapy Networker, 9,* 19–23.

A thought-provoking article citing gender as a universal category of human organization and domination. The author suggests that core family therapy assumptions must be rethought to account for gender and power differences.

Goldner, V. (1988). Generation and gender: Normative and covert hierarchies. *Family Process, 27,* 17–33.

The author argues strongly for considering gender a central category in family theory—an "irreducible category of clinical observation and theorizing," as fundamental an organizing principle of family life as that of generation. She then examines what this understanding means in practice.

Goodrich, T. J. (Ed.). (1991). *Women and power: Perspectives for family therapy.* New York: Norton.

A powerful collection of chapters by the leading feminist thinkers in family therapy provides a searching and challenging analysis of women and power. Combining theoretical discussion with excellent clinical illustrations, this outstanding book is must-reading.

Goodrich, T. J., Rampage, C., Ellman, B., & Halstead, K. (1988). *Feminist family therapy: A casebook.* New York: Norton.

One of the first feminist books in the field, this excellent volume presents the authors' feminist approach to family therapy. Using revealingly honest case illustrations from their own practice, the authors lead us through the complexities, uncertainties, and challenges of giving up old maps and forging new.

Gosling, A., & Zangari, M. E. (in press). Feminist family therapy and the narrative approach: Dovetailing two frameworks for therapy. *Journal of Feminist Family Therapy.*

This excellent article traces the philosophical and theoretical roots of feminist and narrative therapies, explores their similarities and differences, and discusses the possibilities and difficulties of integrating them.

Hare-Mustin, R. T. (1978). A feminist approach to family therapy. *Family Process, 17,* 181–194.

The first to raise feminist concerns in family therapy, this pioneering article examines the unquestioned reinforcement of traditional gender roles in practice and the application of feminist principles to family therapy practice.

Hare-Mustin, R. T. (1994). Discourses in the mirrored room: A postmodern analysis of therapy. *Family Process, 33,* 19–35.

This fascinating article examines three dominant gender discourses (the male sex-drive discourse, the permissive discourse, and the marriage-between-equals discourse), and how they shape the content of therapeutic conversations. The author recommends therapist self-reflexivity as a means to challenge oppressive discourses and remain open to alternative, marginalized ones. Highly recommended.

Jacobson, N. S. (1983). Beyond empiricism: The politics of marital therapy. *American Journal of Family Therapy, 11,* 11–24.

An excellent discussion of the political issues inherent in therapy in general and behavioral marital therapy (BMT) in particular. Jacobson identifies the processes through which traditional values and roles oppressive to women are inadvertently reinforced in BMT and makes specific recommendations for changing them.

Jaggar, A. M., & Rothenberg, P. S. (Eds.). (1984). *Feminist frameworks: Alternative theoretical accounts of the relations between women and men* (2nd ed.). New York: McGraw-Hill.

This edited volume offers an extremely helpful organization of major feminist theories. Excellent selections of lively and instructive readings are provided.

James, K., & MacKinnon, L. (1990). The "incestuous family" revisited: A critical analysis of family therapy myths. *Journal of Marital and Family Therapy, 16,* 71–88.

An excellent feminist critique of family therapy literature on incest. The authors identify pervasive myths in the literature, which result in blaming the victim and obscuring the dynamics of power and gender, and propose criteria for developing an adequate clinical account of incest. Important reading.

James, K., & McIntyre, D. (1983). The reproduction of families: The social role of family therapy? *Journal of Marital and Family Therapy, 9,* 119–129.

An excellent early article providing a scholarly analysis of family therapy's failure to respond to critical analyses of the family or to consider the socioeconomic and political contexts of family functioning. An incisive critique of systems theory.

Jenkins, A. (1990). *Invitations to responsibility: The therapeutic engagement of men who are violent and abusive.* Adelaide, South Australia: Dulwich Centre Publications.

This wonderful little book is a gold mine of ideas for working with men who abuse their partners or sexually abuse children. It provides both a theoretical framework for understanding violence and abuse, and detailed guidelines for therapy, including exhaustive lists of narrative questions that invite men to greater responsibility. Highly recommended.

Kamsler, A. (1991). Her-story in the making: Therapy with women who were sexually abused in childhood. In M. Durrant & C. White (Eds.), *Ideas for therapy with sexual abuse.* Adelaide, South Australia: Dulwich Centre Publications.

An extremely helpful article that integrates feminist and narrative ideas in working with adult survivors of sexual abuse. The author examines problematic aspects of dominant cultural stories about both long-term effects of child sexual assault and traditional approaches to therapy. She then outlines ideas for an alternative approach.

Kliman, J. (1994). The interweaving of gender, class, and race in family therapy. In M. P. Mirkin (Ed.), *Women in context: Toward a feminist reconstruction of psychotherapy.* New York: Guilford Press.

This particularly insightful and articulate article clearly explicates the complex interactions of culture, class, and gender in clients' lives and provides helpful examples of family therapy across contexts. Illuminating.

Lerner, H. G. (1985). *The dance of anger: A women's guide to changing the patterns of intimate relationships.* New York: Harper & Row.

A helpful guide for women on dealing with anger in important relationships. Filled with strategies for using anger productively to change and develop relationships, as well as to define oneself, this book is a valuable resource for both clients and therapists. Recommended.

Luepnitz, D. A. (1988). *The family interpreted: Feminist theory in clinical practice.* New York: Basic Books.

A comprehensive feminist analysis and critique of eight leading approaches to family therapy. The author also presents a historical perspective on family structures and forms, and explores psychoanalytic theory as an appropriate conceptual source for feminist family therapy. Informative reading.

McGoldrick, M., Anderson, C., & Walsh, F. (Eds.). (1988). *Women in families: A framework for family therapy.* New York: Norton.

A very useful collection of articles by leading feminist therapists on a wide range of issues of concern to women in families and in therapy.

Meth, R. L., & Pasick, R. S. (1990). *Men in therapy: The challenge of change.* New York: Guilford Press.

The authors describe how gender stereotypes and dysfunctional gender-role prescriptions inhibit men's development and limit their lives, and explore ways to engage and work with men in therapy. Although not feminist (the focus is on gender socialization and its consequences, not on power), this book provides a helpful elaboration of gender issues in men's lives.

Mirkin, M. P. (Ed.). (1994). *Women in context: Toward a feminist reconstruction of psychotherapy.* New York: Guilford Press.

A groundbreaking collection of papers that explore how race, class, ethnicity, gender, and sexual orientation shape women's lives and experience. The authors transform thinking about women and therapy by powerfully articulating the need to understand women in sociopolitical context and challenging us to become aware of the interaction of gender with other forms of oppression. Required reading.

Roth, S. (1985). Psychotherapy with lesbian couples: Individual issues, female socialization, and the social context. *Journal of Marital and Family Therapy, 11,* 273–286.

An extremely helpful guide to understanding the particular issues and experiences confronting lesbian couples and to working with them in therapy. Strongly recommended.

Sheinberg, M., & Penn, P. (1991). Gender dilemmas, gender questions, and the gender mantra. *Journal of Marital and Family Therapy, 17,* 33–44.

A discussion of the dilemmas posed by the social constructions of gender and their problematic effects on intimate relationships. The authors also describe the use of gender questions and the gender mantra as clinical techniques to encourage alternative, more accurate constructions. Interesting and useful.

Taggart, M. (1985). The feminist critique in epistemological perspective: Questions of context in family therapy. *Journal of Marital and Family Therapy, 11,* 113–126.

A highly theoretical discussion of the feminist critique of systemic epistemology. The author argues that feminist thought enriches and expands systems theory by challenging it to include broader contexts and thus become more truly systemic.

Walters, M., Carter, B., Papp, P., & Silverstein, O. (1988). *The invisible web: Gender patterns in family relationships.* New York: Guilford Press.

Four leading women in family therapy apply a gender analysis to their clinical practice. Filled with clinical dialogue and examples, the authors provide a helpful exploration of gender patterns in family relationships and share their experience in applying feminist ideas to their practice.

Weiner, J. P., & Boss, P. (1985). Exploring gender bias against women: Ethics for marriage and family therapy. *Counseling and Values, 30,* 9–23.

The authors cast gender issues in family therapy in ethical terms and call for affirmative action in both theory and training. Most valuable are their ethical guidelines for reducing gender bias in family therapy.

Wheeler, D. (1989). Faulty fathering: Working ideas on the treatment of male incest perpetrators. *Journal of Feminist Family Therapy, 1,* 27–48.

An excellent article that argues for individual therapy with male incest perpetrators in conjunction with group therapy and as a prerequisite to couple or family work. The author discusses ways to establish a strong therapeutic alliance with the offender, redefine power in his life, and expand his capacity for empathy and responsibility in relationships. Highly recommended.

Wheeler, D. (1990). Father–daughter incest: Considerations for the family therapist. In M. P. Mirkin (Ed.), *The social and political contexts of family therapy.* New York: Gardner.

A very helpful description of a feminist approach working with incest. The author addresses the therapeutic needs of all family members and provides clear guidelines for working with different members and subsystems, as well as an overall map of therapy. Highly recommended.

Wheeler, D., Avis, J. M., Miller, L., & Chaney, S. (1988). Rethinking family therapy education and supervision: A feminist model. In M. McGoldrick, C. Anderson, & F. Walsh, (Eds.), *Women in families: A framework for family therapy.* New York: Norton.

The authors delineate perceptual, conceptual, and executive skills in a feminist approach to family therapy, as well as methods for teaching them. Tables of skills make the article unique.

REFERENCES

Allen, J., & Laird, J. (1990). Men and story: Constructing new narratives in therapy. In M. Bograd (Ed.), *Feminist approaches for men in family therapy.* New York: Harrington Park Press.

Almeida, R., & Bograd, M. (1990). Sponsorship: Men holding men accountable for domestic violence. In M. Bograd (Ed.), *Feminist approaches for men in family therapy.* New York: Harrington Park Press.

American Psychological Association Task Force (1975). Report of the task force on sex bias and sex-role stereotyping in psychotherapeutic practice. *American Psychologist, 30,* 1169–1175.

Anderson, H., & Goolishian, H. (1988). Human systems as linguistic systems: Evolving ideas about the implications for theory and practice. *Family Process, 27,* 371–393.

Anderson, H., & Goolishian, H. (1992). The client is the expert: A not-knowing approach to therapy. In S. McNamee & K. Gergen (Eds.), *Therapy as social construction.* London: Sage.

Ault-Riche, M. (Ed.). (1986). *Women and family therapy.* Rockville, MD: Aspen Systems.

Ault-Riche, M. (1988). Teaching an integrated model of family therapy: Women as students, women as supervisors. In L. Braverman (Ed.), *Women, feminism and family therapy.* Binghamton, NY: Haworth.

Avis, J. M. (1985). The politics of functional family therapy: A feminist critique. *Journal of Marital and Family Therapy, 11,* 127–138.

Avis, J. M. (1986). *Training and supervision of feminist-informed family therapy.* Unpublished doctoral dissertation, Purdue University, West Lafayette, IN.

Avis, J. M. (1989a). Integrating gender into the family therapy curriculum. *Journal of Feminist Family Therapy, 1,* 3–26.

Avis, J. M. (1989b). Reference guide to feminism and family therapy. *Journal of Feminist Family Therapy, 1,* 94–100.

Avis, J. M. (1991). Power politics in therapy with women. In T. J. Goodrich (Ed.), *Women and power.* New York: Norton.

Avis, J. M. (1992). Violence and abuse in families: The problem and family therapy's response. *Journal of Marital and Family Therapy, 18,* 223–230.

Avis, J. M., & Turner, J. (1996). Feminist lenses in family therapy research: Gender, politics, and science. In D. H. Sprenkle & S. M. Moon (Eds.), *Research methods in family therapy.* New York: Guilford Press.

Avis, J. M., Lero, D., & Guldner, C. (1992). *Meeting the challenge: Educating professionals for child sexual abuse treatment. Final report of a national study.* Ottawa, Ontario, Canada: Health and Welfare.

Black, L., & Piercy, F. P. (1991). A feminist family therapy scale. *Journal of Marital and Family Therapy, 17,* 111–120.

Bograd, M. (1984). Family systems approaches to wife battering: A feminist critique. *American Journal of Orthopsychiatry, 54,* 558–568.

Bograd, M. (Ed.). (1990). *Feminist approaches for men in family therapy.* New York: Harrington Park Press.

Bograd, M. (1992). Values in conflict: Challenges to family therapists' thinking. *Journal of Marital and Family Therapy, 18,* 245–256.

Braverman, L. (Ed.). (1988). *Women, feminism and family therapy.* Binghamton, NY: Haworth.

Caplan, P. J. (1985). *The myth of women's masochism.* New York: Dutton.

Caplan, P. J., & Hall-McCorquodale, I. (1985). Mother-blaming in major clinical journals. *American Journal of Orthopsychiatry, 55,* 345–353.

Chaney, S. (1986). *The development of a feminist family therapy rating scale.* Unpublished doctoral dissertation, Purdue University, West Lafayette, IN.

Chaney, S., & Piercy, F. (1988). A feminist family therapist behavior checklist. *American Journal of Family Therapy, 16,* 305–318.

Chodorow, N. (1978). *The reproduction of mothering: Psychoanalysis and the sociology of gender.* Berkeley: University of California Press.

Dienhart, A., & Avis, J. M. (1990). Men in therapy: Exploring feminist-informed alternatives. In M. Bograd (Ed.), *Feminist approaches for men in family therapy.* New York: Harrington Park Press.

Dienhart, A., & Avis, J. M. (1994). Working with men in family therapy: An exploratory study. *Journal of Marital and Family Therapy, 20,* 397–417.

Dinnerstein, D. (1976). *The mermaid and the minotaur: Sexual arrangements and human malaise.* New York: Harper & Row.

Ehrenreich, B., & English, D. (1978). *For her own good: 150 years of the experts' advice to women.* Garden City, NY: Anchor Books.

Farrell, W. (1986). *Why men are the way they are.* New York: McGraw-Hill.

Flax, J. (1990). *Thinking fragments: Psychoanalysis, feminism, and postmodernism in the contemporary west.* Berkeley: University of California Press.

Ganley, A. (1990). Feminist therapy with male clients. In M. Bograd (Ed.), *Feminist approaches for men in family therapy.* New York: Harrington Park Press.

Goldner, V. (1985a). Feminism and family therapy. *Family Process, 24,* 31–47.

Goldner, V. (1985b). Warning: Family therapy may be dangerous to your health. *Family Therapy Networker, 9,* 19–23.

Goodrich, T. J. (1991). *Women and power: Perspectives for family therapy.* New York: Norton.

Goodrich, T. J., Rampage, C., Ellman, B., & Halstead, K. (1988). *Feminist family therapy: A casebook.* New York: Norton.

Greene, B. (1994). Diversity and difference: Race and feminist psychotherapy. In M. P. Mirkin (Ed.), *Women in context: Toward a feminist reconstruction of psychotherapy.* New York: Guilford Press.

Greenglass, E. R. (1982). *A world of difference: Gender roles in perspective.* New York: Wiley.

Gurman, A. S., & Klein, M. H. (1984). Marriage and the family: An unconscious male bias in behavioral treatment? In E. A. Blechman (Ed.), *Behavior modification with women.* New York: Guilford Press.

Haig, C. (1988). *Mother-blaming in major family therapy journals: A content analysis.* Unpublished masters thesis, University of Guelph, Ontario.

Hare-Mustin, R. T. (1978). A feminist approach to family therapy. *Family Process, 17,* 181–194.

Hare-Mustin, R. T. (1979). Family therapy and sex-role stereotypes. *The Counseling Psychologist, 8,* 31–32.

Hare-Mustin, R. T. (1980). Family therapy may be dangerous for your health. *Professional Psychology, 11,* 935–938.

Hare-Mustin, R. (1994). Discourses in the mirrored room: A postmodern analysis of therapy. *Family Process, 33,* 19–35.

Hartman, H. (1984). The unhappy marriage of Marxism and feminism: Toward a more progressive union. In A. M. Jaggar & P. S. Rothenberg (Eds.), *Feminist frameworks: Alternative theoretical accounts of the relations between women and men* (2nd ed.). New York: McGraw-Hill.

Jacobson, N. S. (1983). Beyond empiricism: The politics of marital therapy. *American Journal of Family Therapy, 11,* 11–24.

Jaggar, A. M., & Rothenberg, P. S. (Eds.). (1984). *Feminist frameworks: Alternative theoretical accounts of the relations between women and men* (2nd ed.). New York: McGraw-Hill.

James, K. (1984). Breaking the chains of gender. *Australian Journal of Family Therapy, 5,* 241–248.

James, K., & MacKinnon, L. (1990). The "incestuous family" revisited: A critical analysis of family therapy myths. *Journal of Marital and Family Therapy, 16,* 71–88.

James, K., & McIntyre, D. (1983). The reproduction of families: The social role of family therapy? *Journal of Marital and Family Therapy, 9,* 119–129.

Jenkins, A. (1990). *Invitations to responsibility: The therapeutic engagement of men who are violent and abusive.* Adelaide, South Australia: Dulwich Centre Publications.

Kliman, J. (1994). The interweaving of gender, class, and race in family therapy. In M. P. Mirkin (Ed.), *Women in context: Toward a feminist reconstruction of psychotherapy.* New York: Guilford Press.

Laird, J. (1994). Lesbian families: A cultural perspective. In M. P. Mirkin (Ed.), *Women in context: Toward a feminist reconstruction of psychotherapy.* New York: Guilford Press.

Lamb, S. (1991). Acts without agents: An analysis of linguistic avoidance in journal articles of men who batter women. *American Journal of Orthopsychiatry, 61,* 250–257.

Layton, M. (1984). Tipping the therapeutic balance: Masculine, feminine or neuter? *Family Therapy Networker, 8,* 21–27.

Lerner, H. G. (1986). *The creation of patriarchy.* New York: Oxford University Press.

Lerner, H. G. (1985). Dianna and Lillie: Can a feminist still like Murray Bowen? *Family Therapy Networker, 9*(6), 36–39.

Lerner, H. G. (1988). Is family systems theory really systemic? A feminist communication. *Journal of Psychotherapy and the Family, 3*(4), 47–63.

Libow, J. A. (1986). Training family therapists as feminists. In M. Ault-Riche (Ed.), *Women and family therapy.* Rockville, MD: Aspen Systems.

Libow, J. A., Raskin, P. A., & Caust, B. L. (1982). Feminist and family systems therapy: Are they irreconcilable? *American Journal of Family Therapy, 10,* 3–12.

Luepnitz, D. (1988). *The family interpreted: Feminist theory in clinical practice.* New York: Basic Books.

Miller, J. B. (1976). *Toward a new psychology of women.* Boston: Beacon Press.

McGoldrick, M., Anderson, C., & Walsh, F. (Eds.). (1988). *Women in families: A framework for family therapy.* New York: Norton.

Meth, R. L., & Pasick, R. S. (1990). *Men in therapy: The challenge of change.* New York: Guilford Press.

Mirkin, M. P. (Ed.). (1994). *Women in context: Toward a feminist reconstruction of psychotherapy.* New York: Guilford Press.

Nichols, M. (1994). Therapy with bisexual women: Working on the edge of emerging cultural and personal identities. In M. P. Mirkin (Ed.), *Women in context: Toward a feminist reconstruction of psychotherapy.* New York: Guilford Press.

Penfold, P. S., & Walker, G. A. (1983). *Women and the psychiatric paradox.* Montreal: Eden Press.

Pressman, B. (1994). Violence against women: Ramifications of gender, class, and race inequality. In M. P. Mirkin (Ed.), *Women in context: Toward a feminist reconstruction of psychotherapy.* New York: Guilford Press.

Reinharz, S. (1992). *Feminist methods in social research.* New York: Oxford University Press.

Sinclair, J. (Ed.). (1986). *Collins English language dictionary.* New York: Harper Collins.

Taggart, M. (1985). The feminist critique in epistemological perspective: Questions of context in family therapy. *Journal of Marital and Family Therapy, 11,* 113–126.

Tamasese, K., & Waldegrave, C. (1993). Cultural and gender accountability in the "Just Therapy" approach. *Journal of Feminist Family Therapy, 5,* 29–45.

Thorne, B. (1982). Feminist rethinking of the family: An overview. In B. Thorne & M. Yalom (Eds.), *Rethinking the family: Some feminist questions.* New York: Longman.

Walters, M., Carter, B., Papp, P., & Silverstein, O. (1988). *The invisible web: Gender patterns in family relationships.* New York: Guilford Press.

Weiner, J. P., & Boss, P. (1985). Exploring gender bias against women: Ethics for marriage and family therapy. *Counseling and Values, 30,* 9–23.

Weingarten, K. (1991). The discourses of intimacy: Adding a social constructionist and feminist view. *Family Process, 30,* 285–305.

Weingarten, K. (1992). A consideration of intimate and non-intimate interactions in therapy. *Family Process, 31,* 45–59.

Wheeler, D. (1985). *The theory and practice of feminist-informed family therapy: A Delphi study.* Unpublished doctoral dissertation, Purdue University, West Lafayette, IN.

Wheeler, D. (1989). Faulty fathering: Working ideas on the treatment of male incest perpetrators. *Journal of Feminist Family Therapy, 1,* 27–48.

Wheeler, D., Avis, J. M., Miller, L. A., & Chaney, S. (1988). Rethinking family therapy education and supervision: A feminist model. In M. McGoldrick, C. Anderson, & F. Walsh (Eds.), *Women in families: A framework for family therapy.* New York: Norton.

White, M. (1992). Men's culture, the men's movement, and the constitution of men's lives. *Dulwich Centre Newsletter, 3–4,* 1–21.

White, M. (1994). *The politics of therapy: Putting to rest the illusion of neutrality.* Presentation to the Narrative Ideas and Therapeutic Practice Conference, Vancouver, British Columbia.

Woodard, C. (1991). *Gender as a social variable in family therapy research: A content analysis.* Unpublished master's thesis, University of Guelph, Ontario.

10

Cultural Issues
in Family Therapy

LISA ARONSON FONTES
VOLKER THOMAS

ATTENTION TO CULTURAL issues in family therapy resulted from recognition of the limitations of earlier family therapy approaches, which discussed families in isolation from their cultural contexts. This attention to culture may be seen as a radical change of focus for the field, or as a natural extension of the outward rippling inherent in family therapy itself, which emerged from a recognition of the limitations of individual approaches. In each case, perspectives shifted dramatically when the lenses were widened. The results have been striking.

Today, the once-radical propositions of multicultural theorists are considered core learnings. In 1988, the Commission on Accreditation for Marriage and Family Therapy Education required that accredited training programs "demonstrate that ethnicity and gender are taught throughout the entire curriculum or that there are two separate courses offered addressing these issues" (Commission on Accreditation for Marriage and Family Education, 1988). The American Family Therapy Academy (AFTA) has highlighted cultural issues in its magazine and in annual conferences, including the 1995 conference on issues of social class, the 1994 conference on power and privilege, the 1993 conference on social, cultural, and economic diversity, and others.

The early works on culture in family therapy focused on applications of existing therapy models to previously overlooked groups, highlighting the culture of the clients. The next wave of works highlighted the culture of the therapists as well, and the dynamic interplay between therapist and client cultures. More recent works frequently discuss the Western European and White North American biases of the models themselves (and, indeed, of the models of all the social sciences; Tamasese & Waldgrave, 1993, p. 30). Although the first step in considering cultural issues in family therapy involved avoiding pathologizing ethnic minority families, and this remains an important and largely unrealized goal, the cutting edges of writing on culture and family therapy today go several steps further: They consider the biases in theory and practice built into the central ideas of the field.

Entire books have been written about culture and family therapy, and there is still much left to say. This review, then, is necessarily partial. Due to space considerations, we will not be able to address thoroughly any particular way of defining culture (e.g., along lines of ethnicity or sexual orientation) or any particular cultural group (e.g., West Indians or lesbians). Instead, we will map out some of the major ways the field of family therapy has handled cultural issues and discuss key concepts, clinical interventions, training tools, and research implications. We will also describe some of the key resources in the field. Although this chapter cannot be complete in its coverage, we do hope it alerts readers to some of the essential issues of culture in family therapy and points them toward prime resources for continuing their exploration of this area.

Goldner (1989) has written that "gender and gendering are not secondary mediating variables affecting family life; they construct family life in the deepest sense" (p. 56). The same may be said about culture: who is and is not considered family; the meaning of "family"; role obligations for family members; and how power and resources handled in the family are constructed through cultural beliefs and behaviors. Attention to issues of culture in family therapy can no more be considered "extra" or "specialized" or "optional" than attention to family communication. Cultural issues are present for all families (and therapists and researchers) at all times. The extent to which therapists harness their power and potential depends on their knowledge, comfort, and commitment to this area.

CULTURAL SPECIFICITY AND MULTICULTURALISM

Most writings on culture in family therapy may be characterized as falling into one of two groups, which we will call the culture specific and the multicultural. The first and larger group consists of the rapidly expanding body of writings that tell therapists how to do family therapy with members of specific groups. Most of these works define groups along racial or ethnic lines (e.g., Boyd-Franklin, 1989; McGoldrick, Giordano, & Pearce, 1982). Recently, cultural groups have been defined along increasingly diverse parameters, including gender (Bograd, 1990; McGoldrick, Anderson, & Walsh, 1989), sexual orientation (*Family Therapy Networker*, 1991; Perez, 1996), age (Atwood & Ruiz, 1993), ability (Seligman & Darling, 1989) religion (Stander, Piercy, MacKinnon, & Helmeke, 1994), social class (Inclan, 1990), and others. These works typically include historical, sociological, and cultural information, and suggest techniques which seem to "fit well" with people from the specific group in question. These works are often written with the assumption that the reader is from a group other than the one discussed. The culture-specific writings are like travel guides for the therapist who is about to tread into relatively unknown territory: They include history, a map of typical relationships and balances of power, a phrase book, guidelines as to the use of time and space, and typically some information on how to avoid offending clients through ignorance or common errors of etiquette. These works advise therapists to attend to therapist–client differences in values, gender roles, discipline practices, and expression of affect. Each of these works describes a group in such a way that the therapist will feel less lost and may be less likely to pathologize certain practices that are normative for members of the group.

The culture-specific writings are often quite practical, "how-to" manuals for working with members of specific groups. They have been praised as "dehomogenizing" the field of family therapy by raising awareness of differences that may be attributable to ethnicity, race, or other group characteristics; however, they have also been criticized for perpetuating the "myth of sameness" by overemphasizing the level of "sameness" among families sharing similar cultural backgrounds (Hardy, 1989, p. 21).

It is wise to consult the culture-specific family therapy guidelines but not consider them recipe books for work with any specific family. Families and individuals within families, adhere to and reject typical cultural norms for their group. They do this to varying degrees, depending on factors such as degree of acculturation, idiosyncratic individual and family history, social class, and identification group. For example, members of a given Mexican American family may identify themselves primarily as Catholics, Californians, professionals, and Democrats. The country of their ancestors may be peripheral to their felt identity and the way they live their lives. Learning about "the Chinese American family" or "the lesbian family" or "the family with deaf parents" from a description of typical characteristics should never interfere with a therapist's ability to know and join with a particular family that, un-doubtedly, has developed a culture of its own (Lappin, 1983).

Multicultural writings differ from those that are culture specific in that they are not geared to the discussion of one particular group. They advise therapists to adopt a culturally sensitive approach to all clients, including those who appear to be members of the therapist's own group(s). These writings prescribe a frame of mind and an approach that is flexible and inclusive enough to work well with diverse families. The therapist is frequently described as an anthropologist and the clients as cultural guides in *all* families (Lappin, 1983; Schwartzmann, 1983). Multicultural advocates caution that culture-specific information can sometimes blind the therapist to the human issues that undergird the family's problems or make the therapist favor a cultural frame when other ways of construing the issue might be more productive (Falicov, 1988). Schwartzmann (1983) suggests that we make sense of data provided by the family from the "inside out" rather than relying on generalities about families from specific groups from the "outside in" (p. 140).

Multicultural works include discussion of concepts that affect diverse groups, including cultural transition (Landau, 1982), acculturation (Sluzki, 1979), historical/generational sequences (Breunlin, Schwartz, & Mac Kune-Karrer, 1992), cultural fit (Breunlin et al., 1992), cultural matching between therapist and client (Fontes, 1995), and discrimination (Saba & Rodgers, 1989). Several multicultural works focus on approaches to specific problems, such as sexual abuse (e.g., Fontes, 1993, 1995), or life stages, such as adolescence (e.g., Mirkin, 1992).

Multicultural works frequently advise the therapist to embark on a journey of cultural self-discovery. Knowing one's own values, positions, and assumptions and their origin, and understanding that these are not absolutes, is considered an essential step for the therapist who hopes to be culturally sensitive. Multicultural works frequently stress that therapy does not involve just the client's culture, but also the culture of the therapist, the culture of the agency or institution where the therapy is practiced, the dominant culture of the society where the therapist and client work together, and the culture of therapy itself. Therapists are also cautioned not to assume that therapy will be "easy sailing" or free of cultural issues simply because the therapist and client seem to come from the same group. Sharing the same ethnic or other identity group origin can lead therapist and client to assumptions of sameness and understanding that might not be warranted (e.g., the therapist assumes that because he or she and the client are both Puerto Rican, they share values and experiences, and therefore fail to inquire about ways in which the client's life growing up in New York may differ from his or her own experiences growing up on the island; or the therapist assumes that he or she understands a Mormon family because he or she is also a Mormon, but elements of a shared background make it difficult for the therapist to see how the family's values and dreams differ from his or her own).

KEY CONCEPTS

Acculturation. "Acculturation is an accommodation process that occurs when groups from two distinct cultures are in contact over a sustained period of time" (Berry, 1980, as cited in Breunlin et al., 1992, p. 206). Most commonly, acculturation is used to describe the process through which members of an immigrant group adjust to the norms of their new land. Theorists often describe the acculturation process as consisting of predictable stages, which Jalali and Boyce (1980) have enumerated as follows: (1) isolation and alienation from the new culture while rigidly adhering to one's own cultural norms; (2) denigrating and rejecting the old culture by changing style of dress, eating habits, values, and sometimes names; (3) uneven adaptation by different family members, leading to polarization and conflict in the family; and (4) integration to the host culture while preserving elements of the old culture. Issues of acculturation are most obvious when working with immigrant groups, but they are also relevant for members of racial and religious minority groups, sexual minority groups, and others who may daily face questions related to their degree of belonging to the dominant culture. When working with a family from a minority group, it is important for the therapist to assess the degree to which various family members have taken on the customs, language, values, and behaviors of the dominant culture. Immigrant families frequently experience stress related to acculturation. Children often acculturate faster than their parents, through their facility in learning the language and culture of their host country, and family members who work usually acculturate more rapidly than those who stay at home. Those who acculturate faster are frequently blamed for abandoning the old ways and dishonoring the ancestors. Those who are slow to acculturate are frequently seen as stubborn or stuck in the past. It can be helpful to normalize the stressors of the acculturation process and make explicit the acculturation differences that have emerged in a given family. Families can be helped to develop rituals to maintain or recover their distinct traditions and rituals that mark their new life circumstances.

Biculturalism. Minority families and individuals frequently find themselves needing recognition, acceptance, and membership in at least two worlds, one of which is usually the dominant or mainstream society. Examples of these are Black and White, gay and straight, deaf and hearing. People who are bicultural have the ability to step back and forth between two worlds, adjusting temporarily to the norms of each. Aspects of biculturalism include the ability to speak and understand the language, demonstrate appropriate affect and body language, and gain acceptance in both worlds. Although members of minority groups are frequently expected to be bicultural (e.g., Puerto Rican therapists are expected to demonstrate their ability to speak standard English in their work with European American clients, as well as cultural proficiency in working with Latino clients; gay therapists are expected to be familiar with aspects of heterosexual culture, including dating, marriage, and sexuality), members of the dominant group are rarely expected to be bicultural (e.g., European American therapists are rarely expected to learn Black English or African American customs in order to work more effectively with African American clients). Although it is not practical for therapists who work with clients from numerous groups to become culturally fluent in all the groups, it is advisable for therapists to become as familiar as possible with the language, customs, values, political struggles, and arts of the major groups in their catchment area. The process of becoming bicultural involves more than just reading culture-specific therapy information; it also requires extended cultural immersion through friendships, partaking in rituals, eating the food, enjoying the arts, and understanding the social constraints of people from the other group.

Class. There are various ways of defining social or economic class, ranging from social status or income level to one's relationship to the means of production. Kliman (1994) presents a four-step "historical materialist" model for defining the classes:

> (1) the ruling class (or wealthiest households), (2) the petite bourgeoisie (or "upper-middle-income" and "middle-income" households), (3) the proletariat or working class (including "lower-middle-income" and "working-poor" households), and (4) the poor. Inclan and Ferran (1990) have divided the poor into these subgroups: (recently) unemployed; chronically unemployed (at least 5 years in 7), who hold mainstream values about work and education; and the underclass or "lumpenproletariat," who make their living illegally or otherwise on the fringes of society. (p. 29)

Social class as one of the matrices that make up culture is largely ignored in family therapy, except for occasional discussions of poor clients. U.S. therapists and family therapy researchers often participate in the "denial of differential access to resources and power (allocated differentially by gender and culture within each class)" which is common in the United States (Kliman, 1994). Class is one of the primary dividers of society, separating the haves and have-nots in regard to many resources, including therapy itself. In addition to determining material wealth, class also largely shapes beliefs, values, and behaviors, that is, culture.

Cross-cultural therapy. All therapy in which the therapist and client(s) are not from the same identification group is considered cross-cultural. Although this term is most commonly used to refer to therapy in which there are ethnic differences between the therapist and the clients, it may be helpful to recognize the cross-cultural nature of therapy in which therapist–client differences are based on race, religion, sexual orientation, class, age, and even gender.

Culture. The shared meanings, symbols, and values of a people (Rosenthal, 1986) or shared beliefs, values, history, and customs of a people, comprise the people's culture. Falicov (1988) defines culture as "those sets of shared world views and adaptive behaviors derived from simultaneous membership in a variety of contexts" (p. 336).

Diversity. Currently, this term does not just refer to the mere acceptance or acknowledgment of differences among people, but also implies a respect and even celebration of these differences as a source of richness (Gonzalez-Calvó, 1993, p. x). The concept of diversity lacks an analysis of power.

Dominant group. Those who hold the most power in society or in a given situation by virtue of economic affluence, judicial favoritism, greatest access to resources, greater comfort with the language and customs of the institutions, and those who are portrayed in the media as typical, average, or generic ("unhyphenated") may be seen as members of the dominant group. An individual may be dominant in one area yet not in another (e.g., a *White* working-class Jewish lesbian). Although there are, indeed, nested hierarchies of oppression, it is clear that some are more salient and more dangerous than others in general and in specific situations. For example, although White French Canadians may experience some teasing at school about their ethnic origin, they are unlikely to fear police brutality because of it. Another example might be an Irish American female therapist who is afraid to stroll alone at night after a conference because of her gender. She is unlikely to be approached by hotel security and asked what she is doing on the hotel premises, as might an African American male therapist (McGoldrick, 1994). It is frequently uncomfortable for therapists, trainees, and others to recognize the ways in which they are dominant and privileged in society. This analysis is absolutely essential if therapists and trainees are to understand their clients' experiences of oppression and privilege.

Empowerment. Frequently used in the literature on therapy with members of oppressed groups, empowerment refers to the process by which individuals, communities, and families gain mastery over their lives (Sotomayor, 1991, p. xxi). Therapists act as agents of empowerment when they help clients access resources within themselves, their communities, and society; when they impart skills and knowledge that will help clients become more active in determining their future; when they help clients recognize and activate their own strengths; and when they encourage clients to define their own needs, determine their own goals, and actively choose from the available resources in the course of therapy. Empowerment leads to felt and actual mastery by the individual, family, and community. Activating self-help and mutual-help networks in families and communities are keys to empowerment in family therapy.

Ethnicity. Ethnicity reflects a set of commonalities transmitted over generations by the family and reinforced by the surrounding community (McGoldrick, 1982). Ethnicity fulfills a need for a sense of belonging and may include elements of race, religion, and national origin. For many people, it defines the sense of "we" (the in-group) and "they" (others or the out-groups). *Identity group.* The group(s) with whom we feel most closely identified comprise our identity groups. There are three dimensions to this definition: (1) an endogenous aspect, or how individuals or families define themselves; (2), an exogenous aspect, or how others define these individuals or families; and (3) a factual aspect, or the objective aspects of the group such as language, cultural history, or specific behaviors.

Minority. People who are numerically less than half of the social group in question are considered minorities. Usually while members of minority groups suffer from greater discrimination, prejudice, and economic hardship, there are exceptions to this, as when Blacks who are a numerical majority in South Africa are clearly subjugated by a relatively small group of Whites, or when women who are in a numerical majority in the United States are clearly at an economic and social disadvantage as compared to men as a group.

Power. Power is the capability to access and mobilize material and knowledge resources. In families, power is won and maintained in many ways. Among these, it may be ascribed by the family's culture because of one's gender role or age; it may be given because of one's earning power; and it may be maintained through instilling respect or fear in others. In society, power is unequally distributed among people partially based on their class, profession, race, gender, age, sexual orientation, degree of physical ability, and ethnicity. In the therapy session, therapists have more power than clients due to their familiarity with the setting and norms of therapy, the fact that they are being paid, and their ability to shake off the problem by ending the session (Goldner, 1993).

Race. Although appearing to be a biological term referring to visible human features such as skin color and hair texture, the concept of race is largely socially constructed and contains highly political elements. In most family therapy literature, when race is not explicitly denoted, it is assumed that the people in question are White (Hardy & Lazsloffy, 1994). Whites are usually and mistakenly considered generic, the default option, the people without a race. This tendency to ignore the racial grouping of Whites obscures the privileges obtained by Whites by virtue of their skin color.

KEY CLINICAL SKILLS

Improving clinical skills related to cultural issues in family therapy involves changes in cognitions, affect, and behavior. To distinguish between the cognitive and affective aspects of cultural competence, we separately describe cultural awareness and sensitivity.

Cultural awareness. Learning about clients' cultural backgrounds (e.g., ethnicity, social class, sexual orientation, religion) increases the therapist's awareness of cultural issues as they relate to the therapeutic process. Heightened awareness expands the context of therapy from merely relational to contextual. Therapy broadens from a focus on how clients' relationships affect their well-being and vice versa, to considering how cultural contexts affect these relationships, the clients' sense of self, and the therapy process (Hardy & Laszloffy, 1995).

Sensitivity. Although curiosity and awareness reflect cognitive skills, cultural sensitivity is primarily an affective skill. Being culturally sensitive means respecting one's self and others as cultural beings, maintaining one's cultural curiosity, appreciating one's cultural uniqueness as well as cultural diversity among people, and keeping one's heart open to similarities and differences among people from diverse cultural backgrounds. Unprovoked emotional reactions to members of specific cultural groups, such as fear, mistrust, revulsion, adoration, or pity, are signs of reduced cultural sensitivity. They limit therapists' awareness and effectiveness and must be addressed in training and supervision.

Cultural curiosity. Cultural curiosity describes therapists' openness to clients' cultural backgrounds and who they are as cultural beings. It is rooted in therapists' openness to their own cultural backgrounds and willingness to experience themselves as cultural beings. Curiosity is a quality that is innate to children as they explore and discover the world around them without passing judgment. When the therapist is not familiar with the client's world but is willing to explore and discover it, the therapist uses respectful curiosity as a guiding tool to learn more about the client's cultural background.

Social analysis. Analyzing one's own and clients' social contexts helps therapists foster their cultural curiosity, increase their awareness, and improve their sensitivity and effectiveness (Breunlin et al., 1992; Ehrenreich, 1983). Analyzing historical and sociocultural factors as they play out in client's lives and in the therapy process is a grossly underestimated clinical skill among family therapists. When therapists engage in this analysis, they model for clients ways to view themselves as historically situated cultural beings. This is a powerful therapeutic tool that can help clients release feelings of shame or blame for circumstances that may be at least partially due to economics, oppression, or other social forces that are beyond their control.

INTERVENTION SKILLS

Many of the skills identified in the literature are culture specific and are described as being particularly useful for working with clients from a specific cultural group. The previously mentioned cognitive and affective preparation sets the stage for the following four broad categories of intervention skills: (1) empowering clients; (2) making cultural issues explicit; (3) finding a cultural fit between family and therapist; and (4) co-creating new stories.

Empowering clients. A universally agreed upon goal of family therapy is to empower clients. Clients usually feel empowered when the therapist puts their presenting problem in a cultural context, acknowledges them as cultural beings, and understands and confirms their life dilemmas as embedded in social circumstances, cultural norms, and values. This is particularly key for clients who belong to oppressed groups (e.g., clients living in poverty, gay men and lesbians, African Americans). Culturally aware and sensitive therapists use various interventions to empower their clients along cultural lines. These interventions may include but are not limited to (1) encouraging clients to value and be proud of their cultural backgrounds; (2) fostering self-esteem by acknowledging clients' cultural uniqueness; (3) validating clients' cultural values and experiences; (4) encouraging clients to preserve and express their cultural traditions and practices; (5) acknowledging the strengths of clients' cultures; (6) acknowledging clients' bicultural competence; and (7) acknowledging the social forces (such as discrimination, racism, and homophobia) that may have led them to positions of reduced power in society and contributed to their presenting issues.

Making cultural issues explicit. Therapists can make errors of two kinds in regard to making pertinent cultural issues explicit. Expanding on Hardy and Laszloffy's (1994, p. 19) writings on race, we can consider alpha errors as those that occur when a therapist assumes incorrectly that culture is central to the presenting problem, and beta errors as those that occur when culture is central to the presenting problem but is ignored or dismissed as unrelated. Lack of familiarity with cultural issues can lead to both types of errors. When therapists have correctly determined that culture is central to the presenting problem, making this explicit can transform the course of therapy. Placing the presenting problem in the appropriate cultural context and putting it into words with and for the clients deconstruct many client problems as contextual rather than internal. Interventions of this sort may include (1) defining the presenting problem within the context of cultural values and practices; (2) openly discussing the clients' and therapist's cultural backgrounds, norms, and practices (Hardy & Laszloffy, 1995; White & Tyson-Rawson, 1995); (3) challenging stereotypical cultural behaviors and attitudes; (4) placing the presenting problem within the context of societal pressures on the clients because of their cultural identity; and (5) modeling alternative cultural practices in the relationship between therapist and clients, including openly discussing similarities and differences in their respective backgrounds.

Building a cultural fit between client and therapist. A cultural fit between client and therapist does not require that the client and therapist have the same cultural background. Cultural fit implies the creation of a comfortable setting and relationship wherein the client feels welcome, respected, validated, and understood (Fontes, 1995). The therapeutic setting and specific interventions must be experienced as "user-friendly" by the client. Services, paperwork, and outreach should be readily available in the client's language and fit the schedules, finances, and geographic location of the client population. When there is cultural fit, clients feel that the therapist truly cares about their well-being, a situation that can be elusive when therapy is conducted over a cultural divide. Through a variety of small and large choices, the therapist creates an environment where clients feel "It's okay to be me here." The validation offered by culturally competent professionals can begin to ease the crushing of the soul caused by oppression and by the difficult issues that often pull clients into therapy (e.g., abuse, violence, abandonments, addictions, failures, losses, and conflicts, among others).

Respect and openness, not sameness, constitute cultural fit. Specific interventions aimed at achieving cultural fit include (1) curiously inquiring about the client's cultural background by using contextual questions and statements (Breunlin et al., 1992) that acknowledge the therapist's cultural background; (2) acknowledging the ways in which therapist–client differences and similarities impact on the therapy; (3) modeling nonoppressive therapeutic practices by creating a collaborative relationship between client and therapist; and (4) being open to redesigning therapy so its fits the clients' ways of being. This last step may include adjusting the treatment unit to include members of the extended family or community, incorporating rituals or spirituality into sessions, using time flexibly, and framing the therapeutic work so that it makes sense to the clients (e.g., it may be discussed as a form of education, a medical or spiritual intervention, community support, and so on).

Therapists should try to be flexible within their given limits to maximize the possibility of cultural fit. For example, Fulani (1988) found that adding a drop-in component to her clinic for low-income minority families in Harlem reduced the problem of no-shows. For cultural reasons, some clients may prefer longer sessions, or may prefer to incorporate members of the clergy or friends or extended family into therapy. Unless there are counterindications, therapists are wise to collaborate with clients in adjusting "standard" therapy (which emerges from a given culture) into practices that fit the clients' life situations. This does *not* mean totally disregarding boundaries or in other ways compromising the integrity of the therapy. Deviations from standard practice should be clinically appropriate and carefully considered. Offering a wider variety of services (e.g., group, individual, couple, or family treatment; psychodynamic, behavioral, medical or narrative models) may increase the likelihood that clients will be able to find a therapy that fits with their worldview within a given agency. Clearly, not all therapists can work well with all clients, and not all clients accept working with all therapists. The reasons may be cultural, developmental, personal, or historical, and should be honored whenever possible.

→ *Co-creating new stories.* Roberts (1994) has written movingly about the use of stories in family therapy: "We cannot always control what happens to us in our lives, but we can control how we make meaning of it—by when, where, and how we tell the story and explain its significance" (p. 56). Stories can be used to help clients affirm their reality, which often differs from "the party line" or "the official story," particularly for members of oppressed groups who may feel invisible or denigrated in the narratives that are dominant in schools or in the media. Their cultural stories may be repressed, silenced, distorted, co-opted, or told stereotypically. Many cultural narratives are lost because of migration, loss, trauma, and/or dislocation. (Roberts, 1994, p. 132). The deliberate telling of stories in therapy can be empowering, particularly for clients from oppressed groups.

Using stories in therapy can help clients release themselves from patterns that are bound by narratives that are no longer useful. For instance, couples often create narratives around incidents of battering that make these incidents seem acceptable within their relationship (Hydén, 1994). Elements of these stories can be cultural (e.g., the husband "has to" respond to his wife's taunts with a slap because he is hot-blooded). Storytelling can be a nonjudgmental approach to facilitating change. Techniques for helping clients create new stories include playing with time (e.g., "How would you describe this dilemma in five years?"), creating invisible witnesses ("When you begin to fight, picture your Godmother sitting in the room. What would she say?"), and adjusting place ("How would this incident have been different if you were all still in Puerto Rico?").

Storytelling is a common practice in all cultures, therefore, the narrative therapies may hold special promise for cultural fit with clients from diverse backgrounds.

SELF-OF-THERAPIST ISSUES AND CLINICAL INTERVENTION

To intervene effectively, therapists must know themselves, including their biases, values, and beliefs; strengths and weaknesses in relating to others; communications skills and deficits; habitual degree of warmth and empathy; trigger issues; and comfort with boundaries. The core of the therapist's intervention repertoire is self-knowledge and use of self. Culturally aware and sensitive therapists must know themselves as cultural beings and understand the historical/cultural origins of their beliefs and the relativity of these beliefs. Culturally self-aware and sensitive therapists use appropriate self-disclosure with regard to cultural background and cultural identity. They will not feel forced to use a cultural frame where it is not most useful, nor will they ignore cultural issues as they arise (for a fascinating discussion of when gay and lesbian couples need attention to issues related to their sexual orientation, and when other frames are most useful, see Perez, 1996). Although therapists, like others, may feel ambivalent about their cultural heritages, they are well-advised to learn to accept themselves as cultural beings who create a self-identity out of a selective acceptance, casting off, and re-creation of tradition. The therapist who was raised as a Jew may now be a Buddhist, the therapist who was born in Korea may have been adopted into a New England family and feel like more of a Yankee than a Korean—each of us reflects a variety of cultures related to our ethnicity, class, gender, sexual orientation, generation, and other factors. Therapists who are comfortable with themselves as cultural beings can serve as better role models for clients. In other words, intensive self-of-therapist work is considered crucial for developing clinical skills and becoming a culturally aware and sensitive therapist. This self-of-therapist work cannot stop when therapists know who they are and understand their position in society. Therapists must also face how they respond to people from their own and other groups, and how this may impact on therapy.

TEACHING TOOLS AND TECHNIQUES

Course Work

Didactic course work raises cultural awareness in many training programs. Some programs integrate information on cultural issues into their general coursework, whereas other programs offer one or more courses devoted solely to topics such as gender, social class, ethnicity, religion, race, and sexual orientation. We have found a combination of both approaches most effective. Although it is crucial to take the time to address cultural issues in a separate course, these issues are relevant to all practice and theory classes and should not be neglected simply because there is a separate course dedicated to this area. One doctoral program declared that during the sixth class meeting of every course in every semester, the class would cover issues of culture, thus guaranteeing that discussions of culture would occur in all courses (including assessment, theory, and specialized therapies). Professors who did not feel fully qualified to lead the discussions often simply supplied the reading materials and followed the students' lead.

Although the main focus of the course work is on raising trainees' cultural awareness, a second training goal is to increase trainees' cultural sensitivity, related to self-knowledge. The following exercises are excellent examples how therapists can become more culturally sensitive by exploring their own cultural backgrounds and biases.

1. *Cultural genogram.* Hardy and Laszloffy (1995) developed the cultural genogram as a training tool to increase trainees' cultural awareness and sensitivity. In preparing their cultural genogram, trainees define their own culture of origin, identify organizing principles, and address pride and shame issues associated with their culture of origin. Trainees create their own symbols and use colors for different cultural groups to enhance the visual effects of the genogram. They prepare Cultural Framework Charts (CFCs), providing additional cultural information to aid in the interpretation of the genogram. The cultural genogram is a powerful and respectful tool to use with trainees, making cultural issues explicit on a cognitive and emotional level. It fosters trainees' understanding of their own cultural backgrounds and prepares them to work more effectively with clients' cultural backgrounds.

2. *Gendergram.* Although White and Tyson-Rawson (1995) designed the gendergram as a therapeutic tool for working with clients, therapy trainees can also profit greatly from constructing their own gendergram. The gendergram connects the trainee's life-cycle stages, gender roles, patterns, and themes with life events that were salient for the trainee's gender identity development. A gendergram contains same-sex and other-sex parts that highlight gender identity development across life-cycle stages. It helps trainees explore and challenge their perceptions of gender as they relate to their family of origin and thus raises gender awareness and sensitivity. Trainees who do both the cultural genogram and the gendergram can link the two, exploring the ways gender and culture have shaped their experience.

3. *Popular media.* Trainees can be asked to read fiction or watch movies about people from a culture other than their own and then conduct an assessment or design an intervention for that family using a specific theory. For example, students can be asked to write a structural assessment of a

family as portrayed in a novel (adapted from Janine Roberts, private communication, 1987). Students can then discuss their work together, with the classroom declared an attack-free zone, so they can speak freely about their ignorance or biases regarding the members of the group portrayed in the novel. Knowing that the family is fictional permits trainees to take risks and speak freely, which is often difficult when first encountering families that differ culturally from their own in a clinical situation.

Many of the materials discussed in the "Key Books, Chapters, and Articles" section are used in courses on cultural issues in family therapy. We would like to call particular attention to Falicov (1988), Preli and Bernard (1993), Roberts (1993), and Skowron (1995), which contain excellent exercises for leading students and trainees in exploring various dimensions of culture and therapy.

INCLUDING CULTURE IN THERAPY

It is important to apply cultural awareness and sensitivity to all therapeutic processes, whether these issues are explicit or implicit, and central or peripheral to the presenting problem. Culture-specific information as well as multicultural sensitivity training can prepare therapists to create a culturally safe therapeutic environment that encourages clients to bring their full selves into the therapy room. The cultural genogram and the gendergram are not only useful training tools, but can also be used directly with clients as therapeutic interventions. They engage the therapist and clients in a culturally sensitive approach to therapy, thus creating a context that reaches beyond traditional family therapy approaches.

A comprehensive approach to including cultural issues in therapy has been proposed by Breunlin et al. (1992) in their Multicultural Metaframework, where they include the following aspects of culture: economics, education, ethnicity, religion, gender, age, race, minority–majority status, regional background. (Sexual orientation is noticeably absent from this list, other than its inclusion in the minority–majority status category). The framework encourages therapists to address all cultural aspects as they are brought into therapy by both the client and therapist.

We encourage therapists to do the following: (1) Consider including cultural aspects in the conceptualization of all cases; (2) assess the most salient aspects of the client's culture, and address them early in therapy to create a culturally safe therapy environment; (3) consider the cultural contexts when framing the presenting problem and establishing treatment goals; (4) design interventions that are consistent with the client's cultural background; (5) openly address the therapist's cultural background in relation to the client's, acknowledging differences and similarities and utilizing these as resources to increase cultural awareness and sensitivity, where pertinent.

Culture in Supervision

Based on the notion of the isomorphism between therapy and supervision, the same suggestions made for therapy also apply to supervision. When conceptualizing cases, it is crucial to focus not only on the cultural context of the therapy session (e.g., cultural similarities and differences between client and therapist; the cultural climate of the agency) but also in the supervision session (e.g., cultural similarities and differences between supervisee and supervisor; the cultural climate of the training setting). The latter may influence how each conceptualizes the case and their roles in relation to each other, and thus must be addressed in supervision.

For example, an Asian trainee frequently professed ignorance of the next steps to take in therapy, turning to her supervisor for advice in a way that seemed obsequious and developmentally inappropriate to the Jewish supervisor. When the supervisor initiated a discussion of each of their cultural expectations regarding the supervisory relationship, pressure was relieved and the two were able to work productively together. The supervisor and trainee also discussed the way their shared upper-middle-class background might lead them to ignore some of the economic constraints that were affecting the working-class client family.

The supervisor and supervisee should explore cultural issues on the supervision level and the therapy level simultaneously. This will create a culturally safe environment that allows for the individual and collective blossoming of the clients, the therapist, and the supervisor. Once a safe environment has been created, the different forms of supervision provide a variety of possibilities to include cultural issues in the supervision process.

Live Supervision

Live supervision may be used to address cultural issues directly as they emerge in therapy. The supervisor can model for the therapist when and how to explore cultural issues and how to create a culturally safe therapeutic environment. Supervisors who are more familiar with the client's cultural background than the therapist may occasionally use live supervision as an opportunity to serve as a cultural guide (e.g., suggesting to a therapist working with a Puerto Rican family that he or she inquire about the influence of the extended family on the problem). At times, it may be advisable for a therapist to engage the services of a supervisor or consultant from the client's culture and consult the relevant culture-specific treatment literature. With some creativity, live supervision can be used to describe the family's cultural dilemmas in a nonjudgmental way. For example, with a reflecting team approach, the treatment team can describe to a family how they see diverse members caught in the process of acculturation.

Video Supervision

Video supervision allows for intense reflection on therapy sessions by stepping in and out of the therapy process. Being able to interrupt the therapy process when stopping the videotape provides opportunities for supervisors and supervisees to increase their cultural awareness and sensitivity. For example, they can watch a tape of a therapist who ignores cultural issues in therapy and role-play how they could identify and address these issues. When watching a videotape of a supervisee exploring the clients' cultural background, the emerging information can be analyzed in the context of the therapist's cultural genogram and gendergram. Role plays and discussions of alternatives can help therapists answer questions such as the following: What different cultural expectations does each member of a couple bring to their relationship and to therapy? What are the unspoken cultural tensions between client and therapist as they emerge during the session, and how might they be addressed? How do interventions on the videotape reflect culturally sensitive therapy goals, and how could they be modified?

Case Consultation

Case consultation provides additional opportunities to focus on the supervisee's ability to acknowledge culture in conceptualizing cases. Including cultural issues in case consultation raises supervisees' cultural awareness and changes their conceptual approach to therapy. This can be done in different ways:

1. The supervisor may present a case history that does not incorporate salient cultural aspects in its conceptualization and ask the supervisee to discuss the case from a multicultural perspective, exploring how the presenting problem may be related to cultural issues, and developing culturally appropriate treatment goals and interventions.

2. When presenting one of his or her own cases, the supervisee may be asked to comment on the influence of his or her own cultural background on the work.

3. In group supervision, group members may give the presenting supervisee feedback on their perceptions of cultural similarities and differences between the client, the therapist, and the supervisor, and how these influence the supervision and therapy processes. The group may also process each member's cultural norms around group participation and alter its

format according to the preferences of the supervisee who is presenting a case. An open, respectful, nonconfrontational group discussion creates and facilitates the kind of safe supervision environment that is most helpful for discussing culturally sensitive issues and raising cultural awareness and sensitivity among group members.

CONSIDERING CULTURE IN RESEARCH

Traditionally, family therapy research has focused on the White, middle class couples and families who most commonly self-refer to private practices and family therapy institutes (Gurman & Kniskern, 1991; Pinsof, 1991). Research in family therapy will change drastically when issues affecting culture, such as race, ethnicity, religion, class, and sexual orientation, are more fully considered. Discussions of culture and family therapy have reflected the split between research and practice. Early writings on cultural issues and family therapy focused solely on clinical issues. For example, the McGoldrick et al. (1982) classic book on ethnicity and family therapy does not include a chapter devoted solely to research issues, and most chapters do not discuss research implications. Extensive family therapy research into cultural issues is long overdue. We recommend the following steps: First, acknowledging the importance of cultural issues in family therapy necessitates a shift in research participants. Theoretical model–oriented outcome studies cannot be conducted with exclusively White convenience samples while neglecting the cultural context of family therapy across theoretical models and approaches. Second, outcome studies can no longer generalize the treatment efficacy unless cultural variables are included and/or controlled for. It is crucial to include cultural variables in determining outcome factors for therapy.

Third, we must recognize the political dimension inherent in all research. Therapy and research/science are socially constructed concepts. Research is funded by those in power. Modern social science reflects the values and norms of the dominant culture, and its research is often conducted, either consciously or unconsciously, in the interests of that dominant culture. For example, research with members of oppressed groups is often designed to demonstrate the effectiveness of a given intervention in reducing a supposed pathology, rather than demonstrating a cultural strength or the need for structural change to reduce oppression. Current research may boost the reputation of family therapy but is not necessarily the most useful research for the participants. In addition, research is rarely used to empower the participants directly; rather, it elevates the careers and reputations of those who conduct the research. Researchers who are part of the dominant culture usually apply their cultural views when conducting research with members of their own and other cultural groups. Even those researchers who are not members of the dominant group by birth (although almost anyone who has become a researcher has ascended into the dominant social class!) have usually learned research methods and paradigms which support the status quo. It is important to recognize this division of interests between researchers and research subjects and their respective cultural contexts and make appropriate shifts in research methods. For example, traditional empirical approaches using standardized quantitative methods may not always be sufficient for culturally sensitive research in family therapy. Research methods are sorely needed that take the cultural contexts of all participants (clients and therapists) and researchers into account.

The following research questions should be explored:

1. How can the cultural awareness and sensitivity of therapists be raised, and how can the increase be evaluated?
2. How are the therapist's cultural awareness and sensitivity related to therapy outcome?
3. How can cultural fit between therapist and client be evaluated, and how does the fit influence therapy outcome?
4. What is the impact of process variables such as "empowering clients," "making cultural issues explicit," and "finding a cultural fit between client and therapist" on treatment outcome?
5. How does didactic course work focusing on cultural issues affect therapists' cultural awareness and sensitivity, and how can that be evaluated?
6. Are the cultural and gender genograms valuable measures for assessing the therapist and client's cultural background and gender socialization, respectively, and how can they be used most effectively to increase cultural awareness and sensitivity?
7. Can family therapy help clients overcome the damaging effects of racism, sexism, homophobia, and other forms of oppression, and how can this be evaluated?
8. With which presenting problems and which clients should cultural issues be made explicit, and how can therapists be trained to determine this?
9. How does the inclusion of cultural issues in supervision affect supervisee development and therapy outcome, and how can these be evaluated?
10. How can supervision be used most effectively to raise the supervisee's cultural awareness and sensitivity, and how can this be evaluated?
11. Do certain therapy techniques, modalities, or theories "fit" better with clients from specific groups?

12. How central to therapy are issues of therapist–client cultural difference and sameness, and in what ways do these affect the therapy process?

13. How do cultural issues intersect with the stage of the family life cycle, individual development, and other normative processes in families?

14. How can family therapy researchers be recruited from a variety of cultural groups? How does researcher identity affect the focus of research, the methodologies employed, the results obtained, and the dissemination of the findings?

15. What are the most effective ways to help trainees overcome racism, ageism, ableism, xenophobia, homophobia, and other biases that might hinder their work with clients from diverse groups?

16. What are the special issues facing families in which members come from a variety of cultural groups (e.g., interracial couples, families with cross-ethnic adoptions, families with both hearing and deaf members, families with members with various class backgrounds or sexual orientations)?

Exploring these research questions requires a variety of quantitative and qualitative research methods. Most of them are exploratory in nature; others concern measurement. The answers to these questions will improve the field's vision of the role of culture in research, therapy, supervision, and family life in general.

CONCLUSION

When we incorporate cultural issues into family therapy, we enhance the optimistic, liberating potential of our field. As we widen our lenses in this way, we must make changes that will feel uncomfortable at first to some. But just as when we buy a new pair of glasses, we will soon get used to seeing more clearly. We trust that the field of family therapy will similarly adjust to considering cultural issues in theory, training, clinical work, and research.

KEY BOOKS, CHAPTERS, AND ARTICLES

Almeida, R. V. (Ed.). (1994). *Expansions of feminist family theory through diversity.* Binghamton, NY: Haworth.

This volume, which was previously published as a special issue of the *Journal of Feminist Family Therapy, 5,* (3–4) 1994, includes chapters by Kenneth Hardy,

Lillian Comas-Díaz, Eliana Korin, Rhea Almeida, Monica McGoldrick, and other major theorists on issues of diversity in family therapy. Korin's application of the ideas of Paulo Freire to clinical practice is particularly noteworthy, pointing a path from personal and familial change to social action.

Breunlin, D. C., Schwartz, R. C., & Mac Kune-Karrer, B. (1992). Unifying diverse parameters: The multicultural framework. In *Metaframeworks: Transcending the models of family therapy*. San Francisco: Jossey-Bass.

In this chapter, the authors critique the field of family therapy and the social structure of the United States from a multicultural perspective. The chapter is built around the twin concepts of cultural transition in its historical or generational context and "degree of fit" between the majority and the minority group, the immigrant and the host society, or the family and the therapist. The chapter offers ideas about potential generational and gender differences in immigrant groups, which therapists can use in their work with people from various backgrounds. The chapter also includes questions about multicultural issues—some focusing on the family and others on the therapist—that can be used as bases for discussions in the classroom or therapy session.

Boyd-Franklin, N. (1989). *Black families in therapy: A multisystems approach*. New York: Guilford Press.

In this classic text, Boyd-Franklin offers a broad conceptual overview and detailed practical suggestions for working with Black families in therapy. In the first section, the cultural contexts of Black families are discussed, including racism, extended family patterns, role flexibility, and religion. The second section covers major treatment theories, issues, and interventions, including the therapist's use of self, a critique of major family therapy approaches, and a step-by-step description of Boyd-Franklin's multisystems approach. The book includes ample and vivid case discussions. The final two sections describe diverse family structures and interventions (e.g., single parent families, Black couples) and implications for training and research.

Brown, L. S., & Rothblum, E. D. (1989). *Fat oppression and psychotherapy: A feminist perspective*. Binghamton, NY: Haworth.

Originally published as a special issue of the journal *Women and Therapy, 8*, this volume includes a variety of articles on fat oppression in psychotherapy. Its articles are varied in their focus and approach. Although not explicitly directed toward family therapists, this book offers an excellent starting point for considering body size as a cultural concern in family therapy.

Comas-Díaz, L., & Greene, B. (Eds.). (1994). *Women of color: Integrating ethnic and gender identities in psychotherapy*. New York: Guilford Press.

This volume presents material relevant to therapists who are working with families of color and have a particular interest in the effects of culture and oppression on girls and women. The book consists of 17 chapters by authors of a variety of backgrounds. Some of these chapters are culture specific (e.g., "Women of the Indian Subcontinent") while others are grouped according to theoretical perspective (e.g., psychodynamic approaches), while still others are organized around special issues (e.g., lesbian women of color).

Falicov, C. J. (1988). Learning to think culturally. In H. A. Liddle, D. C. Breunlin, & R. C. Schwartz, (Eds.), *Handbook of family therapy training and supervision.* New York: Guilford Press.

This chapter offers a complex, textured, and thorough discussion of training in culture and family therapy. In addition to describing ways to teach trainees about culture, the article describes many of the important issues themselves (e.g., how cultural contexts might affect the marital bond). This is essential reading.

Family Therapy Networker. (1993, July/August). The Black middle class: No refuge from racism [Special issue].

In this special issue, Anderson J. Franklin, Kenneth Hardy, Nancy Boyd-Franklin and others discuss African Americans in therapy and in society. This collection of articles is a powerful antidote to so much of the writing about African American families, which collapses issues of race and poverty, thereby falsely presenting African Americans in the United States as monolithic and poor.

Family Therapy Networker. (1991, January/February). Gays and lesbians in therapy [Special issue].

In this special issue, the lives of gay and lesbian people are described, with particular emphasis on their struggles against homophobia in families, in the therapy room, and in society. This issue provides a way for therapists and trainees to begin to learn about some of the challenges facing gay men and lesbians.

Fontes, L. (Ed.). (1995). *Sexual abuse in nine North American cultures: Treatment and prevention.* Newbury Park, CA: Sage.

This collection includes overviews of general cultural issues in addressing issues of sexual abuse, as well as original pieces on the occurrence, prevention, and treatment of sexual abuse in nine cultural groups: African Americans, Anglo Americans, Asian Americans, Cambodians, Puerto Ricans, Jews, Seventh Day Adventists, lesbians, and gay male. Each chapter includes information on the history, culture, traditional views on sexuality and gender roles, and some of the primary oppression issues for members of each group, as well as case histories and practical advice for therapists.

Ham, M. D. (Ed.). (1989). Family therapy with immigrant families [Special issue]. *Journal of Strategic and Systemic Therapies, 8.*

This issue includes culture-specific as well as issue-oriented articles, with information relevant to working with immigrant families from a variety of cultures including Chinese, Southeast Asian, and Central American. Several of the articles include vivid case descriptions as well as theoretical analyses.

Inclan, J. (Ed.). (1990). Working with the urban poor [Special issue]. *Journal of Strategic and Systemic Therapies, 9*(3).

In this issue, five articles address the social context of urban poverty as a backdrop to family therapy. In his article, Inclan presents a detailed training curriculum on understanding Hispanic families, which is ready for use with Latinos or may be adapted to fit the ecological contexts of other groups.

Kliman, J. (1994). The interweaving of gender, class, and race in family therapy. In M. P. Mirkin (Ed.), *Women in context: Toward a feminist reconstruction of psychotherapy.* New York: Guilford Press.

This unusual article addresses the dynamic relationships among gender, class, and race in families and family therapy. Kliman facilitates the demarginalization of multicultural issues in family therapy by discussing race as relevant to Whites as well as Blacks, and gender as relevant to men as well as women. Kliman's attention to class is outstanding.

Leigh, L. A. (1995). The evolving treatment of gender, ethnicity, and sexual orientation in marital and family therapy. *Family Relations, 44,* 359–367.

This article addresses the critique of family therapy as historically oppressive to women in families, racial and ethnic minorities, and gay and lesbian families. It describes three ways in which family therapy may have contributed to the maintenance of an oppressive status quo. The article evaluates the impact of the feminist, multicultural, and gay rights critiques, and areas that warrant further attention.

McGoldrick, M. (Ed.). (1990). Ethnicity and mothers [Special issue]. *Journal of Feminist Family Therapy, 2*(2).

In this issue, the mothering role and dilemmas for mothers from nine different cultures are sketched in brief culture-specific articles. The authors challenge many of the stereotypes about mothers from each group and also explore and reframe as strengths the kernels of truth behind some of the stereotypes.

McGoldrick, M., Giordano, J., & Pearce, J. K. (1996). *Ethnicity and family therapy* (2nd ed.). New York: Guilford Press.

This book contains detailed culture-specific information on working with people from a wide variety of backgrounds, including dozens of ethnic groups within races (e.g., Portuguese, Indonesian), resulting in a greater degree of specificity than is available anywhere else. The overview and introduction of ecological models remain as important today as they were when the first edition was written over a decade ago. This new edition is improved in its attention to the dynamic interrelationships among culture, class, gender, and racial issues.

Preli, R., & Bernard, J. M. (1993). Making multiculturalism relevant for majority culture graduate students. *Journal of Marital and Family Therapy, 19,* 5–16.

This article should be consulted by every training program at the beginning of every semester. It describes ways to alert White graduate students to the relevance of culture in their own lives. It provides exercises to help students understand the complexity of their multiple cultural identities, as well as ways to sensitize them to the extent to which they have identified with the majority culture. It is both a complex, textured, theoretical piece and a practical how- to guide for working with students.

Roberts, J. (Ed.). (1993). *Honoring and working with diversity in family therapy.* (Available from the American Family Therapy Academy, 2020 Pennsylvania Avenue, N.W., #273, Washington, DC 20006; 202-994-2776.)

This resource packet consists of a variety of articles, lists of bibliographic materials organized by topic (e.g., gay and lesbian issues), training exercises, and conceptual models (e.g., the umbrella model of oppression) to be used in therapist training and, to a lesser extent, in the therapy room. Some of the materials are culture specific (e.g., Miguel Hernández & Jaime Inclan's "Working with Hispanic Families in Therapy"), whereas others are related to diversity issues more generally (e.g., Bailey Jackson, & Rita Hardiman's "Model of Oppression/Liberation Identity Development"). This resource packet is an excellent starting-off point for trainers and instructors committed to facilitating exploration of multicultural issues.

Saba, G. W., Karrer, B. M., & Hardy, K. V. (1989). *Minorities and family therapy.* Binghamton, NY: Haworth.

This collection, previously published as a special issue of the *Journal of Psychotherapy and the Family,* 6(1–2), 1989, sets out to substitute deficit approaches to minority families with discussions of the strengths of minority families. The book includes key culture-specific articles (e.g., a piece by Terry Tafoya on Native Americans and family therapy), as well as discussions of issues that can affect families from a variety of minority backgrounds (e.g., Hardy's oft-cited piece on the theoretical myth of sameness).

Skowron, E. A. (1995). *Instructor's manual for Nichols and Schwartz's family therapy: Concepts and methods* (3rd ed.). Boston: Allyn & Bacon.

The manual includes several excellent suggestions for small-group discussions and role plays on different aspects of culture (e.g., ethnicity, race and class, sexual orientation).

Tamasese, K., & Waldegrave, C. (1993). Culture and gender accountability in the "just therapy" approach. *Journal of Feminist Family Therapy,* 5(2), 29–45.

This article introduces and describes the issue of "accountability" of people from dominant groups (e.g., men, Whites) to people from subjugated groups, focusing on the interactions among professionals and the organizational structure of agency settings, rather than on contacts with clients. The article is based on struggles within a multicultural agency in New Zealand and is relevant for all who wish to create more just, egalitarian, and nurturing environments for mental health workers from all backgrounds.

REFERENCES

Atwood, J. D., & Ruiz, J. (1993). Social constructionist therapy with the elderly. *Journal of Family Psychotherapy, 4*(1), 1–32.

Bograd, M. (Ed.). (1990). *Feminist approaches for men in therapy.* Binghamton, NY: Haworth.

Boyd-Franklin, N. (1989). *Black families in therapy: A multisystems approach.* New York: Guilford Press.

Breunlin, D. C., Schwartz, R. C., & Mac Kune-Karrer, B. (1992). *Metaframeworks: Transcending the models of family therapy.* San Francisco: Jossey-Bass.

Commission on Accreditation for Marriage and Family Therapy Education (1988). *Manual on accreditation.* Washington, DC: Author.

Ehrenreich, B. (1983). *The hearts of men.* New York: Anchor Press.

Facundo, A., Nuttal, E., & Walton, J. (1994). Culturally sensitive assessment in schools. In P. Pedersen & J. C. Carey, (Eds.), *Multicultural counseling in schools: A practical handbook.* Boston: Allyn & Bacon.

Falicov, C. J. (1988). Learning to think culturally. In H. A. Liddle, D. C. Breunlin, & R. C. Schwartz, *Handbook of family therapy training and supervision.* New York: Guilford Press.

Fontes, L. (1993). Considering culture and oppression: Steps toward an ecology of sexual child abuse. *Journal of Feminist Family Therapy, 5*(1), 25–54.

Fontes, L. (Ed.). (1995). *Sexual abuse in nine North American cultures: Treatment and prevention.* Newbury Park, CA: Sage.

Fulani, L. (Ed.). (1988). *The psychopathology of everyday racism and sexism.* New York: Harrington Park Press.

Goldner, V. (1989). Generation and gender: Normative and covert hierarchies. In M. McGoldrick, C. M. Anderson, & F. Walsh (Eds), *Women in families: A framework for family therapy.* New York: Norton.

Goldner, V. (1993). Power and hierarchy: Let's talk about it. *Family Process, 32*(2), 157–162.

Gonzalez-Calvó, J. T. (1993). Introduction. In J. T. Gonzalez-Calvó (Ed.), *Gender: Multicultural perspectives.* Dubuque, IA: Kendall/Hunt.

Gurman, A. S., & Kniskern, D. P. (1991). Family therapy outcome research: Knowns and unknowns. In A. S. Gurman & D. P. Kniskern (Eds.), *Handbook of family therapy* (Vol. 1). New York: Brunner/Mazel.

Hardy, K. V. (1989). The theoretical myth of sameness: A critical issue in family therapy treatment and training. In G. W. Saba, B. M. Karrer, & K. V. Hardy (Ed.), *Minorities and family therapy.* Binghamton, NY: Haworth.

Hardy, K. V., & Laszloffy, T. A. (1994) Deconstructing race in family therapy. *Journal of Feminist Family Therapy, 5*(3–4), 5–33.

Hardy, K. V., & Laszloffy, T. A. (1995). The cultural genogram: Key to training culturally competent family therapists. *Journal of Marital and Family Therapy, 21*(3), 227–237.

Hydén, M. (1994). *Woman battering as marital act: The construction of a violent marriage.* New York: Oxford University Press.

Inclan, J. (Ed.). (1990). Working with the urban poor [Special issue]. *Journal of Strategic and Systemic Therapies, 9*(3).

Jalali, B., & Boyce, E. (1980). Multicultural families in treatment. *International Journal of Family Psychiatry, 1,* 475–484.

Kliman, J. (1994) The interweaving of gender, class, and race in family therapy. In M. P. Mirkin (Ed.), *Women in context: Toward a feminist reconstruction of psychotherapy.* New York: Guilford Press.

Landau, J. (1982). Therapies with families in cultural transition. In M. McGoldrick, J. Giordano, & J. K. Pearce (Eds.), *Ethnicity and family therapy.* New York: Guilford Press.

Lappin, J. (1983). On becoming a culturally conscious family therapist. In C. J. Falicov (Ed.), *Cultural perspectives in family therapy.* Rockville, MD: Aspen Publications.

McGoldrick, M. (1982). Ethnicity and family therapy: An overview. In M. McGoldrick, J. Giordano, & J. K. Pearce (Eds.), *Ethnicity and family therapy.* New York: Guilford Press.

McGoldrick, M. (1994). Family therapy: Having a place called home. *Journal of Feminist Family Therapy, 5*(3–4), 127–156.

McGoldrick, M., Anderson, C. M., & Walsh, F. (Eds.). (1989). *Women in families: A framework for family therapy.* New York: Norton.

McGoldrick, M., Giordano, J., & Pearce, J. K. (1982). *Ethnicity and family therapy.* New York: Guilford Press.

McGoldrick, M., Giordano, J., & Pearce, J. K. (1996). *Ethnicity and family therapy* (2nd ed.). New York: Guilford Press.

McGoldrick, M., Preto, N. G., Hines, P. M., & Lee, E. (1991). Ethnicity and family therapy. In A. S. Gurman & D. P. Kniskern, *Handbook of family therapy* (Vol. 2). New York: Brunner/Mazel.

Mirkin, M. P. (1992). Female adolescence revisited: Understanding girls in their sociocultural contexts. *Journal of Feminist Family Therapy, 4*(2), 43–60.

Perez, P. (1996). Tailoring a collaborative, constructionist approach for the treatment of same sex couples. *Family Journal, 4*(1).

Pinsof, W. M. (1991). Family therapy process research. In A. S. Gurman & D. P. Kniskern, *Handbook of family therapy* (Vol. 1). New York: Brunner/Mazel.

Preli, R., & Bernard, J. M. (1993). Making multiculturalism relevant for majority culture graduate students. *Journal of Marital and Family Therapy, 19,* 5–16.

Roberts, J. (Ed.). (1993). *AFTA resource packet: Honoring and working with diversity in family therapy.* (Available from the American Family Therapy Academy, 2020 Pennsylvania Avenue, N.W., #273, Washington, DC 20006.)

Roberts, J. (1994). *Tales and transformations: Stories in families and family therapy.* New York: Norton.

Rosenthal, C. J. (1986). Family supports in later life: Does ethnicity make a difference? *The Gerontologist, 26*(1), 9–24.

Saba, G. W., & Rodgers, D. V. (1989). Discrimination in urban family practice:

Lessons from poor minority families. In G. W. Saba, B. M. Karrer, & K. V. Hardy (Eds.), *Minorities and family therapy.* Binghamton, NY: Haworth.

Schwartzmann, J. (1983). Family ethnography: A tool for clinicians. In C. J. Falicov (Ed.), *Cultural perspectives in family therapy.* Rockville, MD: Aspen Publications.

Seligman, M., & Darling, R. B. (1989). *Ordinary families, special children: A systems approach to childhood disability.* New York: Guilford Press.

Skowron, E. A. (1995). *Instructor's manual for Nichols and Schwartz "Family therapy: Concepts and methods"* (3rd ed.). Boston: Allyn & Bacon.

Sluzki, C. E. (1979). Migration and family conflict. *Family Process, 18,* 379–390.

Sotomayor, M. (1991). Introduction. In M. Sotomayor (Ed.), *Empowering Hispanic families: A critical issue for the '90s.* Milwaukee: Family Service America.

Stander, V., Piercy, F., MacKinnon, D., & Helmeke, K. (1994). Spirituality, religion and family therapy: Competing or complimentary worlds. *American Journal of Family Therapy, 22*(1), 27–41.

Tomasese, K., & Waldgrave, C. (1993). Culture and gender accountability in the "Just Therapy" approach. *Journal of Feminist Family Therapy, 5*(2), 29–45.

White, M. B., & Tyson-Rawson, K. J. (1995). Assessing the dynamics of gender in couples and families. *Family Relations, 44,* 253–260.

11

Other Family Therapies

FRED P. PIERCY
JOSEPH L. WETCHLER
LORNA L. HECKER

Each chapter in this book deals with a different family therapy theory or domain. A variety of other family therapies have had a significant impact on the field's development. In this chapter we will provide both an introduction to and key resources on eight additional approaches to family therapy. This chapter has two major sections. The first contains those theories of historical significance in the field that have had few new contributions in the last several years. This section includes (1) multiple-family group therapy; (2) multiple impact therapy; (3) marital group therapy; (4) network therapy; and (5) Gerald Zuk's triadic therapy.

In the second section, several theories are somewhat new to the field. Others are older. All have had a significant impact during the last few years. This section contains (1) internal family systems therapy; (2) the psychoanalytic family therapies; and (3) psychoeducational family therapy. Inclusion in one section or another is not a sign of superiority of ideas, but rather reflects the amount of recent work in that theory.

THEORIES OF HISTORICAL IMPORTANCE

Multiple-Family Group Therapy

Introduction to the Therapy

Multiple-family group therapy (MFGT) involves the treatment of several families together within regularly scheduled therapy sessions. Cotherapists typically act as active facilitators to improve communication, encourage insight into problematic interactions, and restructure family relationship patterns. MFGT has been used on both an inpatient and an outpatient basis by theoretically diverse therapists working with families with a wide range of symptomatic behaviors. The person most closely associated with MFGT, however, is Laqueur (1966, 1972a, 1972b, 1976).

Generally, MFGT combines many of the advantages of both family and group therapy. Families learn indirectly from other families through analogy, indirect interpretation, and modeling (Laqueur, 1976). Also, the therapist creates a supportive context to try new behaviors and develop more flexible roles (Gritzer & Okun, 1983). The families themselves sometimes serve as "cotherapists," in that they often confront members of other families more effectively and powerfully than the therapist. When families hear from other families, they are less likely to deny feedback. They are also more likely to hear the message (McFarlane, 1982).

Key Books, Chapters, and Articles

Benningfield, A. B. (1978). Multiple family therapy systems. *Journal of Marriage and Family Counseling, 4,* 25–34.

The author provides a table that organizes over 40 reports on MFGT in terms of population, setting, and conclusions or outcomes of the report. She then discusses the role of the therapist and implications for research, as well as other topics covered more thoroughly in the Strelnick (1977) review.

Durell, V. G. (1988). Adolescents in multiple family group therapy in a school setting. In W. M. Walsh & N. J. Giblin (Eds.), *Family counseling in school settings.* Springfield, IL: Thomas.

This chapter presents a case study of a multiple-family group in a school setting for families with adolescent boys with school-focused problems. The chapter focuses on issues pertaining to establishing the group, the role of the leader, and the evolution of the group.

Gritzer, P. H., & Okun, H. S. (1983). Multiple family group therapy: A model for all families. In B. B. Wolman & G. Stricker (Eds.), *Handbook of family and marital therapy.* New York: Plenum Press.

This well-written chapter includes a comprehensive description of MFGT as applied to outpatient settings, providing a useful preparation for conducting an

MFGT group when read in conjunction with the Leichter and Schulman (1972, 1974) articles and the McFarlane (1982) chapter.

Laqueur, H. P. (1966). General systems theory and multiple family therapy. In J. H. Masserman (Ed.), *Handbook of psychiatric therapies.* New York: Grune & Stratton.

This brief, pithy chapter is devoted to each of the MFGT theories and their interface. This information is not available in such detail in the other Laqueur writings.

Laqueur, H. P. (1972a). Mechanisms of change in multiple-family therapy. In C. J. Sager & H. S. Kaplan (Eds.), *Progress in group and family therapy.* New York: Brunner/Mazel.

Unique to this chapter are excellent clinical illustrations of the 11 mechanisms of change in MFGT as conceptualized by Laqueur.

Laqueur, H. P. (1972b). Multiple-family therapy. In A. Ferber, M. Mendelsohn, & A. Napier (Eds.), *The book of family therapy.* Boston: Houghton Mifflin.

This chapter provides a straightforward description of how a MFGT therapist introduces families, leads a group, and responds to absenteeism. Also provided are examples of interaction in an MFT group and a comparison of successful and unsuccessful cotherapy.

Laqueur, H. P. (1976). Multiple family therapy. In P. J. Guerin (Ed.), *Family therapy: Theory and practice.* New York: Gardner.

This is an important chapter. It clearly articulates Laqueur's chief concepts. Topics covered include the history and description of MFGT, its theoretical framework, the process and mechanisms of change, and goals and results. Particularly interesting is Laqueur's summary of the structure of disturbed and healthy families. Of considerable help is the lucid description of several MFGT interventions.

Laqueur, H. P., & LaBurt, H. A. (1973). Multiple family therapy: Questions and answers. In D. Block (Ed.), *Techniques of family psychotherapy: A primer.* New York: Grune & Stratton.

This chapter offers much of the same information contained in the Laqueur (1976) chapter; however, its question-and-answer format and the section on the typical problems in the conduct of a group are unique.

Laqueur, H. P., Wells, C. F., & Agresti, M. (1969). Multiple-family therapy in a state hospital. *Hospital and Community Psychiatry, 20,* 13–19.

This article offers the most comprehensive description of Laqueur's actual work at a state hospital; however, it does not include a description of his research study.

Leichter, E., & Schulman, G. L. (1972). Interplay of group and family treatment techniques in multi-group family therapy. *International Journal of Group Psychotherapy, 22,* 167–176.

After working several years as cotherapists in outpatient MFGT, the authors articulate their own thinking about process and goals. They have found one of the greatest values of MFGT to be the interaction between members across family boundaries. For example, an adolescent can practice differentiation first with adults who are not his or her parents. The authors provide numerous examples of their concepts from their own clinical practice.

Leichter, E., & Schulman, G. (1974). Multi-family group therapy: Multidimensional approach. *Family Process, 13*(1), 95–110.

Case examples are used to illustrate the dynamics and process of outpatient MFGT. This is an excellent article and would be useful for anyone about to initiate outpatient MFGT.

McFarlane, W. R. (1982). Multiple-family therapy in the psychiatric hospital. In H. T. Harbin (Ed.), *The psychiatric hospital and the family.* New York: Spectrum.

This lucid chapter is by an author who practices MFGT in an inpatient setting. McFarlane believes that groups made up of nonpsychotic clients need to be run differently from those made up of psychotic clients. He provides guidelines for managing both. Also, the author discusses nine mechanisms for change "unique" to MFGT. The author also outlines five problems that result from the institutionalization of the psychotic client and reviews how MFGT can make them better.

Paul, N. L., Bloom, J. D., & Paul, B. B. (1981). Outpatient multiple family group therapy—why not? In L. R. Wolterg & M. L. Aronson (Eds.), *Group and family therapy.* New York: Brunner/Mazel.

The participating families are well described. The authors include transcripts of sessions to demonstrate the impact on others in the group when hidden critical historical material is revealed. Norman Paul is the therapist of the group. A worthwhile chapter.

Strelnick, A. H. (1977). Multiple family group therapy: A review of the literature. *Family Process, 16*, 307–325.

This review is neatly organized into subsections that include origins, methods, development of the group, goals, themes, and mechanisms of change. The author also provides comparisons of MFGT with group and individual family therapy, as well as an evaluation of outcome.

Multiple-Impact Therapy

Introduction to the Therapy

Robert MacGregor and his colleagues (MacGregor et al., 1964) developed multiple-impact therapy (MIT) as a means of having a maximum impact on families with a disturbed adolescent in crisis. These highly motivated families would come long distances to the University of Texas Medical Branch in Galveston, Texas, and spend several days in intense therapy with a large team of professionals. The team typically included psychologists, psychiatric residents, social workers, and trainees, who would meet with family members individually and in various combinations in order to assess and treat problematic aspects of a family's functioning. On the second afternoon of these sessions, a team–family conference was held, in which findings were reviewed, recommendations were made, and follow-up sessions scheduled for several months later.

During the 2 days of sessions, the team would attempt to examine and strengthen the parents' marital relationship and focus intensely on parent–adolescent communication patterns. Beyond helping families develop insight into their problems and restructure their relationship patterns, the MIT process took family members through a powerful emotional experience that jolted them toward more open system functioning. The experience often resulted in better communication, greater acceptance of differences, clearer hierarchies and boundaries, and a resolve to look toward the future for more creative, growth-producing ways of functioning (MacGregor, 1972; Richie, 1971).

MIT is not practiced extensively today, perhaps because of the considerable time, expense, and number of professional staff members needed to implement it, as well as its lack of empirical support. Another barrier may be conceptual. Many therapists believe that families need time between sessions to assimilate learning and to facilitate a transfer of gains to real-life situations. Nonetheless, the historical significance of MIT to the field of family therapy is considerable, and many of the assumptions and procedures implemented in MIT are still applicable to other forms of family therapy.

Key Books, Chapters, and Articles

Garrison, C., & Weber, J. (1981). Family crises intervention using multiple impact therapy. *Social Casework, 62,* 585–593.

In this study, MIT was employed to (1) reduce the time lag between family crisis onset and professional intervention; (2) minimize removal of children from the family; (3) provide quicker, more intensive treatment than traditional methods; and (4) encourage more effective cooperation among agencies involved with a particular family. Representatives from each caregiving agency formed a team that met with the family for a day and then divided responsibilities so as to be allied with different family members for the following month. The reported results of this cooperation are encouraging.

MacGregor, R. (1967). Progress in multiple impact theory. In N. W. Ackerman, F. L. Beatman, & S. N. Sherman (Eds.), *Expanding theory and practice in family therapy.* New York: Family Service Association.

In this chapter, MacGregor defines MIT as a freeing up of natural processes in the family, as opposed to an insight-oriented therapy. He gives a historical perspective on this treatment modality, as well as a look at the underlying theory and techniques used to change a "closed" family system into an "open" one.

MacGregor, R. (1972). Multiple impact psychotherapy with families. In G. D. Erickson & T. P. Hogan (Eds.), *Family therapy: An introduction to theory and technique*. Monterey, CA: Brooks/Cole.

This is perhaps the most complete explication of MIT offered by MacGregor. He expands his earlier works by discussing how to incorporate the contributions of relevant community personnel into the treatment team's impact. The results of a 2-year study suggest that disturbed adolescents and their families may be better thought of as developmentally arrested then as requiring a particular diagnostic category for the acting-out child.

MacGregor, R., Riche, A. M., Serrano, A. C., Schuster, F. P., McDonald, E. C., & Goolishian, H. A. (1964). *Multiple impact therapy with families*. New York: McGraw-Hill.

This volume represents the authors' initial, formal evaluation of their MIT experiences with 62 adolescents and their families over a 3-year period. The treatment team was designed to spend 2–3 days with a family for 6–8 hours per day. The study confirmed hypotheses that extreme behavior in an adolescent was related to extreme behavior on the part of at least one parent and found that the approach increased flexibility of roles in 49 of the 62 families examined. Today's researchers would consider this study to be "descriptive" at best.

Richie, A. (1971). Multiple impact therapy: An experiment. In J. Haley (Ed.), *Changing families: A family therapy reader*. New York: Grune & Stratton.

This reprint of Richie's 1960 article gives an overall description of how MIT was done at the Youth Development Project of the University of Texas Medical Branch at Galveston, Texas. This article lacks a discussion of theoretical underpinning but reflects much of the excitement over what was, at the time, a new treatment procedure.

Marital Group Therapy

Introduction to the Therapy

Although a variety of authors have written about marital group therapy, their rationales vary considerably. Proponents have identified such advantages as (1) facilitation of communications; (2) relief of guilt, shame, and embarrassment through observing other couples with similar problems; (3) cost; (4) reality testing aided by group feedback; (5) identification by group members of inappropriate behaviors and expectations; (6) development of insight and skills through observation of other couples; (7) group support that encourages ventilation and change, and reduces fear of reprisal; (8) differentiation from marital symbiosis; (9) identification and interruption of counterproductive "games"; (10) the isomorphism between group and couple interactions (Alger, 1976; Coche, 1995; Coche & Coche, 1990; Framo, 1973; Lieberman & Lieberman, 1986; Linden, Goodwin, & Resnik, 1968). In essence, the marital group becomes a "third family" that gives each couple an opportunity for growth (Leichter, 1973).

Marital group formats and procedures also vary widely. Alger (1976), for example, discusses his own creative uses of role playing, family choreography, and videotape feedback. Framo (1973) has at least one session with each group member and his or her family of origin, whereas Liberman, Wheeler, and Sanders (1976) advocate behavioral communication skills training in their couples groups. In contrast, Coche and Coche (1990) propose a 1-year, closed-group format that emphasizes experiential and systems concepts, and Neimeyer (1987) utilizes a live supervision team acting as a "Greek chorus."

Coche (1995) believes that marital group activity takes place at multiple levels. Therapists can intervene at the personal level of each group member, the couple level, the interpersonal relationships between various group members, the whole group, or any combination of the aforementioned.

Various psychoanalytic therapists have identified potential disadvantages of the marital group format (see Boas, 1962; Gottlieb & Pattison, 1966; Linden et al., 1968). For example, complications in the development of the essential transference neurosis within the marital group format have been thought to lead to a dilution of transference reactions (Boas, 1962). Additional fears include the potential for acting out within the group and the strengthening of marital defenses. However, these psychoanalytic criticisms do not appear to have a substantive basis, either empirically or in therapeutic practice (Gurman, 1971).

Framo (1973) has summed up the enthusiasm of many marital group therapy proponents in stating that marital group therapy is "probably the treatment of choice for dealing with marital problems" (p. 96). However, others advise that leaders admit higher functioning couples (Lieberman & Lieberman, 1986) and omit those with overt psychosis (Coche & Coche, 1990) to enhance a successful group experience. As with other marital and family therapies, more empirical support clearly is needed to substantiate claims of effectiveness (Marett, 1988).

Key Books, Chapters, and Articles

Alger, I. (1976). Multiple couples therapy. In P. J. Guerin (Ed.), *Family therapy: Theory and practice*. New York: Gardner.

In this chapter, Alger does a good job of covering many of the important issues in couples group therapy from an eclectic framework. Topics include the indications for use of couples group therapy, stages of evolution in the group, the therapist's role, size and structure of the group, and specialized techniques.

Arieli, A. (1981). Multicouple group therapy of alcoholics. *International Journal of the Addictions, 16,* 773–782.

This article presents the author's experience in the treatment of alcoholics in a marital group format. The author cites the interactional nature of alcoholism and speaks of how the issues are highlighted in the group format.

Blinder, M. G., & Kirschenbaum, M. (1967). The technique of married couple group therapy. *Archives of General Psychiatry, 17,* 44–52.

This article presents a theoretical and practical approach to their "married couples group therapy," based on treating the interpersonal marital relationship. The authors believe that mate selection is based on the fulfillment of neurotic needs. They discuss the curative aspects of the group, as well as positive therapeutic interventions.

Boas, C. V. E. (1962). Intensive group psychotherapy with married couples. *International Journal of Group Psychotherapy, 12,* 142–153.

This article presents the author's early experiences with a marital couples group. Boas discusses the positive effects of breaking away from psychoanalytic "taboos" regarding seeing married couples together in a group. This is an excellent historical article in its reflection of the excitement that existed when marital group therapy first began.

Burton, G. (1962). Group counseling with alcoholic husbands and their nonalcoholic wives. *Marriage and Family Living, 24,* 56–61.

This early article discusses the profit gained in working with alcoholics in a group marital format. The author emphasizes the need to analyze the interpersonal relationship of these couples and make these interactions the focus of change in treatment.

Coche, J. (1995). Group therapy with couples. In N. S. Jacobson & A. S. Gurman (Eds.), *Clinical handbook of couple therapy.* New York: Guilford Press.

In this chapter, the author provides a synopsis of her model, plus an excellent discussion of the theoretical, technical, and clinical issues involved in couples group treatment.

Coche, J., & Coche, E. (1990). *Couples group psychotherapy: A clinical practice model.* New York: Brunner/Mazel.

This excellent book provides detailed instructions for utilizing the authors' model of couples group therapy. They provide theoretical rationales and technical advise on such issues as preparing couples for group, establishing ground rules, assessing outcome, and handling problems. Included in this book is a small study by the authors on the effectiveness of their model.

Flint, A. A., Jr., & MacLennan, B. W. (1962). Some dynamic factors in marital group psychotherapy. *International Journal of Group Psychotherapy, 12,* 355–361.

This article presents common characteristics observed in six marital therapy groups. The authors present the group process in terms of five specific stages and describe such pertinent aspects of treatment dynamics as (1) the marital partner in the therapeutic role, (2) the relationship of the couple to the group, and (3) the relationship of the couple to the therapist.

Framo, J. L. (1973). Marriage therapy in a couples group. In D. A. Bloch (Ed.), *Techniques of family psychotherapy: A primer.* New York: Grune & Stratton.

This excellent overview of Framo's approach to couples group therapy is must-reading. Many important issues are presented, such as therapeutic rationale, selection of couples, session structure, and group process. In keeping with Framo's orientation toward family-of-origin theory, he gives attention to helping couples recognize patterns in their marriages that stem from their respective families of origin.

Gottlieb, A., & Pattison, E. M. (1966). Married couples group psychotherapy. *Archives of General Psychiatry, 14,* 143–152.

This article maintains that many of the early psychoanalytic fears of seeing couples together in a group are unfounded. The authors give special attention to the positive aspects of the group in facilitating the couples' growth. Also, they discuss the breaking up of symbiosis in disturbed marital relationships.

Gurman, A. S. (1971). Group marital therapy: Clinical and empirical implications for outcome research. *International Journal of Group Psychotherapy, 21,* 174–189.

This is an excellent review of the literature on couples group therapy through 1970. In the section on theoretical and clinical implications, Gurman discusses the early psychoanalytic controversy over whether to include spouses in group therapy. Gurman also raises the question of whether group marital goals should stress individual or interactional change. In the assessment section, he critically examines the research to date and makes recommendations for future research.

Leichter, E. (1962). Group psychotherapy with married couples: Some characteristic treatment dynamics. *International Journal of Group Psychotherapy, 12,* 154–163.

In this article, the author highlights several interactional dynamics that couples enact in marital group therapy. Particularly interesting topics include the use of the spouse as an alter ego to facilitate treatment, negative reactions spouses may have to changes in their mates, and how marital group therapy helps diminish symbiotic marital ties.

Leichter, E. (1973). Treatment of married couples groups. *Family Coordinator, 22,* 31–42

The author discusses the differences between couples group therapy and treatment groups in which participants are not related. He places special emphasis on the need to have homogeneous groups based on marital stages, due to the unique problems that exist at each stage. The author demonstrates how the group serves a curative function for problematic marriages in each of these stages.

Liberman, R. P., Wheeler, E., & Sanders, W. (1976). Behavioral therapy for marital disharmony: An educational approach. *Journal of Marriage and Family Counseling, 2,* 383–395.

In this article, the author presents a good example of the behavioral approach to marital group therapy. This brief treatment model employs 8–10 highly structured sessions focused on (1) improving communication skills, (2) enhancing pleasing interactions, and (3) introducing contingency-contracting skills.

Lieberman, E. J., & Lieberman, S. B. (1986). Couples group therapy. In N. S. Jacobson & A. S. Gurman (Eds.), *Clinical handbook of marital therapy.* New York: Guilford Press.

This interesting chapter covers such important issues as selection of group members, logistics of leading a couples group, and the principles of couples group therapy. This is a good first source for those wishing to learn about this model.

Linden, M. E., Goodwin, H. M., & Resnik, H. (1968). Group psychotherapy of couples in marriage counseling. *International Journal of Group Psychotherapy, 18,* 313–324.

This article is one of the first by group marital therapists to state that in most instances of marital discord, the problem is relational. The authors state that their goal is to improve interpersonal relationships rather than to change individual character. Furthermore, the authors discuss selection of clients, therapist qualities, and other important therapeutic issues.

Marett, K. M. (1988). A substantive and methodological review of couples group therapy outcome research. *Group, 12,* 241–246.

This review focuses on effectiveness research on couples group therapy from 1976 to the present. He provides suggestions for future studies.

Neimeyer, G. J. (1987). Marital role reconstruction through couples group therapy. In R. A. Neimeyer & G. J. Neimeyer (Eds.), *Personal construct therapy casebook.* New York: Springer.

This chapter presents a couples group format based on personal construct theory and incorporating a live supervision team functioning as a "Greek chorus." The chapter primarily utilizes a case study format following the progress of one short-term couples group.

Neubeck, G. (1954). Factors affecting group psychotherapy with married couples. *Marriage and Family Living, 16,* 216–220.

This classic study examined whether treating married couples in a group would have a positive or a negative effect on the therapy. Several factors were found that both enhanced and inhibited the therapeutic process. In analyzing these factors, the author concludes that the advantages of group therapy outweigh the disadvantages.

Occhetti, A. E., & Occhetti, D. R. (1981). Group therapy with married couples. *Social Casework, 62,* 74–79.

The authors present an existentialist approach to marital group therapy, succinctly discussing such issues as group impact on a couple, types of couples appropriate for group therapy, and specific techniques. Particularly useful is the presentation regarding the roles of the cotherapy team and the importance of the pregroup interview.

Ohlsen, M. M. (1979). *Marriage counseling in groups.* Champaign, IL: Research Press.

This basic text, written for marriage counselors and prospective clients, presents an introduction to counseling couples in groups. The author provides sections on selecting couples, starting up the group, couples' exercises, and termination.

Papp, P. (1976). Brief therapy with couples groups. In P. Guerin (Ed.), *Family therapy: Theory and practice.* New York: Gardner.

This chapter presents an excellent example of a brief strategic approach to couples group therapy. Papp uses choreography in the group, with follow-up tasks designed to alter repetitive cycles of marital interaction. She provides case studies with informative commentary on the use and rationale of these techniques.

Papp, P. (1980). The use of fantasy in a couples' group. In M. Andolfi & I. Zwerling (Eds.), *Dimensions of family therapy.* New York: Guilford Press.

In this chapter Papp presents a structured format for a couples group based on an interactional theory of marriage. Family choreography is used to discover each couple's reciprocal sequences of behaviors and to intervene accordingly.

Papp, P. (1982). Staging reciprocal metaphors in a couples group. *Family Process, 21,* 453–467.

In this interesting article, Papp presents an approach to couple therapy in which the technique of couples choreography is used to help married couples define and act out their patterns of behavior in metaphorical terms.

Perelman, J. (1960). Group treatment of married couples: A symposium. *International Journal of Group Psychotherapy, 10,* 136–142.

This classic article deals with the author's first attempts at including marital couples in a group therapy format. The author discusses the pitfalls he experienced and points out several important lessons he learned—most notably that, despite psychoanalytic doubts, couples can be seen together effectively in a group.

Network Therapy

Introduction to the Therapy

Network therapy is a procedure for intervening in families in crisis and is associated with the work of Ross Speck, Carolyn Attneave, and Uri Rueveni. In network therapy, a therapeutic team (usually two or three individuals) assembles no fewer than 40 members of the social network of the family in crisis, in order to use the therapeutic force of this network in a systematic way. The networking process aims to break destructive patterns of family relationships and provide support for alternative options (Rueveni, 1979; Speck & Attneave, 1971).

A therapeutic team typically meets with a network for about six 3- to 4-hour sessions (Speck & Attneave, 1971). The leader's role is that of a director and facilitator who can be both charismatic and self-effacing, and can mobilize the resources of the group. The members of the therapeutic team are often from different generations and support the networking process in a variety of ways (Speck & Attneave, 1971).

The leader typically uses a series of encounter/sensitivity techniques to shake up the system and encourage change. Change occurs by setting in motion the forces of healing within the network. The leader encourages the network's members to support one another by strengthening bonds, opening channels of communication, and generally enabling the social network to nurture and sustain the individual in crisis. This approach implies a basic faith in the ability of human beings to support one another in crises (Speck & Attneave, 1971, 1973).

Speck and Attneave (1973) have identified the six phases of the networking process as retribalization, polarization, mobilization, depression, breakthrough, and exhaustion–elation, and have outlined the therapist's role and the dynamics of the group associated with each of these phases. The basic agent of change in network therapy, however, is not so easy to categorize and objectify. Speck and Attneave (1971, 1973) have termed it the "network effect"—a euphoric connectedness to others that they liken to the emotions created by religious revival meetings, tribal healing ceremonies, peace marches, and contemporary rock concerts. They maintain that the group atmosphere generated within a social network, as well as the resources of the network members, can help bring about change better than a professional therapist alone. Rueveni (1979), however, warns that family network intervention should be reserved for times of difficult family crises and should not be considered a substitute for other forms of therapy. Network therapies have recently been used for problems with adolescent disturbance (Reed, 1989), substance abuse (Galanter, 1993a, 1993b), cult involvement (Sirkin & Rueveni, 1992), and racial stress (Freeman, 1993).

Key Books, Chapters, and Articles

Attneave, C. (1969). Therapy in tribal settings and urban network intervention. *Family Process, 8,* 192–210.

By providing a case example of a naturally evolved Indian clan, Attneave shows the effects of network therapy. She then compares, contrasts, and evaluates the use of network therapy with naturally evolved groups and with therapist-created groups in an urban setting. She also discusses the network therapist's role as facilitator (as opposed to leader).

Attneave, C. (1976). Social networks as the unit of intervention. In P. J. Guerin (Ed.), *Family therapy: Theory and practice.* New York: Gardner.

In this well-written chapter, Attneave addresses many of the important issues related to network therapy. She discusses practical issues, such as how to map a family network, whom to include in therapy, and how to use network therapy as a preventive mental health tool.

Bishop, S. M. (1984). Perspectives on individual–family–social network interrelations. *International Journal of Family Therapy, 6,* 124–133.

Bishop urges family therapists to expand their focus of assessment and intervention to the larger social network of the family. In his rationale, Bishop attempts to bridge network theory with mainstream family therapy theory. The author also presents different ways in which networking approaches may be used.

Erickson, G. D. (1975). The concept of personal network and clinical practice. *Family Process, 14,* 487–498.

Erickson brings together the emerging strands of network practice to form a conceptual framework for network analysis. He discusses topics such as the characteristics that make up a network, a rationale for clinicians to think in terms of a client's personal network, and the characteristics of a client's network that appear to be indicators that network therapy is the treatment of choice.

Erickson, G. D. (1984). A framework and themes for social network interventions. *Family Process, 23,* 187–198.

In this article, Erickson presents his hypothesis that the networks of psychiatric clients tend to be truncated in comparison to those of normal individuals. He further states that it is important to assess a client's network to identify the nature of the truncation and what type of network therapy is required. He also presents a framework of network types and treatment modalities.

Galanter, M. (1993). Network therapy for addiction: A model for office practice. *American Journal of Psychiatry, 150,* 28–36.

The author presents a model of network therapy adapted for the treatment of substance abuse. It is based more on psychodynamic and behavioral components than traditional network therapy. Several clinical vignettes are included that illustrate this method.

Garrison, J. (1974). Network techniques: Studies in the screening–linking–planning conference method. *Family Process, 13,* 337–353.

This often-cited article is a good example of network therapy used in a brief, problem-solving manner. The author stresses the use of positive connotation and the avoidance of pathology. Garrison provides in-depth case studies to exemplify the use of this method with crisis and chronic hospitalized cases.

Hemly van der Velden, E. M., Halevy-Martini, J., Rulf, L. L., & Schoenfeld, P. (1984). Conceptual issues in network therapy. *International Journal of Family Therapy, 6,* 68–81.

This interesting article presents three concepts developed by the authors while engaged in a project to study and conduct network therapy. The concepts discussed are (1) the achievement of a balanced network to create change, (2) the technique of polarizing the network against the team, and (3) the development of a "multiconductor" model of team leadership.

Reed, C. Y. (1989). Marriage by arrangement: A metaphor for one particular use of network therapy. *Journal of Adolescence, 12,* 279–294.

This article describes the use of the author's model of network therapy with adolescent problems. This model is more structured than traditional network therapy; Reed includes time lines and tasks, as well as an interesting literature review in which the author discusses some of the theoretical changes that have taken place within network therapy over the years.

Rueveni, U. (1977). Family network intervention: Mobilizing support for families in crisis. *International Journal of Family Counseling, 5,* 77–83.

This article provides a brief overview of network therapy, including its process, phases, goals, and strategies. Rueveni also presents short summaries of cases to demonstrate the variety of crisis situations he has treated and their subsequent outcomes. In all, this is a good introduction to network therapy.

Rueveni, U. (1979). *Networking families in crisis.* New York: Human Sciences Press.

This straightforward and readable book is a "cookbook" for the family therapist who wants to know more about networking. The author does a good job of presenting detailed case studies. He also gives ample space to a review of network research, the process of network intervention, and the therapist's role, as well as network techniques. This book provides a good, in-depth description of network therapy.

Rueveni, U. (Ed.). (1984). Application of networking in family and community [Special issue]. *International Journal of Family Therapy, 6*(2).

This special issue of the *International Journal of Family Therapy* is an excellent source of recent innovations in network therapy, as well as information on its application to specific client populations.

Rueveni, U., & Winer, M. (1976). Network intervention of disturbed families: The key role of the network activists. *Psychotherapy: Theory, Research and Practice, 13,* 173–176.

This brief article demonstrates, by way of case presentation, the importance of network activists—the volunteers who actively help create and implement the solutions generated by the assembled network. This article also emphasizes that nonfamily members of the network may play as important a role in network therapy as the family members themselves.

Sirkin, M. I., & Rueveni, U. (1992). The role of network therapy in the treatment of relational disorders: Cults and *folie à deux. Contemporary Family Therapy, 14,* 211–224.

In this article, the authors discuss cult involvement as a relational disorder. They propose network therapy as a means of helping individuals break from cults.

They include an overview of the stages of network therapy and a case example that exemplifies how network therapy was used as part of the treatment for one young man.

Speck, R. V. (1967). Psychotherapy of the social network of a schizophrenic family. *Family Process, 6,* 208–214.

In this often-cited article, Speck discusses the important role that nonmembers of the nuclear family play in the maintenance of a schizophrenic pattern and in its resistance to change. Also, Speck presents an initial report regarding the use of network therapy with a schizophrenic family and its network. This is an interesting article.

Speck, R. V., & Attneave, C. A. (1971). Social network intervention. In J. Haley (Ed.), *Changing families: A family therapy reader.* New York: Grune & Stratton.

This excellent chapter looks at many important issues in network therapy. Included are important pragmatic issues, such as (1) makeup of a network team, (2) goals of the network team, and (3) initiating the network process, as well as a theoretical discussion of the effects of social networks on individuals. Although the chapter is very informative, no citations of other works are given.

Speck, R. V., & Rueveni, U. (1969). Network therapy—A developing concept. *Family Process, 8,* 182–191.

This article presents network therapy as a developing mode of treatment. The reader is able to feel much of the authors' excitement and energy as they struggle with this emerging treatment modality. The focus of the article is on the techniques used as the authors treat schizophrenics' family networks. An important concept discussed is that of creating a new curative synthesis in the family network by creating polarities.

Gerald Zuk's Triadic Family Therapy

Introduction to the Therapy

Zuk defines two basic types of values and views all interactive processes in terms of these dichotomous male–female value sets. He calls the values most characteristic of males in our society "discontinuous" (e.g., adherence to structure, instrumentality, law and order, and rational process) and those more characteristic of females "continuous" (e.g., nurturance, empathy, aesthetics).

Zuk (1975, 1979) says that much of pathogenic family relating results from imbalances or conflicts between these sets of values. These conflicts can also occur in the interfaces between marriage partners, between parents and children, and between family members and the outer society.

One of Zuk's (1975, 1979) overriding impressions is that much pathogenic relating results from the overemphasis on continuous values and underemphasis on discontinuous values that result from what he sees as the overinvolvement of mothers with their children and the isolation and alienation of fathers from child rearing and family life in modern society. Children reaching adolescence have not sufficiently learned the values of discontinuity and therefore are ill prepared to assume adult roles and responsibility in society.

In his later writings, Zuk (1975, 1978, 1979) addresses the need for societywide changes involving sex roles and ethnic groups to enhance functioning at all systemic levels.

The "go-between" process, for which Zuk is primarily recognized, outlines the methods by which therapists get families to enact pathogenic patterns and then strategically intervene by acting as either go-between (negotiator), side-taker (shifter of the balance of relating), or celebrant (empowered representative for the family) to disrupt their dysfunctional relating (Zuk, 1966, 1967, 1968, 1971, 1975, 1981). Zuk (1966) sees all pathogenic family behavior as occurring in triads, with two parties drawing in a third in an attempt to resolve conflict or stress. Zuk (1967, 1968) asserts that there is no way for the therapist to stay outside this process, as the family system will automatically move to incorporate him or her. Therefore, the therapist must respond according to a rational scheme. The therapist will act as side-taker or go-between, representing continuous or discontinuous values, depending upon which side he or she takes (Zuk, 1979). Change in triadic family therapy is directed at the process by which the family relates. The focus of therapy is not on the content of family issues, although content will be used as a lever if deemed useful. Outcome is achieved when the pathogenic process is eliminated or reduced to the point where the symptom is relieved (Zuk, 1971, 1975, 1981).

Triadic family therapy, then, is therapy that utilizes the concepts of group process for assessment and intervention in disturbed families (Zuk, 1966). The focus is on coalitions, alliances, and cliques, and the process is one of mediation and side-taking. The go-between process occurs when the therapist initiates the enactment of conflict between two principals, intensifies that conflict and begins movement of a third party into the role of go-between, engages in a process of negotiation of roles and positions, and finally induces a change in positions and roles that the therapist determines is more functional. This results in reduction or elimination of symptoms (Zuk, 1966, 1967, 1968, 1971, 1975, 1981). Zuk's (1988) recent work has focused on defining family conflict cycles, the interactional nature of thought disorders (1989), and termination in the process of family therapy (1993).

Key Books, Chapters, and Articles

Garrigan, J. J., & Bambrick, A. F. (1977). Family therapy for disturbed children: Some experimental results in special education. *Journal of Marriage and Family Counseling, 3,* 83–93.

This article reports the results of a study employing Zuk's go-between process with families of emotionally disturbed children. Specific results included a reduction of the identified patients' symptoms in the classroom and home, and the enhancement of mutually experienced empathic understanding and congruence in the marital dyads.

Garrigan, J. J., & Bambrick, A. F. (1979). New findings in research on go-between process. *International Journal of Family Therapy, 1,* 76–85.

This article reports on a follow-up study of emotionally disturbed children treated in family therapy using Zuk's go-between process. Positive gains were found to have persisted over 2 years after therapy, with a concomitant reduction in symptoms and improvement in functioning. This study also found that single-parent, mother-only families were less responsive to treatment than intact families.

Zuk, G. H. (1965). On the pathology of silencing strategies. *Family Process, 4,* 32–49.

In this article Zuk examines a form of pathogenic relating in which various members of a family silence other family members by either verbal or nonverbal cues. These strategies, when used often, may induce psychoses in certain family members. Silencing strategies may also be employed by family members and patients to keep the therapist from discovering key family issues.

Zuk, G. H. (1966). The go-between process in family therapy. *Family Process, 5,* 162–178.

In this classic article, Zuk discusses the rationale for the use of the go-between process in family therapy. He gives a theoretical rationale and provides detailed examples. This article is clearly written and will help the reader understand Zuk's therapeutic techniques.

Zuk, G. H. (1967). The side-taking function in family therapy. *American Journal of Orthopsychiatry, 38,* 553–559.

Zuk focuses specifically on the use of side-taking as a therapeutic maneuver to disrupt pathogenic relating on the part of the family in treatment. He discusses the inevitability of the therapist's taking sides in family therapy, as well as the difference between side-taking that alters pathogenic relating and side-taking that reinforces it.

Zuk, G. H. (1968). When the family therapist takes sides: A case report. *Psychotherapy: Theory, Research and Practice, 5,* 24–28.

This transcribed family interview provides an excellent illustration of therapeutic side-taking. Zuk, engaging in the go-between process, breaks up the pathogenic relating in a triad by siding with one member against the others.

Zuk, G. H. (1971). Family therapy. In J. Haley (Ed.), *Changing families: A family therapy reader.* New York: Grune & Stratton.

This chapter represents a comprehensive overview of Zuk's methods and theory. Zuk gives many details of the methods and techniques for engaging in the go-between process with families and shows how this process fits his theoretical framework.

Zuk, G. H. (1975). *Process and practice in family therapy.* Haverford, PA: Psychiatry and Behavior Science Books.

This book presents Zuk's theory of family therapy and family process. Zuk makes ample use of transcripts of family interviews and speaking engagements. He also clearly presents his ideas on continuity and discontinuity values in families.

Zuk, G. H. (1976). Family therapy: Clinical hodgepodge or clinical science. *Journal of Marital and Family Counseling, 2,* 299–303.

Zuk sets forth a summary of his perspective on family therapy for the purpose of examination, evaluation, and research. It is a concise recounting of his basic principles, which he regards as a theory of family therapy. In so presenting them, he invites others to test his ideas through research.

Zuk, G. H. (1979). Value systems and psychopathology in family therapy. *International Journal of Family Therapy, 1,* 133–151.

Zuk elaborates on the two value types into which he sees most values in families falling: continuity and discontinuity. These two conflictual value types polarize in relationships comprising males versus females, older versus younger generations, and the nuclear family versus society. Zuk discusses the inevitability of encountering these value differences and the importance of being aware of them in therapy.

Zuk, G. H. (1981). *Family therapy: A triadic based approach* (rev. ed.). New York: Human Sciences Press.

This book includes several of Zuk's key articles. It provides an in-depth look at Zuk's conceptualization of family process, family pathology, and the use of the go-between process as a treatment technique. This book is extremely useful in that it captures the development of Zuk's theoretical ideas over time.

Zuk, G. H. (1988). The conflict cycle in families and therapy. *Contemporary Family Therapy, 10,* 145–153.

This article presents a 4-stage model of family conflict: (1) eruption of the dispute; (2) parties begin to accuse each other; (3) individuals react with shame, guilt, and denial; and (4) the parties move toward reparation, reconciliation, or retaliation.

Zuk, G. H. (1993). The reach of systems theory: A clinician's retrospective, 1984–1993. *Contemporary Family Therapy, 15,* 259–284.

This excellent article provides a detailed summary of Zuk's recent work. It focuses on the interactional nature of blaming in families, his 4-stage model of conflict, the connection between delusions and learning, and termination in family therapy.

THEORIES OF RECENT IMPORTANCE

Internal Family Systems Therapy

Introduction to the Therapy

In internal family systems therapy (IFST), Richard Schwartz (1987, 1995) applies family systems ideas to intrapsychic process. This is a systemic therapy that focus on intrapsychic dynamics and their interface with the family and larger systems.

The core tenet of IFST is that the mind is a multiplicity-oriented entity (Goulding & Schwartz, 1995). An individual's mind, Schwartz contends, is comprised of many subpersonalities or "parts." Each part is believed to be a personality in its own right. Different parts take on various tasks for an individual. When an individual is relatively problem-free, the mind appears to be more unified in nature, with different parts moving into prominence virtually unnoticed. It is when a person experiences specific traumas that their parts become polarized and more noticeable (Breunlin, Schwartz, & Mac Kune-Karrer, 1992; Schwartz, 1995).

Overseeing the interactions of the various parts is the self. The self assumes the leadership role when dealing with both internal and external problems. This is not an authoritarian leadership, but is more benevolent and nurturing. The self acts like an orchestra conductor, in that it brings out the strengths in the various parts and encourages them to take the lead at appropriate times (Schwartz, 1995). Furthermore, the self serves to mediate disagreements among the various parts. When the self is in the lead, balance and harmony pervade the internal family system (Breunlin et al., 1992; Schwartz, 1988).

In cases where there is severe trauma to an individual, such as physical or sexual abuse, the self appears weak to the other parts and eventually is subsumed by them (Goulding & Schwartz, 1995; Schwartz, 1992, 1995). This is more of a means to protect the self than an insurrection. Various parts now vie to take the lead. At this point, the internal family system is in a state of imbalance and polarization. The various parts fall into three classes: exiles, managers, and firefighters (Goulding & Schwartz, 1995; Schwartz, 1995).

Exiles are those parts of the internal family system that encompass the experience of the trauma (Goulding & Schwartz, 1995; Schwartz, 1992). They are like scared children wanting to share their pain and be nurtured. They are constantly trying to bring painful memories to the surface to be dealt with by the individual. The managers and firefighters fear that exposure to the exiles' pain will cause the self to be overwhelmed and lose all ability to lead. The managers take on the role of helping the individual cope with daily tasks at home and work. They also serve to keep the exiles at bay (Goulding & Schwartz, 1995; Schwartz, 1995). In cases when the exiles push through the managers' defenses, the firefighters are brought in to stop the impending crisis. Unfortunately, this is often done through symptomatic behavior such as bulimic, alcoholic, or compulsive activities (Schwartz, 1995).

Therapy comprises helping the individual to again place the self in a leadership position. The self then helps the exiles share their pain with the internal family system. By the self taking the leadership role, the managers and firefighters are able to take on more aspects of their personalities, and the system goes back into balance (Goulding & Schwartz, 1995; Schwartz, 1995).

Various internal parts can be constrained through family and community relationships. In those cases, the therapist may have to work with the parts of other family members and significant others (Schwartz, 1988, 1995). As IFS therapy is collaborative and works at the pace of the individual, it can be a long-term treatment. At present, IFST has generated a good deal of enthusiasm among some family therapists but little research supporting its efficacy.

Key Books, Chapters, and Articles

Breunlin, D. C., Schwartz, R. C., Mac Kune-Karrer, B. (1992). *Metaframeworks: Transcending the models of family therapy.* San Francisco: Jossey-Bass.

Metaframeworks is a model that attempts to transcend the schools of family therapy by combining them into six metaframeworks: self, interaction, organization, development, culture, and gender. The internal family systems model comprises the "self" metaframework. This book presents the internal family systems model and how it interfaces with the other metaframeworks in assessment and therapy.

Goulding, R. A., & Schwartz, R. C. (1995). *The mosaic mind: Empowering the tormented selves of child abuse survivors.* New York: Norton.

This excellent book provides a in-depth discussion of the internal family systems model in the treatment of abuse. The authors provide detailed presentations on the various parts and their interaction. Especially interesting is the use of verbatim transcripts from the therapy with one client to exemplify the points of the model.

Schwartz, R. C. (1987, March/April). Our multiple selves: Applying systems thinking to the inner family. *Family Therapy Networker, 11,* 25–31, 80–83.

This key article applies family systems concepts to intrapsychic process. Schwartz discusses how he came to think in terms of the mind as a multiplicity-oriented entity and presents the initial concepts of internal family systems.

Schwartz, R. C. (1988, November/December). Know thy selves. *Family Therapy Networker, 12,* 21–29.

This article provides an overview of internal family systems and how it can be used in couple therapy. It discusses the interface between intrapsychic process and couples interaction.

Schwartz, R. C. (1992, May/June). Rescuing the exiles. *Family Therapy Networker*, *16*, 33–37, 75.

In this article, Schwartz reveals how memories of abuse exist as exiled parts of the individual. He discusses how the self needs to be accessed to embrace these exiled parts to eventually lead to balance in the internal family system of abuse survivors.

Schwartz, R. C. (1995). *Internal family systems therapy*. New York: Guilford Press.

This is the foundational text on internal family systems therapy. It presents the core concepts of the model and how they apply to assessment and treatment. The book is especially noteworthy for the detailed discussion of problems and issues that practitioners will face using this approach. Readers will be interested in the discussion of how this model fits with other multiplicity-oriented models in mental health.

Psychoanalytic Family Therapies

Nathan Ackerman, Murray Bowen, Lyman Wynne, Theodore Lidz, Ivan Boszormengi-Nagy, Carl Whitaker, Don Jackson, and Salvador Minuchin had two things in common: They were pioneers in the field of family therapy, and they were all psychoanalytically trained. (And, yes, they are also all men.) Some of these pioneers held on to their psychoanalytic roots, but most in the 1960s and 1970s followed the lead of Minuchin and Jackson, seeing psychodynamic thinking as blinders that decontextualized the individual (Nichols & Schwartz, 1995). Although there are some remnants of Freud's drive psychology within family therapy, two psychoanalytic theories appear to be most integrated in the field: Adlerian family therapy and object relations family therapy.

Adlerian Family Therapy

A tradition that grew out of reaction against Freud's lack of emphasis on context is Adlerian family therapy. Although Adler was a psychoanalyst, there are many overlaps between Adlerian theory and systems theory. Adler (cf. 1931, 1964) has made important contributions to psychotherapy and the roots of family therapy. Adler, a student of Freud, challenged Freud's lack of emphasis on social elements and offered a theory of psychodynamics rooted in social relationships. Adler's work was a precursor to family therapist beliefs that pathology is influenced by family conflict (Broderick & Schrader, 1991). Although Adlerian therapy is a cognitive theory, Adler believed that cognitions are based on thinking, feeling, and behavior. One of Adler's students, Rudolph Dreikurs, helped develop Adlerian theory throughout the United States (cf. Dreikurs, 1947, 1953). Adlerian thought has developed in the marriage enrichment and marital counseling arena (cf. Carlson & Dinkmeyer, 1987; Dinkmeyer & Carlson, 1984; Dinkmeyer & Dinkmeyer, 1982; Freeman, Carlson, & Sperry, 1993; Slavik, Carlson, & Sperry, 1992; Sperry & Carlson, 1991), and in the parent education area (Dinkmeyer & McKay, 1976, 1983).

Sherman and Dinkmeyer (1987) have adapted Adlerian principles to family therapy. Some principles directly overlap with systems theory, such as the belief that movement in one part of the system creates movement in another. Adlerians also have a holistic view of people. They believe that the conscious and unconscious mind, physical body, mental capacities, and emotions are all part of one system moving toward a "goal." All behavior is purposeful. Adlerians, like systemic family therapists, are not interested in blame.

Sherman and Dinkmeyer (1987) have adopted Adler's notion that goals are related to feeling significant and belonging. Behavior is also designed to overcome feelings of inferiority left over from childhood; these feelings are often based on faulty perceptions. Thus, the family therapist must know the perceptions of each family member to help change occur. Likewise, one's position (birth order) in the family is not as important as the *meaning* the position has to the person. Adlerians also believe that social interest is a measure of mental health.

Object Relations Family Therapy

Fairbairn (1952) contends that a fundamental motive of human life is the development of satisfying (human) object relationships. According to Fairbairn, a child must deal with a mother, who is largely experienced as good, who meets the child's needs. Yet, at times, the child is frustrated when the mother does not meet his or her needs or desires. (Later theorists, incidentally, substitute "nurturing figure" for "mother.") Because the child cannot leave the relationship due to his or her dependency, nor can the child control the mother, the child must construct an inner psychological world that makes these contradicting aspects of mother less threatening. Fairbairn refers to this process as "splitting" of the mother into good and bad objects. This splitting allows the child to maintain his or her dependency on mother, without feeling constantly threatened (Cashdan, 1988). The good object (the rewarding aspects of mother) is an internal representation that allows the child to feel loved. The bad object (the frustrating or hostile aspects of mother) is an internal representation that causes the child to feel unloved.

These good and bad objects make up psychological "introjects" that may be integrated into the personality or projected onto another person.

These introjects and projections unconsciously influence one's relationships (Framo, 1970).

Henry Dicks (1963, 1967) was one of the first to apply Fairbairn's (1952) object relations concepts to marriage. Dicks (1963) stated that distressed marriages are characterized by "mutual attribution and projection . . . with each spouse perceived to a degree as an internal object" (p. 126). Dicks's conceptualizations are useful in understanding why many neurotic "cat-and-dog" marriages stay together but seem impervious to change. Each spouse's ego identity (which includes both good and bad objects) is, in effect, preserved by having one or more bad objects split off onto his or her partner. In other words, each spouse disowns his or her own bad-object introjects and thus needs the other to accept the projection of these introjects. Each begins to subtly conform to the inner role model of the other in a collusive manner. Dicks (1963) believed that this collusive process continues because both spouses hope for integration of lost introjects by finding them in the other. Resulting unconscious marital bargains (cf. Sager, 1976) may take many forms (e.g., "You be my courage, and I will be your support," "You be tender, and I will be strong"). The distressed marriage, then, represents a total personality that, according to Dicks, is problematic. Therapists employing object relations theory attempt in various ways to help couples own their introjects and begin seeing their spouses for the people they really are and not projected parts of themselves.

Examples of approaches that integrate object relations with family therapy include Scharff's model of object relations family therapy (J. Scharff, 1991; D. Scharff, 1991a; Scharff & Scharff, 1987), object relations couple therapy (D. Scharff, 1991b; Scharff & Scharff, 1991) and its extensions (cf. D. Scharff, 1982; Scharff & Scharff, 1994) as well as Samuel Slipp's work (1980, 1984, 1988, 1991). In addition, although he integrates many eclectic techniques, Framo (1981) draws from Fairbairn's object relations theory and Dicks' marital interaction theory in his marital therapy with spouses' families of origin.

Key Books, Chapters, and Articles

Ackerman, N. (1958). *The psychodynamics of family life: Diagnosis and treatment of family relationships.* New York: Basic Books.

This key work by a family therapy pioneer remains an important contribution for understanding the psychodynamics of family life. Ackerman presents a schema for integrating the individual self and the social self. This is a truly influential, pioneering work.

Bentovim, A., & Kinston, W. (1991). Focal family therapy: Joining systems theory with psychodynamic understanding. In A. S. Gurman & D. P. Kniskern (Eds.), *Handbook of family therapy* (Vol. 2). New York: Brunner/Mazel.

These authors bring the best of both worlds of systems and psychodynamic understanding into a model they call "focal family therapy." This model also emphasizes the role of trauma on intrapsychic, interpersonal, and transactional aspects of individuals and families. This is a must-read integration chapter for those interested in systems and psychodynamic integration.

Dicks, H. V. (1963). Object relations theory and marital status. *British Journal of Medical Psychology, 36,* 125–129.

In this classic article, Dicks extends the object relations theory of Klein, Fairbairn, and Guntrip to the study of marital relationships. Dicks describes marriage as a mutual process of attribution or projection, with each spouse perceived to a degree as an internal object. This article is well written and provides an excellent general background for viewing marriages in terms of object relations theory, so often mentioned by Framo, Williamson, Bowen, and others.

Dicks, H. V. (1967). *Marital tensions.* New York: Basic Books.

In this important volume, Dicks applies Fairbairn's object relations concepts to the understanding and treatment of marital dysfunction.

Fairbairn, W. R. D. (1952). *An object-relations theory of the personality.* New York: Basic Books.

This key work in object relations theory had a significant influence on the later work of Dicks, Bowen, Framo, Williamson, and others. Although it is steeped in ponderous psychoanalytic terminology, its influence on the field makes it required reading for those interested in the role of object relations in psychopathology.

Friedman, L. J., & Pearce, J. K. (Eds.). (1980). *Family therapy: Combining psychodynamic and family systems approaches.* New York: Grune & Stratton.

This book is a fine attempt to show that psychodynamic approaches can be integrated with family systems theory. Of particular note are the chapters by L. J. Friedman on integrating object relations theory with family therapy, and S. Slipp on symbiotic survival pattern, which integrates psychoanalytic theory with family systems theory. The authors provide case examples and techniques, as well as a chapter on integrating ethnicity within family therapy.

Gurman, A. S. (1981). Integrative marital therapy: Toward the development of an interpersonal approach. In S. H. Budman (Ed.), *Forms of brief therapy.* New York: Guilford Press.

Gurman argues for an integrative form of marital therapy, including blending familiar family therapy approaches with psychodynamic understanding. Gurman argues that only psychodynamic views can incorporate the complex nature of intimate relationships.

Jacobs, E. H. (1991). Self psychology and family therapy. *American Journal of Psychotherapy, 45*(4), 483–498.

This is an interesting therapeutic application mixing systems theory with

Kohut's self psychology. The author discusses narcissistic family systems and provides treatment examples blending self psychology with family therapy.

Kirschner, D. A., & Kirschner, S. (1986). *Comprehensive family therapy: An integration of systemic and psychodynamic treatment models.* New York: Brunner/Mazel.

This book details theory and treatment of "comprehensive family therapy," first developed by Arthur Stein. This text integrates systems theory. The author provides excellent case examples.

Lidz, T. (1992). *The relevance of the family to psychoanalytic theory.* Madison, CT: International Universities Press.

Lidz unravels some psychoanalytic theory and then reknits it in a way that includes the role of the family and attachment. This is a well-written book, emphasizing the best of Freud and Lidz.

Nichols, M. P. (1987). *The self in the system: Expanding the limits of family therapy.* New York: Brunner/Mazel.

Nichols acknowledges that, in an attempt to depart from its psychoanalytic roots, the field of family therapy inadvertently blinded itself to the individual. Nichols discusses how trends such as quick-fix "techniquism" and overly abstract thinking in systems theory have obliterated the individual. He proposes "interactional psychodynamics" as a treatment model, whereby the interaction of the personal and family dynamics is circular. With this book, Nichols has helped family therapy reintegrate individual dynamics. This is one of the most important works of the 1980s.

Sander, F. M. (1979). *Individual and family therapy: Toward an integration.* Northvale, NJ: Jason Aronson.

Sander was trained as a psychoanalyst, *and* by Nathan Ackerman. Thus, this book contains unique blends of theory and practice.

Scharff, J. S. (Ed.). (1991). *Foundations of object relations family therapy.* Northvale, NJ: Jason Aronson.

This edited volume is a great resource for understanding object relations theory and its usefulness to family therapy. The authors emphasize different aspects of object relations. Yet a coherent whole emerges, which allows the reader to understand the application of each chapter to the family. There is a good history of object relations family therapy. In addition, the authors provide concrete suggestions for working with more difficult clients, including borderlines, narcissists, and incest cases.

Scharff, J. S., & Scharff, D. E. (1991). *Object relations couple therapy.* Northvale, NJ: Jason Aronson.

The Scharff draw on Fairbairn and Klein's object relations theories, as well as Freudian theory, in this special brand of object relations couple therapy. They discuss couple and sex therapy, and manage to clarify the fuzzy concept of projective identification.

Sherman, J. R., & Dinkmeyer, D. (1987). *Systems of family therapy: An Adlerian integration*. New York: Brunner/Mazel.

In this book, the authors skillfully compare and contrast Adlerian individual psychology with family systems theories and models. The authors assert that Adlerian theory can be used as a theoretical base for synthesizing contemporary family therapy models. They explain Adlerian principles and apply them to various family problems. Four guest authors illustrate the use of Adlerian concepts by integrating them with family therapy models such as Satir's the MRI interactional view, strategic family therapy, and structural family therapy. Another strength is the authors' attention to historical contexts of both individual psychology and family therapy.

Slipp, S. (1984). *Object relations: A dynamic bridge between individual and family treatment*. Northvale, NJ: Jason Aronson.

Slipp was one of the first in the United States to integrate systems theory with object relations theory. This is the foundational work of this integration. Slipp also integrates intergenerational theory in looking at the transmission through generations of psychic trauma. This is a unique and interesting text.

Slipp, S. (1988). *The technique and practice of object relations family therapy*. Northvale, NJ: Jason Aronson.

This book reflects further clinical application of Slipp's integration of psychoanalysis and family therapy. Slipp reviews object relations theory and systems theory. He also discusses an object relations family therapy in which he describes dysfunctional family patterns from an object relations typology. His detailed case studies make it easier for the reader to see how he or she might apply object relations family therapy.

Stewart, R. H., Peters, T. C., Marsh, S., & Peters, M. J. (1975). An object relations approach to psychotherapy with marital couples, families, and children. *Family Process, 14*(2), 161–178.

In this article, the authors use object relations concepts to understand marital and family problems, as well as various dynamics between therapist and client. They present countertransference, for example, as a legitimate way to help the therapist understand the projected splits of his or her client. This is a good introduction to the role of object relations concepts in family therapy.

Will, D., & Wrate, R. M. (1985). *Integrated family therapy: A problem-centered psychodynamic approach*. New York: Tavistock.

This book presents an integrated approach to family therapy based on the McMaster model of family therapy, psychoanalytic family therapy, and structural family therapy. The resulting problem-centered psychodynamic family therapy (PCPFT) is a directive model, which has experiential and cognitive (i.e., insight) dimensions. The authors believe that rather than just labeling family dysfunction, psychoanalysis can be used to help explain the etiology of the dysfunction and provide families with insight to promote change. The approach is very clear and compelling.

Psychoeducational Family Therapy

Introduction to the Therapy

The psychoeducational programs presented here are based on a specific medical model called the "stress diathesis model." Within this model, psychoeducational family therapists strive to give families education/information about the medical management of the patient's physical or mental illness (Levant, 1990). Proponents of this model include Anderson, Hogarty, and Reiss (1986), Falloon, Boyd, McGill, Razoni, Moss, and Gilderman (1982), and Goldstein (1981). This model was developed in part in reaction to family therapists who saw the family as the "cause" of the illness, especially in the case of schizophrenia. This trend was typified by the double bind theory of schizophrenia (Bateson, Jackson, Haley, & Weakland, 1956), as well as others who labeled family pathologies (Lidz, Fleck, & Cornelison, 1965; Selvini Palazzoli, Boscolo, Cecchin, & Prata, 1978; Wynne, Ryckoff, Day, & Hirsch, 1958) as etiological factors in schizophrenia. Anderson et al. (1986) have questioned these findings and have spearheaded the use of psychoeducation for schizophrenics and their families.

Family psychoeducation was developed to deal with the fact that antipsychotic drugs used alone are less effective than when the family is also involved in treatment. Psychoeducation also recognizes the fact that families must care for a family member plagued by chronic brain impairment (McFarlane, 1991). The goal of the Anderson et al. (1986) approach is to prevent symptom relapse. While acknowledging being in the "stress diathesis" treatment camp of schizophrenia, Anderson et al. (1986) also acknowledge that environmental factors play a part in schizophrenic relapse rates. The psychoeducational model was developed to give families education, support, information, and coping mechanisms to deal with the schizophrenic member (Anderson, 1983). They use multiple family groups to facilitate community reentry, social and vocational rehabilitation, and a stronger social network (McFarlane, 1991, 1992, 1994).

Pychoeducational models also acknowledge the need, in most cases, for medication for the patient. The models also integrate the importance of affect in treatment, usually in terms of "expressed emotion" (EE), originally studied by Brown, Monck, Carstairs, and Wing (1962). EE has three components: critical comments (CC), hostility (H), emotional overinvolvement (EOI; Vaughn, 1989; Leff & Vaughn, 1985). Relatives of patients who are high on EE express hostility, a rejecting attitude, or high emotional overinvolvement. Many studies have linked relapse rates in schizophrenia to high EE in families (cf. Koenigberg & Handley, 1986; Leff & Vaughn, 1981; Moline, Singh, Morris, & Meltzer, 1985; Nuechterlein, Snyder, & Mintz, 1992; Vaughn, Snyder, Jones, Freeman, & Falloon, 1984). (High EE has also been linked to higher relapse rates for depression and bipolar disorder; see Mueser & Glynn, 1995). Some have objected to the categorizations and implicit blame within the construct of EE (Hatfield, 1990; Lefley, 1992). To review the impact of expressed emotion, see Leff and Vaughn (1985); Hatfield, Spaniol, and Zipple (1987); Kanter, Lamb, and Loeper (1987), and Lefley (1992).

A parallel construct, similar to EE, that some have integrated into psychoeducational treatment models is "parental affective style" (AS; Doane, Falloon, Goldstein, & Mintz, 1985; Doane, West, Goldstein, Rodnick, & Jones, 1981). High AS indicates the parent has been critical, guilt inducing, or intrusive with their child, and is also linked to higher relapse rates for schizophrenia.

Key Books, Chapters, and Articles

Anderson, C., Hogarty, G., & Reiss, D. J. (1986). *Schizophrenia and the family: A practitioner's guide to psychoeducation and management.* New York: Guilford Press.

This pivotal book describes the rationale for accepting the "stress diathesis" model of managing schizophrenia, while simultaneously steering clear of independent psychological, biological, or environmental determinism. The authors present their psychoeducational model for managing schizophrenia. It includes a detailed survival-skills workshop for families, managing reentry of the schizophrenic member into society, and rehabilitation on social and vocational levels. The treatment model is detailed, with ample case examples.

Atkinson, J. M., & Coia, D. A. (1995). *Families coping with schizophrenia: A practitioner's guide to family groups.* New York: Wiley.

In this book, the authors detail expressed emotion research in schizophrenia, and note models and historical trends. The authors also present psychoeducational programs for relatives and catalogue the emotional issues for caregivers. They also discuss self-help groups, and detail, session by session, educational groups for relatives. This book couples practical advice with compelling research. It includes a wonderful chapter in which the authors discuss ethical issues and political quagmires in work with schizophrenics and their families.

Clarkin, J. F. (1989). Family education. In A. S. Bellack (Ed.), *A clinical guide for the treatment of schizophrenia.* New York: Plenum Press.

In this chapter, Clarkin discusses family education for schizophrenia. In it, they review empirical studies of psychoeducation and give the clinician guidelines for treatment/psychoeducation.

Doane, J. A., Falloon, I. R. H., Goldstein, M. J., & Mintz, J. (1985). Parental affective style and the treatment of schizophrenia. *Archives of General Psychiatry, 42,* 34–42.

This randomized, controlled study linked parental affective style with relapse rates in schizophrenia. Family-based intervention reduced negative AS and relapse rates for schizophrenics compared to individual intervention.

Goldstein, M. J., & Miklowitz, D. J. (1995). The effectiveness of psychoeducational family therapy in the treatment of schizophrenic disorders. *Journal of Marital and Family Therapy, 21,* 361–376.

This important article provides a comprehensive review of the research on the effectiveness of psychoeducational family therapy in the treatment of schizophrenia. It provides an excellent starting point for studying this area.

Hatfield, A. B. (Ed.). (1994). *Family interventions in mental illness.* San Francisco: Jossey-Bass.

In this edited book, Hatfield presents family education and psychoeducation as a means to help treat severe mental illness. The author reviews research, theory, and practice on various topics such as schizophrenia, bipolar disorder, and cultural application of family psychoeducation. Hatfield also discussed behavioral family management and multiple family groups. This is an excellent psychoeducational resource book.

Hogarty, G. E. (1993). Prevention of relapse in chronic schizophrenic patients. *Journal of Clinical Psychiatry, 54*(Suppl. 3), 18–23.

Hogarty's research supports the need for both antipsychotic medication and psychosocial therapy for patients suffering from schizophrenia. Hogarty advocates creating a stimuli-controlled environment, therapeutic sensitivity to expressed emotion, minimal drug dosing, psychoeducation, resource management, and a treatment plan for schizophrenia management.

Hogarty, G. E., Anderson, C. M., Reiss, D. J., Kornbluth, S. J., Greenwald, D. P., Javna, C. D., & Madonia, M. J. (1986). Family psychoeducation, social skills training, and maintenance chemotherapy in the aftercare of schizophrenia. *Archives of General Psychiatry, 43,* 633–642.

In this important research, the authors used psychoeducation to reduce high expressed emotion in order to prevent relapse in schizophrenia.

Keefer, J., & Koritar, E. (1994). Essential elements of a family psychoeducation program in the aftercare of schizophrenia. *Journal of Marital and Family Therapy, 20,* 369–380.

This article gives the basics of a family psychoeducational program used in Montreal, based on 10 years work with schizophrenics and their caregivers. Elements of the program include universal service, crisis intervention, social functioning of the patient and family, 2-year continuity of care postdischarge, and the role of the family clinician.

Leff, J., & Vaughn, C. (1985). *Expressed emotion in families: Its significance for mental illness.* New York: Guilford Press.

This landmark book reflects a shift from focusing on the etiology of schizophrenia to focusing on factors that influence the progression of schizophrenia. Family theorists initially asked, "What factors are responsible for the first appearance of schizophrenia" (p. 3). Leff and Vaughn represent, in their book, a paradigm shift to the clinical focus of the research question: "Given that this individual suffers from schizophrenia, what factors make his or her illness worse or improve it?" (p. 3). Expressed emotion is part of the answer to this question, and is the focus of this book.

Lefley, H. P., & Wasow, M. (Eds.). (1994). *Helping families cope with mental illness.* Langhorne, PA: Harwood Academic Publishers/Gordon & Breach Science Publishers.

This edited book includes many important issues in the treatment of families experiencing chronic mental illness. Authors present research on expressed emotion as well as single and multiple family psychoeducational research. Contributors also discuss ethical and cultural issues in treatment.

McFarlane, W. R. (Ed.). (1983). *Family therapy in schizophrenia.* New York: Guilford Press.

This edited work represents some of the early movement in the field toward psychoeducation in schizophrenia. Early research on expressed emotion is included.

McFarlane, W. R. (1991). Family psychoeducational treatment. In A. S. Gurman & D. P. Kniskern (Eds.), *Handbook of family therapy* (Vol. 2). New York: Brunner/Mazel.

This is a meaty chapter on the psychoeducational approach for families of patients suffering from schizophrenia. McFarlane's model is based on the medical model; that is, he gives education to client families about schizophrenia to help them cope with the disease. McFarlane also discusses expressed emotion and his detailed treatment outline.

Mueser, K. T., & Glynn, S. M. (1995). *Behavioral family therapy for psychiatric disorders.* Boston: Allyn & Bacon.

In this text, the authors thoroughly describe how to apply behavioral family therapy to psychiatric disorders, including schizophrenia, affective disorders, and anxiety disorders. Of particular note is the chapter on family education. Also, the appendix provides useful educational handouts on the psychiatric disorders.

Papolos, D. F. (1994). The family psychoeducational approach: Rationale for a multigenerational treatment modality for the major affective disorders. In D. F. Papolos & H. M. Lachman (Eds.), *Genetic studies in affective disorders: Overview of basic methods, current directions, and critical research issues.* New York: Wiley.

Papolos advocates educational programs for high-risk families. Highlights include genetic findings and implications for treatment.

Shields, C. G., Franks, P., Harp, J. J., McDaniel, S. H., & Campbell, T. L. (1992). Development of the Family Emotional Involvement and Criticism Scale (FEICS). A self-report measure of expressed emotion. *Journal of Marital and Family Therapy, 18,* 395–407.

These researchers have developed a self-report measure of expressed emotion in extended families of adults. Its two subscales include Intensity of Emotion (EI), and Perceived Criticism (PC). Preliminary reliability estimates range from .74 to .82. High levels of EE negatively impact individuals and families.

REFERENCES

Adler, A. (1931). *What life should mean to you.* Boston: Little, Brown.

Adler, A. (1964). *The problems of neurosis.* New York: Harper & Row.

Alger, I. (1976). Multiple couple therapy. In P. J. Guerin (Ed.), *Family therapy: Theory and practice.* New York: Gardner.

Anderson, C. (1983). A psychoeducational program for families of patients with schizophrenia. In W. R. McFarlane (Ed.), *Family therapy in schizophrenia.* New York: Guilford Press.

Anderson, C., Hogarty, G., & Reiss, D. J. (1986). *Schizophrenia and the family: A practitioner's guide to psychoeducation and management.* New York: Guilford Press.

Bateson, G., Jackson, D. D., Haley, J., & Weakland, J. (1956). Toward a theory of schizophrenia. *Behavioral Science, 1,* 51–264.

Boas, C. V. E. (1962). Intensive group psychotherapy with married couples. *International Journal of Group Psychotherapy, 12,* 142–153.

Breunlin, D. C., Schwartz, R. C., Mac Kune-Karrer, B. (1992). *Metaframeworks: Transcending the models of family therapy.* San Francisco: Jossey-Bass.

Broderick, C. B., & Schrader, S. S. (1991). The history of professional marriage and family therapy. In A. S. Gurman & D. P. Kniskern (Eds.), *Handbook of family therapy* (Vol. 2). New York: Brunner/Mazel.

Brown, G. W., Monck, E. M., Carstairs, G. M., & Wing, J. K. (1962). Influence of family life on the course of schizophrenic illness. *British Journal of Psychiatry, 16,* 55–68.

Carlson, J., & Dinkmeyer, D. C. (1987). Adlerian marriage therapy. *American Journal of Family Therapy, 15,* 326–332.

Cashdan, S. (1988). *Object relations therapy: Using the relationship.* New York: Norton.

Coche, J. (1995). Group therapy with couples. In N. S. Jacobson & A. S. Gurman (Eds.), *Clinical handbook of couple therapy.* New York: Guilford Press.

Coche, J., & Coche, E. (1990). *Couples group psychotherapy: A clinical practice model.* New York: Brunner/Mazel.

Dicks, H. (1963). Objects relations theory and marital studies. *British Journal of Medical Psychology, 36,* 125–129.

Dicks, H. (1967). *Marital tensions.* New York: Basic Books.

Dinkmeyer, D., & Carlson, J. (1984). *Training in marriage enrichment.* Circle Pines, MN: American Guidance Service.

Dinkmeyer, D., & Dinkmeyer, J. (1982). Adlerian marriage therapy. *Individual Psychology, 38*(2), 115–122.

Dinkmeyer, D., & McKay, G. (1976). *Systematic training for effective parenting.* Circle Pines, MN: American Guidance Service.

Dinkmeyer, D., & McKay, G. (1983). *Systematic training for effective parenting of teens.* Circle Pines, MN: American Guidance Service.

Doane, J. A., Falloon, I. R. H., Goldstein, M. J., & Mintz, J. (1985). Parental affective style and the treatment of schizophrenia: Predicting the course of illness and social functioning. *Archives of General Psychiatry, 42,* 34–42.

Doane, J. A., West, K. L., Goldstein, M. J., Rodnick, E. H., & Jones, J. E. (1981). Parental communication deviance and affective style: Predictors of subsequent schizophrenia spectrum disorders in vulnerable adolescents. *Archives of General Psychiatry, 38,* 679–685.

Dreikurs, R. (1947). The four goals of children's misbehavior. *Nervous Child, 6,* 3–11.

Dreikurs, R. (1953). *Fundamentals of Adlerian psychology.* Chicago: Alfred Adler Institute.

Fairbairn, W. R. D. (1952). *An object-relations theory of the personality.* New York: Basic Books.

Falloon, I. R. H., Boyd, J. L., McGill, C. U., Razoni, J., Moss, H. B., & Gilderman, A. M. (1982). Family management in the prevention of exacerbation of schizophrenia: A controlled study. *New England Journal of Medicine, 306,* 1437–1440.

Framo, J. L. (1970). Symptoms from a family transactional viewpoint. In C. J. Sager & H. S. Kaplan (Eds.), *Progress in family therapy.* New York: Brunner/Mazel.

Framo, J. L. (1973). Marriage therapy in a couples group. In D. A. Bloch (Ed.), *Techniques of family psychotherapy: A primer.* New York: Grune & Stratton.

Framo, J. L. (1981). The integration of marital therapy with sessions with family of origin. In A. S. Gurman & D. P. Kniskern (Eds.), *Handbook of family therapy* (Vol. 1). New York: Brunner/Mazel.

Freeman, C., Carlson, J., & Sperry, L. (1993). Adlerian marital therapy strategies with middle income couples facing financial stress. *American Journal of Family Therapy, 21,* 324–32.

Freeman, E. M. (1993). *Family treatment.* Springfield, IL: Thomas.

Galanter, M. (1993a). Network therapy for addiction: A model for office practice. *American Journal of Psychiatry, 150,* 28–36.

Galanter, M. (1993b). Network therapy for substance abuse: A clinical trial. *Psychotherapy, 30,* 251–258.

Goldstein, M. J. (Ed.). (1981). *New developments in interventions with families of schizophrenics.* San Francisco: Jossey-Bass.

Gottlieb, A., & Pattison, E. M. (1966). Married couples group psychotherapy. *Archives of General Psychiatry, 14,* 143–152.

Goulding, R. A., & Schwartz, R. C. (1995). *The mosaic mind: Empowering the tormented selves of child abuse survivors.* New York: Norton.

Gritzer, P. H., & Okun, H. S. (1983). Multiple family group therapy: A model for all families. In B. B. Wolman & G. Stricker (Eds.), *Handbook of family and marital therapy.* New York: Plenum Press.

Gurman, A. S. (1971). Group marital therapy: Clinical and empirical implications for outcome research. *International Journal of Group Psychotherapy, 21,* 174–189.

Hatfield, A. B. (1990). *Family education in mental illness.* New York: Guilford Press.

Hatfield, A. B., Spaniol, L., & Zipple, A. (1987). Expressed emotion: A family perspective. *Schizophrenia Bulletin, 13,* 221–226.

Kanter, J., Lamb, H. R., & Loeper, C. (1987). Expressed emotion in families: A critical review. *Hospital and Community Psychiatry, 38,* 374–380.

Koenigberg, H., & Handley, R. (1986). Expressed emotion: From predictive index to clinical construct. *American Journal of Psychiatry, 143,* 1361–1373.

Laqueur, H. P. (1966). General systems theory and multiple family therapy. In J. H. Masserman (Ed.), *Handbook of psychiatric therapies.* New York: Grune & Stratton.

Laqueur, H. P. (1972a). Mechanisms of change in multiple family therapy. In C. J. Sager & H. S. Kaplan (Eds.), *Progress in group and family therapy.* New York: Brunner/Mazel.

Laqueur, H. P. (1972b). Multiple family therapy. In A. Ferber, M. Mendelsohn, & A. Napier (Eds.), *The book of family therapy.* Boston: Houghton Mifflin.

Laqueur, H. P. (1976). Multiple family therapy. In P. J. Guerin (Ed.), *Family therapy: Theory and practice.* New York: Gardner.

Leff, J., & Vaughn, C. (1981). The role of maintenance therapy and relatives expressed emotion in relapse of schizophrenia: A two-year follow-up. *British Journal of Psychiatry, 139,* 102–104.

Leff, J., & Vaughn, C. (1985). *Expressed emotion in families: Its significance for mental illness.* New York: Guilford Press.

Lefley, H. P. (1992). Expressed emotion: Conceptual, clinical, and social policy issues. *Hospital and Community Psychiatry, 43,* 591–598.

Leichter, E. (1973). Treatment of married couples groups. *Family Coordinator, 22,* 31–42.

Levant, R. F. (1990). From client-centered family therapy to psychoeducational family programs. In F. W. Kaslow (Ed.), *Voices in family psychology* (Vol. 2). Newbury Park, CA: Sage.

Liberman, R. P., Wheeler, E., & Sanders, W. (1976). Behavioral therapy for marital disharmony: An educational approach. *Journal of Marriage and Family Counseling, 2,* 383–395.

Lidz, T., Fleck, S., & Cornelison, A. R. (1965). *Schizophrenia and the family.* New York: International Universities Press.

Lieberman, E. J., & Lieberman, S. B. (1986). Couples group therapy. In N. S. Jacobson & A. S. Gurman (Eds.), *Clinical handbook of marital therapy.* New York: Guilford Press.

Linden, M. E., Goodwin, H. M., & Resnik, H. (1968). Group psychotherapy of couples in marriage counseling. *International Journal of Group Psychotherapy, 18,* 313–324.

MacGregor, R. (1972). Multiple impact psychotherapy with families. In G. D. Erickson & T. P. Hogan (Eds.), *Family therapy: An introduction to theory and technique.* Monterey, CA: Brooks/Cole.

MacGregor, R., Richie, A. M., Serrano, A. C., Schuster, F. P., McDonald, E. C., &

Goolishian, H. A. (1964). *Multiple impact therapy with families.* New York: McGraw-Hill.

Marett, K. M. (1988). A substantive and methodological review of couples group therapy outcome research. *Group, 12,* 241–246.

McFarlane, W. R. (1982). Multiple-family therapy in the psychiatric hospital. In H. T. Harbin (Ed.), *The psychiatric hospital and the family.* New York: Spectrum.

McFarlane, W. R. (1991). Family psychoeducational treatment. In A. S. Gurman & D. P. Kniskern (Eds.), *Handbook of family therapy* (Vol. 2). New York: Brunner/Mazel.

McFarlane, W. R. (1992). Psychoeducation: A potential model for intervention in family practice. In R. J. Sawa (Ed.), *Family health care.* Newbury Park, CA: Sage.

McFarlane, W. R. (1994). Multiple-family groups and psychoeducation in the treatment of schizophrenia. In A. B. Hatfield (Ed.), *Family interventions in mental illness.* San Francisco: Jossey-Bass.

Moline, R. A., Singh, S., Morris, A., & Meltzer, H. Y. (1985). Family expressed emotion and relapse in schizophrenia in 24 urban American patients. *American Journal of Psychiatry, 142,* 1078–1081.

Mueser, K. T., & Glynn, S. M. (1995). *Behavioral family therapy for psychiatric disorders.* Boston: Allyn & Bacon.

Neimeyer, G. J. (1987). Marital role reconstruction through couples group therapy. In R. A. Neimeyer & G. J. Neimeyer (Eds.), *Personal construct therapy casebook.* New York: Springer.

Nichols, M. P., & Schwartz, R. C. (1995). *Family therapy: Concepts and methods* (3rd ed.). Needham Heights, MA: Simon & Schuster.

Nuechterlein, K. H., Snyder, K. S., & Mintz, J. (1992). Paths to relapse: Possible transactional processes connecting patient illness onset, expressed emotion and psychotic relapse. *British Journal of Psychiatry, 161,* 88–96.

Reed, C. Y. (1989). Marriage by arrangement: A metaphor for one particular use of network therapy. *Journal of Adolescence, 12,* 279–294.

Richie, A. (1971). Multiple impact therapy: An experiment. In J. Haley, (Ed.), *Changing families: A family therapy reader.* New York: Grune & Stratton.

Rueveni, U. (1979). *Networking families in crisis.* New York: Human Sciences Press.

Sager, C. J. (1976). *Marriage contracts and couple therapy.* New York: Brunner/Mazel.

Scharff, D. E. (1982). *The sexual relationship: An object relations view of sex and the family.* London: Routledge & Kegan Paul.

Scharff, D. E. (1991a). *Object relations family therapy.* Northvale, NJ: Jason Aronson.

Scharff, D. E. (1991b). *Object relations couple therapy.* Northvale, NJ: Jason Aronson.

Scharff, J. S. (Ed.). (1991). *Foundations of object relations family therapy.* Northvale, NJ: Jason Aronson.

Scharff, J. S., & Scharff, D. E. (1987). *Object relations family therapy.* Northvale, NJ: Jason Aronson.

Scharff, J. S., & Scharff, D. E. (1991). *Object relations couple therapy.* Northvale, NJ: Jason Aronson.

Scharff, J. S., & Scharff, D. E. (1994). *Object relations therapy of physical and sexual trauma*. Northvale, NJ: Jason Aronson.

Schwartz, R. C. (1987). Our multiple selves: Applying systems thinking to the inner family. *Family Therapy Networker, 10*, 25–31, 80–83.

Schwartz, R. C. (1988). Know thy selves. *Family Therapy Networker, 11*, 21–29.

Schwartz, R. C. (1992). Rescuing the exiles. *Family Therapy Networker, 16*, 33–37, 75.

Schwartz, R. C. (1995). *Internal family systems therapy*. New York: Guilford Press.

Selvini Palazzoli, M., Boscolo, L., Cecchin, G., & Prata, G. (1978). *Paradox and counterparadox*. New York: Jason Aronson.

Sherman, J. R., & Dinkmeyer, D. (1987). *Systems of family therapy: An Adlerian integration*. New York, NY: Brunner/Mazel.

Sirkin, M. I., & Rueveni, U. (1992). The role of network therapy in the treatment of relational disorders: Cults and folie à deux. *Contemporary Family Therapy, 14*, 211–224.

Slavik, S., Carlson, J., & Sperry, L. (1992). Adlerian marital therapy with the passive–aggressive partner. *American Journal of Family Therapy, 20*, 25–35.

Slipp, S. (1980). Interactions between the interpersonal in families and individual intrapsychic dynamics. In J. K. Pearce & L. J. Friedman (Eds.), *Family therapy: Combining psychodynamic and family systems approaches*. New York: Grune & Stratton.

Slipp, S. (1984). *Object relations: A dynamic bridge between individual and family treatment*. Northvale, NJ: Jason Aronson.

Slipp, S. (1988). *The technique and practice of object relations family therapy*. Northvale, NJ: Jason Aronson.

Slipp, S. (1991). *The technique and practice of object relations family therapy*. Northvale, NJ: Jason Aronson.

Speck, R. V., & Attneave, C. A. (1971). Social network intervention. In J. Haley (Ed.), *Changing families: A family therapy reader*. New York: Grune & Stratton.

Speck, R. V., & Attneave, C. A. (1973). *Family networks*. New York: Pantheon.

Sperry, L., & Carlson, J. (1991). *Marital therapy: Integrating theory and technique*. Denver: Love.

Vaughn, C. E. (1989). Expressed emotion in family relationships. *Journal of Child Psychology and Psychiatry, 30*, 13–22.

Vaughn, C. E., Snyder, K. S., Jones, S., Freeman, W., & Falloon, I. R. H. (1984). Family factors in schizophrenic relapse. *Archives of General Psychiatry, 41*, 1169–1177.

Wynne, L., Ryckoff, I., Day, J., & Hirsch, S. (1958). Pseudo mutuality in the family relations of schizophrenics. *Psychiatry, 21*, 205–220.

Zuk, G. H. (1966). The go-between process in family therapy. *Family Process, 5*, 162–178.

Zuk, G. H. (1967). The side-taking function in family therapy. *American Journal of Orthopsychiatry, 38*, 553–559.

Zuk, G. H. (1968). When the family therapist takes sides: A case report. *Psychotherapy: Theory, Research and Practice, 5*, 24–28.

Zuk, G. H. (1971). Family therapy. In J. Haley (Ed.), *Changing families: A family therapy reader.* New York: Grune & Stratton.

Zuk, G. H. (1975). *Process and practice in family therapy.* Haverford, PA: Psychiatry and Behavior Science Books.

Zuk, G. H. (1978). A therapist's perspective on Jewish family values. *Journal of Marriage and Family Counseling, 4,* 103–110.

Zuk, G. H. (1979). Value systems and psychopathology in family therapy. *International Journal of Family Therapy, 1,* 133–151.

Zuk, G. H. (1981). *Family therapy: A triadic based approach* (rev. ed.). New York: Human Sciences Press.

Zuk, G. H. (1988). The conflict cycle in families and therapy. *Contemporary Family Therapy, 10,* 145–153.

Zuk, G. H. (1989). Learning to be possessed as a form of pathogenic relating and a cause of certain delusions. *Contemporary Family Therapy, 11,* 89–100.

Zuk, G. H. (1993). The reach of systems theory: A clinician's retrospective, 1984–1993. *Contemporary Family Therapy, 15,* 259–284.

12

*Family Therapy with Several
Specific Presenting Problems*

FRED P. PIERCY
LISA ARONSON FONTES
GARY H. BISCHOF
YOUNG HEE CHANG

As THE FIELD of family therapy matures, bodies of literature are developing around the family treatment of a number of presenting problems. To illustrate, we have presented in this chapter introductions and annotated bibliographies related to (1) family therapy of drug and alcohol abuse, (2) family therapy for sexual child abuse, (3) family therapy and AIDS, and (4) family systems medicine.

FAMILY THERAPY OF DRUG
AND ALCOHOL ABUSE

A biopsychosocial view of addictions (Donovan, 1988) acknowledges the biological, psychological, and social contributors to abuse and addiction. For example, one's genetic predisposition (biological factor), depression (psychological factor), and peer group (social factor) may all relate to a person's involvement with drugs or alcohol. Various family therapies address the social context of the abuser. The therapist uses family involvement to engage the abuser in treatment, to support him or her in the process of change, and to address psychological factors such as depression. Moreover, the therapist attempts to modify the family's typical behaviors around the abuser's habit in order to break the addictive cycle. Finally, the therapist may address relapse prevention through family intervention and support.

Family therapy for both alcohol and other drug abuse appears to be supported by a growing body of research. For example, in the area of family therapy for alcoholism, various reviews conclude that family therapy is both successful and cost-effective in the treatment of alcoholism (Edwards & Steinglass, 1995; Holder, Longabaugh, Miller, & Rubonis, 1991; O'Farrell, 1993). Edwards and Steinglass (1995) also conclude that secondary factors, such as one's gender and commitment to the marriage, appear to influence the findings of outcome studies. Family therapy, for example, seems to work better when the alcoholic is male, when there is commitment to and/or satisfaction with the marriage, and when there is spousal support for abstinence.

Over the years, a variety of skilled clinicians have described their approach to family therapy with alcoholics (e.g., Berg & Miller, 1992; Davis, 1987; Elkin, 1984; O'Farrell, 1993; Treadway, 1989; Wetchler, McCollum, Nelson, Trepper, & Lewis, 1993). Most emphasize the importance of working collaboratively with 12-step programs such as Alcoholics Anonymous (AA) and Al-Anon, and consider abstinence to be the only appropriate goal for therapy with alcoholics. An exception to this is Berg and Miller's (1992) application of solution-focused therapy to alcoholics. They consider reduced drinking to be an appropriate goal if it is a goal of the clients. They also maintain that many of the more traditional concepts of the disease model (e.g., "Alcohol is a disease"; "Once an alcoholic, always an alcoholic") may, in fact, be counterproductive for many alcoholic clients.

In contrast, Davis (1987) sees many similarities in family therapy and AA. For example, neither ascribes to willpower in the change process, both recognize that others in the family besides the alcoholic are also suffering from the problems of alcoholism, both make use of contact with significant others to facilitate change, and both see family members as potential sources of resistance to change. Similarly, Treadway (1989) believes that family therapists should make use of the powerful effects of AA. He uses the disease concept, for example, as a way of minimizing fault finding and guilt within the alcoholic and his or her family.

Family therapy has also been successfully applied to adult substance abusers. Stanton and Todd (1982), for example, found that structural–strategic family therapy was effective in both eliciting family support and in reducing the drug use of adult heroin users.

Family therapy, though, has been applied more frequently to adolescent substance abusers and appears to be a useful means of addressing adolescent substance abuse (Liddle & Dakof, 1995). This makes sense, given that the family is the central environment of most preadolescents and can remain a powerful influence for many adolescents. Several comprehensive reviews (e.g., Glynn, 1984; Harbin & Mazair, 1975; Stanton, 1979a, 1979b) and reviews of reviews (Glynn, 1981; Stanton, 1978) have chronicled the massive research and theory related to the part played by families in teenage substance abuse. Factors that predict adolescent substance use include family cohesion, degree of parental nurturance and support, parent–child communications, quality of parents' marriage, and quality and consistency of family management procedures. All of these can be directly or indirectly addressed through family therapy.

Specific family therapies for adolescent substance abuse are described in detail in a number of books (e.g., Friedman & Granick, 1990; Szapocznik, Kurtines, and Contributors, 1989; Todd & Selekman, 1991) and articles (Joanning, Thomas, Quinn, & Mullen, 1992; Liddle, Dakof, & Diamond, 1992; Piercy & Frankel, 1989; Szapocznik, Kurtines, Foote, Perez-Vidal, & Hervis, 1986). Although structural and strategic approaches dominated the 1980s (e.g., Piercy & Frankel, 1986; Stanton, 1981), in more recent years family therapists have applied solution-focused therapy (Berg & Gallagher, 1991), social constructionist therapies (Anderson, 1991), and integrative approaches (Henggeler et al., 1991; Liddle et al., 1992) to adolescent substance abuse.

The excellent research of Szapocznik and his colleagues (Szapocznik, Kurtines, Hervis, & Spencer, 1984; Szapocznik et al., 1986, 1989) suggests that systems-oriented family intervention may be just as effective when parents are not directly involved. In fact, some indicators at 6- and 12-month follow-up favor seeing the adolescent alone. Although adolescents seen with their families were beginning to engage in some delinquent behavior and drug use again at follow-up, adolescents seen in one-person family therapy were continuing to reduce their drug use at follow-up and saw their families as more cohesive and less controlling after follow-up than before.

Key Books and Articles

Bepko, C. (Ed.). (1991). *Feminism and addiction*. Binghamton, NY: Haworth.

This edited volume, also published as a special issue of the *Journal of Feminist Family Therapy*, explores addiction and addiction treatment from a feminist perspective. Authors examine through a feminist lens such issues as gender socialization and addiction, codependence, twelve-step programs, and substance abuse treatment and training. Also, several useful feminist clinical models are presented.

Berg, I. K., & Miller, S. D. (1992). *Working with the problem drinker*. New York: Norton.

The authors apply solution-focused therapy to the problem drinker and his or her family. Their approach is clear, respectful, and taps client strengths. In this brave new world of managed care, Berg and Miller's approach has much appeal. Goals are individualized, treatment is short, and therapy is pragmatic. The authors do not adhere to many of the tenets of AA. Still, their interviewing strategies should be useful to therapists from diverse theoretical orientations.

Collins, R. L., Leonard, K. E., & Searles, J. S. (Eds.). (1990). *Alcohol and the family: Research and clinical perspectives.* New York: Guilford Press.

This edited book provides a first-rate review of the research on families and alcoholism. Particularly good are the discussions of genetics, family process, children of alcoholics, and family treatment. The authors provide a balanced view of what is currently known about the more controversial issues pertaining to etiology and treatment of alcoholism.

Davis, D. I. (1987). *Alcoholism treatment.* New York: Gardner.

Davis has an appreciation for family therapy, individual therapy, and AA, and deals directly with many of the issues that have separated systems therapists and those wedded to an AA tradition. He draws from may schools of therapy and provides practical, highly relevant examples. A real bonus is the inclusion of Davis and associates' now classic article, "The Adaptive Consequences of Drinking."

Edwards, M., & Steinglass, P. (1995). Family therapy treatment outcomes for alcoholism. *Journal of Marital and Family Therapy, 21*(4), 475–510.

This article reviews 21 studies of family-involved therapy for alcoholism. The authors conclude that family intervention has a powerful effect in both motivating alcoholics into treatment and in altering drinking behavior through treatment. The authors also conclude that, once the drinker enters treatment, current family models appear to be most effective with males in relationships in which participants are invested and in which partners are supportive of treatment goals. This is a good review article that attempts to explore the ever-elusive specificity question.

Elkin, M. (1984). *Families under the influence.* New York: Norton.

This is an uncommonly clear and engaging book. Elkin does a wonderful job of describing the role of power in the alcoholic system and how this system develops. The last third of the book is a case example of Elkin's work with one family, in which he describes his clinical mistakes and how he learned from them.

Friedman, A. S., & Granick, S. (Eds.). (1990). *Family therapy for adolescent drug abuse.* Lexington, KY: Lexington Books.

Drawing on myriad cases from their clinical practices and research, the contributors share specific techniques regarding how to work with adolescent substance abusers. They also explore how adolescent drug abuse is a result of complex underlying problems that often involve the family. This volume concludes with detailed descriptions and analyses of family therapy conducted with eight families of adolescent substance abusers.

Heath, A. W., & Atkinson, B. J. (1988). Systemic treatment of substance abuse: A graduate course. *Journal of Marital and Family Therapy, 14*(4), 411–418.

The authors provide a useful format and creative strategies for teaching the contributions of family researchers, theorists, and clinicians toward the treatment of substance abuse. Although some of the material cited is now dated, the article itself is still a fine resource for anyone interested in designing a course in family therapy of substance abuse.

Kaufman, E., & Kaufmann, P. (Eds.). (1992). *Family therapy of drug and alcohol abuse* (2nd ed.). Boston: Allyn & Bacon.

In this second edition of their 1979 book, Kaufman and Kaufmann and other well-known experts describe theory and treatment strategies for drug and alcohol problems. There is something for everyone in this volume.

Liddle, H. A., & Dakof, G. (1995). Efficacy of family therapy for drug abuse: Promising but not definitive. *Journal of Marital and Family Therapy, 21*(4), 511–544.

This article presents a critical review of treatment outcome research in the area of family therapy for drug abuse in both adults and adolescents. A number of studies demonstrate that different versions of family intervention can engage and retain drug users and their families in treatment, reduce drug use and other related problems, and enhance certain realms of prosocial functioning. Because of the few controlled studies examined, the authors conclude that the results are "promising but not definitive."

O'Farrell, T. J. (Ed.). (1993). *Treating alcohol problems: Marital and family interventions.* New York: Guilford Press.

Leading clinician-researchers present practical information on research-tested methods for use at different stages of the alcoholism recovery process. Each chapter includes an overview of the specific method and detailed guidelines for implementation. The authors discuss clinical considerations and summarize the current knowledge regarding efficacy. Each chapter also includes a clinical case study.

Stanton, M. D., Todd, T. C., & Associates (1982). *The family therapy of drug abuse and addiction.* New York: Guilford Press.

In this foundational book, the authors report on a large research study in which they applied structural–strategic family therapy to heroin addicts and their families. They clearly and engagingly present their recruitment strategies, therapy model, and a wide range of clinical issues. There is a good deal of clinical wisdom in this book.

Steinglass, P., Bennett, L., Wolin, S., & Reiss, D. (1987). *The alcoholic family.* New York: Basic Books.

This book details the significance of alcohol as a central organizing principle in the day-to-day life and identity of some families. The authors' work reflects well the interactive and mutually enhancing roles of theory, research, and practice. The authors carefully lead the reader through various feedback loops related to their observations, hypotheses, and empirical studies, and conclude by illustrating the treatment implications of their findings. Throughout, they bring their ideas alive with rich case examples.

Szapocznik, J., Kurtines, W., & Contributors. (1989). *Breakthroughs in family therapy with drug-abusing and problem youth*. New York: Springer.

Szapocznik and his colleagues have done some of the most impressive research in the field related to one-person family therapy with adolescent substance abusers. Although this book summarizes some of this research, it is more of a treatment manual that presents the theory and practice of their structural–strategic approach to working with substance abusing adolescents alone in therapy.

Todd, T., & Selekman, M. (1991). *Family therapy approaches with adolescent substance abusers*. Needham Heights, MA: Allyn & Bacon.

This edited book provides a good sense of the ways many family therapies are being applied to substance-abusing adolescents. Therapies represented in this volume include MRI brief therapy, contextual family therapy, solution-focused therapy, intergenerational therapy, Michael White's approach, collaborative family systems therapy, network therapy, and the use of reflecting teams. Moreover, the editors give a good sense of the theoretical and research landscape with their fine integrative overview chapters.

Treadway, D. C. (1989). *Before it's too late: Working with substance abuse in the family*. New York: Norton.

Treadway is a seasoned clinician who masterfully uses case examples to illustrate an integrative, pragmatic therapy for substance abuse. Treadway's therapy is a blend of structural, strategic, and intergenerational therapies. He is also AA-friendly, and uses the disease concept to diffuse fault finding and recrimination in his client families. Treadway's warmth and compassion are obvious throughout and make this book more than a simple treatment manual. At the same time, it provides a superb road map for the practicing clinician.

Weinstein, D. (1992). Alcoholics Anonymous as change agent: Effective Ericksonian psychotherapy. *Journal of Strategic and Systemic Therapies, 11*(1), 33–44.

In this fascinating article, the author describes Alcoholics Anonymous from an Ericksonian perspective. This article makes it clear that AA and strategic family therapy, with its Ericksonian roots, are not that far apart.

FAMILY THERAPY FOR SEXUAL CHILD ABUSE

The sexual abuse of children occurs more frequently and affects a greater variety of families than many of us would care to believe. Therapists can be tempted by the false security of denial, opting to avoid asking the questions that uncover abuse, minimizing the seriousness of the abuse that is disclosed to us, or jumping on the false memory bandwagon and attributing reports of sexual abuse to therapist incompetence rather than actual occurrences.

Despite numerous methodological difficulties in determining exact levels of prevalence (Wyatt & Peters, 1986), we can conservatively say that all family therapists who treat 100 couples or families will work with at least a dozen who are facing issues of sexual abuse, either in their current families or in their families of origin. This is due both to the high general prevalence of sexual child abuse and the higher proportion of sexual child abuse in clinical samples (Peters, Wyatt, & Finkelhor, 1986). Child protection agencies are increasingly contracting family therapists to work with families in which sexual abuse has occurred, to reduce the long-term effects of the abuse and to assure that abuse does not reoccur. In addition, families often seek help for seemingly unrelated presenting problems (e.g., acting-out teenagers, sexual dysfunctions) and—without an adequate assessment—may never reveal their history of sexual child abuse.

Family members are connected by a complex web of history, ideas, and emotions. Thus, entire families are affected by the sexual abuse of a child, its occultation, and its discovery. Recent authors suggest that family therapy can effectively address the family dynamics that may have permitted the abuse to occur, or which result from that abuse and/or its discovery (James & Nasjleti, 1983; Trepper & Barrett, 1989).

The sometimes hidden baggage of childhood sexual abuse often accompanies adults into therapy, even when it is not the presenting complaint. An unprocessed history of childhood sexual abuse is likely to influence couple systems, most particularly in the areas of trust, intimacy, and sexuality. The sexual abuse history may also affect the relationship between the therapist and the clients.

Family Therapists' Role in Family and Societal Intervention

The literature on family therapy approaches to sexual abuse took root firmly in the late 1980s, when the alarmingly widespread nature of sexual child abuse had been confirmed by a variety of prevalence studies (e.g., Russell, 1986) and individual models had been proven inadequate to protect children at risk (Trepper & Barrett, 1989). Family therapy seemed to offer a promising alternative to individual approaches, which may help those who have been victimized resolve the traumatic effects, but often failed to address the pain and confusion of other family members (Maddock & Larson, 1995). Individual interventions were found to leave the victim and other children vulnerable to future abuse by the person who had offended originally and by others. Therapists heard sexual offenders describe their own experiences of childhood victimization and began to write about the intergenerational nature of some sexual abuse (Gilgun, 1991). Family therapy was considered a promising way to "break the cycle" of sexual abuse and stop the process wherein some victims become victimizers.

With notable exceptions, family therapists have not been at the forefront of the research or advocacy movements that aim to protect children from sexual child abuse and promote recovery. This may stem from the perceived incompatibility of family systems and child protection/victim advocacy approaches. Therapists may perceive themselves as having to choose between being on the side of the child or on the side of the family. Some family therapists may view as "antiparent" the terms or attitudes of people in the child protection movement. Conferences on "family violence" may seem to be almost oxymoronic to therapists who have dedicated their lives to enhancing the nurturing potential of families. Without minimizing differences between the family systems and victim advocacy approaches (Maddock & Larson, 1995, pp. 8–9), we advocate for drawing upon the knowledge and resources of both. Family therapists are hopping on one foot when they fail to make use of the many excellent writings, conferences, and networks of victim advocates. Similarly, the victim advocacy movement will be enriched by the increasing participation of family therapists who see family health and functioning as complementary to the recovery and protection of individuals.

Sexual Child Abuse

Sexual abuse may be defined as "any form of coerced sexual interaction between an individual and a person in a position of power over that individual" (Dolan, 1991, p. 1). This power differential may be based on age, size, authority, ability–disability status, numbers (e.g., in gang rape), or social role. The use of intimidation, threat, or a weapon, of course, gives one person power over another.

Incest is sexual contact with someone who would be considered an inappropriate sexual partner because of blood or social ties to the individual or the individual's family (Dolan, 1991). This expanded definition of incest includes not only blood relatives, but also all people who stand in a prolonged relationship of caretaking to a child (e.g., stepparents, baby-sitters, teachers, family friends, clergy, and others). Incest is primarily the betrayal of a relationship, not biology (Gelinas, 1983). Occasionally, sibling incest may not be abusive if there is little age difference between siblings and no violence or coercion, but therapists should beware of situations that look like mutual child play and where, in fact, one sibling is being coerced into participating by the other (Maddock & Larson, 1995). When describing most instances of childhood incest, the term "incestuous abuse" should be used to highlight the power imbalances involved.

Sexual child abuse is a form of sexual abuse in which the victim is a child. It may also be considered a form of child abuse when the maltreatment is enacted sexually. Sexual child abuse describes all acts that involve the sexual use of a child by an adult or by a child who is older or more powerful. These acts may include but are not limited to exhibitionism; sexual fondling of the child by the adult or of the adult by the child; oral, vaginal, or anal intercourse; penetration of the child's orifices with objects; deliberate exposure of a child to pornography; using the child for pornographic purposes; cunnilingus; fellatio; masturbation; practices that are sexually stimulating and disguised as hygiene (Berson & Herman-Giddens, 1994); and observation of a child in a way that makes the child uncomfortable (e.g., spying on a child in the shower). The short- and long-term effects of abuse are not necessarily related to the degree of intrusion into the child's body. Rather, numerous factors have an impact, including the degree of terror surrounding the abuse; the sexual response of the child, the age of the child at the time of the first abusive incident, the presence of supportive others in the child's life, the relationship of the victim to the offender, coping mechanisms used by the child, and the response to the child's first disclosure (Hindman, 1989).

Although most of the literature on sexual abuse refers to situations in which the offender and victim are members of the same family, extrafamilial sexual abuse can also have profound effects on the participants and their families. This area remains relatively neglected in the research and intervention literatures.

Language and Sexual Abuse

Differences in definitions have contributed to conflicts among professionals and clients, and methodological problems in research (Wyatt & Peters, 1986). Often various members of the treatment system hold divergent definitions of what has happened. For example, a mother may say she touched her daughter's labia for hygienic purposes, whereas the daughter experienced her touch as abusive; a grandfather claims to have caressed his grandchildren with the best of intentions, but the district attorney is filing charges of indecent assault on minors; a therapist believes an adolescent brother's prolonged kisses with his prepubertal sister are part of an oversexualized family system, but the family resists this definition; a protective social worker believes a mother is offering tacit approval for her husband's abuse of her child, whereas a family therapist sees a mother who is doing her best to save her marriage; and so on. Family members' lasting understanding of what happened profoundly impacts their views of themselves and of family life in general. These differences in definition are partially co-created in therapy through language. Therefore, it is crucial that therapists pay close attention to the language they use in-session.

No term used to describe the various members of a system organized around abuse (e.g., victim, offender, nonoffending parent) can be considered neutral: Each carries with it implications for how the family will come to derive meaning from the abuse and the interventions. The term "survivor" is preferred by many who work in the child abuse recovery movement as a term that both denotes the severity of the child abuse and the heroism of the person who has made it through. Some people reserve its use for victims of abuse who have been through a deliberate process of recovery. Calling someone a "victim" highlights that this person has been wronged.

Many therapists avoid using all static terms to refer to the people involved in sexual abuse, preferring instead to say "the person who was abused," or referring to people by name. The intention is to avoid the permanence and the global nature of these labels. A person who has been victimized is not only a victim, for example, but may also be a mother, a professional, and a black belt in karate. Similarly, the identity of people who have victimized others cannot be collapsed into a single word, especially if we wish to support their growth and evolution into people who do not abuse.

Basic Goals of Sexual Abuse Treatment

The basic goals for family treatment for sexual child abuse are (1) to prevent further abuse, and (2) to help individual family members and the family as a whole recover from the effects of the abuse that has occurred (this does not mean the family members necessarily stay together). Steps to achieve the first goal often include restricting unsupervised access to children for the person who has offended; a thorough family assessment to uncover other incidents or patterns of inappropriate sexual expression or child abuse; ensuring that the person who offended against the child receives specific treatment for his or her behaviors, takes responsibility for the abusive incidents, and learns ways to prevent him- or herself from abusing again; establishing a supportive network for the child and family to break the isolation that often facilitates sexual abuse and inhibits disclosure; family sessions geared toward increasing support for the person who has been victimized and placing responsibility for the abuse squarely on the shoulders of the person who offended (numerous factors determine if and when the offender is present for these sessions); and sex education for the entire family to learn appropriate avenues for sexual expression. Psychoeducation, individual and group therapies, and network meetings, also often form part of effective treatment for sexual child abuse (Sheinberg, True, & Fraenkel, 1994). Approaches to facilitating individual and family recovery from the effects of abuse range from individually oriented trauma assessment with family support (Hindman, 1989) to Ericksonian hypnosis (Dolan, 1991) to couples work on sexual recovery (e.g., Maltz, 1988) to therapeutic rituals aimed at empowering family members who have experienced sexual child abuse (Adams-Westcott & Isenbart, 1990).

Key Resources

With the vast and varied literature currently available on treating sexual child abuse, this short list of essential works for family therapists is necessarily partial. These works have been chosen to reflect the range of resources available.

Journals

In addition to the general family therapy journals that occasionally address issues of sexual child abuse, family therapists are advised to become familiar with the excellent resources available in the violence prevention movement.

- *Journal of Child Sexual Abuse* (Haworth Press). This quarterly scholarly journal addresses research, treatment, and program innovations for victims, survivors, offenders, families, and communities. Articles are written from medical, legal, judicial, and mental health perspectives.
- *Child Abuse and Neglect* (Pergamon). This monthly scholarly journal publishes research and theoretical ideas on all areas of child abuse and neglect, often including international perspectives.
- *Child Maltreatment* (Sage). This quarterly journal is the official journal of the American Professional Society on the Abuse of Children (APSAC). It provides clear, concise information for professionals involved in all aspects of child maltreatment intervention and research.
- *Violence Against Women* (Sage). This quarterly journal provides a wide range of articles on issues related to violence against women, including sexual child abuse.
- *Journal of Feminist Family Therapy* (Haworth). This quarterly journal frequently publishes feminist perspectives on family interventions for sexual abuse.
- *Journal of Interpersonal Violence* (Sage). This quarterly journal publishes research and occasional theoretical pieces on all forms of interpersonal violence, including sexual child abuse.

Organizations

- American Professional Society on the Abuse of Children (APSAC), 407 South Dearborn, Suite 1300, Chicago, IL 60605 (312-554-0166).
- International Society for the Prevention of Child Abuse and Neglect, 332 South Michigan Avenue, Suite 1600, Chicago, IL 60604 (312-663-3520).

Electronic Mail Lists

The Intimate Violence List, a forum to contact family violence researchers and professionals worldwide, can be reached by sending a message to: listserv@uriacc.edu. In the body of the message write: subscribe INTVIO-L.

A moderated list for child abuse researchers may be reached by writing listproc@cornell.edu. In you message write: subscribe child-maltreatment-research-L.

Additional, related lists are rapidly being created. The Minnesota Higher Education Center against Violence and Abuse maintains an electronic clearinghouse on the World Wide Web that lists a number of related Internet lists. Get to the site by entering: http://www.umn.edu/mincava on any Web browser. Once at the homepage, click on the "News and Discussion" icon for more information.

Key Books and Articles

Barrett, M. J., Trepper, T. S., & Fish, L. S. (1990). Feminist-informed family therapy for the treatment of intrafamily child sexual abuse. *Journal of Family Psychology*, *4*(2), 151–166.

This article elegantly synthesizes feminist theory and family systems therapy, culminating in a description of goals and interventions for feminist-informed treatment of incestuous abuse.

Canavan, M. M., Meyer, W. J., & Higgs, D. C. (1992). The female experience of sibling incest. *Journal of Marital and Family Therapy, 18,* 129–142.

In this review of the literature and compelling presentations of four cases, the authors lay to rest the notion that sibling incest between minor children is less harmful than other forms of sexual child abuse.

Davis, L. (1991). *Allies in healing.* New York: HarperCollins.

This is a support book for partners of people who were abused sexually as children. It offers valuable information for people who may be confused by their partner's behavior related to a history of sexual abuse.

Durrant, M., & White, C. (Eds.). (1990). *Ideas for therapy with sexual abuse.* South Australia: Dulwich Centre Publications.

The Dulwich Centre writers again contribute a fresh, new perspective in this edited volume. The authors identify ways we can approach each family and individual on their own terms, learning about the idiosyncratic meanings and effects of the abuse for them, and working in ways that fit their particular situations and competencies.

Fontes, L. A. (1995). *Sexual abuse in nine North American cultures: Treatment and prevention.* Newbury Park, CA: Sage.

Fontes sets forth frameworks for considering the impact of culture in addressing issues of sexual abuse. Experts on sexual abuse from the following nine cultures offer cultural information, literature reviews, and treatment guidelines for their group: African American; Anglo American; Asian American, Pacific Islander, and Filipino; Cambodian; gay male; Jewish; lesbian; Puerto Rican; and Seventh Day Adventist.

Friedrich, W. N. (1990). *Psychotherapy with sexually abused boys: An integrated approach.* Newbury Park, CA: Sage.

This unusually well-written and practical book provides guidelines for individual, group, and family therapy to treat the disorders of attachment, regulation and self that Friedrich believes lie at the heart of the injury of sexual abuse. It addresses the specific gender messages and sexual acting out that are more likely to affect male victims.

Hindman, J. (1989). *Just before dawn.* Ontario, OR: Alexandria Associates.

This individual-oriented treatment book provides excellent suggestions for working with victims of sexual abuse, including ways to involve their families. It graphically conveys the relationship binds of a child who is abused sexually. The cutesy writing style can be ignored.

Jenkins, A. (1990). *Invitations to responsibility: The therapeutic engagement of men who are violent and abusive.* South Australia: Dulwich Centre Publications.

This book provides theoretical and practical ideas for working with men who have been violent. It suggests ways for therapists to collaborate with the criminal justice system to enhance offenders' motivation and improve therapy outcome.

Wheeler, C. (Ed.). (1989). Special issue on childhood sexual abuse. *Journal of Strategic and Systemic Therapies, 8*(4).

Seven articles in this special issue describe innovative approaches to a variety of childhood sexual abuse situations, including a report on the rapid resolution of the symptoms of an adult incest survivor through Ericksonian hypnosis (Dolan, 1989) and a discussion of structural interventions with a family with incest (Fish & Faynik, 1989).

Maddock, J. W., & Larson, N. R. (1995). *Incestuous families: An ecological approach to understanding and treatment.* New York: Norton.

This book synthesizes diverse writings and contributes some interesting new material in a comprehensive, helpful tome. The authors insist that all family members are in some way affected by incest. Despite frequent disclaimers that all family members are *not* responsible for the abuse that occurred, the case examples seem to suggest that if families in which incest has occurred can be helped to become more "normal" (e.g., the nonoffending wife learns to have orgasms), the likelihood of further abuse is reduced (a dubious suggestion).

Maltz, M. (1991). *The sexual healing journey.* New York: HarperCollins.

This book is written for survivors of sexual child abuse, but also informs professionals of the specifically sexual implications of childhood abuse.

Sheinberg, M., True, F., & Fraenkel, P. (1994). Treating the sexually abused child: A recursive, multimodal program. *Family Process, 33,* 263–276.

This article describes the Ackerman Institute approach to sexual abuse which includes individual, group, and family therapy. A major, unique feature of the approach is a "decision dialogue" in which family members are asked to consider if, how, and with whom to share material that emerges in one modality, enhancing the personal agency of the abused child and encouraging connections among trustworthy family members.

Trepper, T. S., & Barrett, M. J. (1989). *Systemic treatment of incest: A therapeutic handbook.* New York: Brunner/Mazel.

This well-written and highly practical book offers a treatment model for therapists to address ongoing or recently disclosed sexual abuse from a systems perspective.

FAMILY THERAPY AND AIDS

AIDS raises unique challenges for even the most creative and committed family therapists. For example, family therapists must help people living with AIDS and their families both cope with the disease and foster a sense of faith, dignity, hope, and trust. Indeed, pioneering family therapists are facing these challenges with courage, compassion, and ethical and social responsibility.

Increasingly, family researchers and clinicians argue that family therapy is a counseling treatment of choice for people whose lives are touched by AIDS (Landau-Stanton, Clements, & Associates, 1993; Walker, 1991). Family therapists address family fears, cutoffs, secrecy, loyalty issues, generational themes, and family transitional crises brought on by an illness that is both socially stigmatizing and physically debilitating. In addition, family therapists address the effects of racism, poverty, drug use, and societal fears of AIDS (Boyd-Franklin, 1993; Boyd-Franklin, Steiner, & Boland, 1995). An overarching theme is the emphasis on family strengths. Family therapists attempt to empower families. They support existing resources and construct positive narratives to help their clients cope with both living with AIDS and the imminent reality of death (Walker, 1991). Family therapists also increasingly take a broader view by incorporating spirituality, community systems, and culture into their work. Clearly, family therapists must take into account the cultural and political system in which AIDS exists (Landau-Stanton, Clements, & Associates, 1993).

In this work, we must conceptualize "family" in broad terms to include significant relationships of people coping with AIDS. "Family" may include gay or straight couples, a gay man's friendship network, extended family members, professionals, and the intimate network of people who are providing care (Bor & Elford, 1994; Levine, 1994; Miller, Goldman, & Bor, 1994).

AIDS is not selective. Family therapists work with many different groups affected by this disease, shaping therapy in the light of the special needs of each. Treatment will differ depending on the gender, ethnicity, age, and sexual orientation of the client. Some clinician-researchers study parent–child relationships in which the child (Gomez, Haiken, & Lewis, 1995) or adult child (Beckerman, 1994; Dane, 1991) is diagnosed with AIDS. Others explore the special concerns of families in which parents are diagnosed with AIDS (Shiga, Endo, Tobe, & Yanagihara, 1992). Still others examine marital relationships (Black, 1993), partner relationships (Walker, 1991), and extended family members (Boyd-Franklin, 1992).

Families affected by AIDS face many challenges. They must learn to adapt to life with HIV-related symptoms, manage the medical system, establish relationships with the health-care team, make decisions about disclosure, reorganize during crises, and begin the process of planning for illness or death (Walker, 1991). In the broader sense, families also face the challenges of creating meaning in their lives, which may involve spirituality and religion. It may also be important for the person with AIDS to develop a sense of mastery and competency, to grieve the loss of the family identity prior to illness, and to develop a support network to provide care and reduce isolation (Walker, 1991).

Family therapists have explored the role of secrecy in families affected by AIDS (Black, 1993; Walker, 1992). The dynamics of secrets may differ depending on the ethnicity of the family (Boyd-Franklin, 1993; Boyd-Franklin, Aleman, Jean-Giles, & Lewis, 1995). There are also many confidentiality and duty-to-warn issues in AIDS-related therapy, which may lead to legal and ethical concerns for family therapists (Walker, 1991; Schlossberger & Hecker, 1996).

Various therapies have been used with individuals and families affected by AIDS, including Bowenian (Ackerman, 1989); family systems (Boyd-Franklin, Aleman, Steiner, Drelich, & Norford, 1995); multisystems (Boyd-Franklin & Boland, 1995); centripetal and centrifugal (Britton & Zarski, 1989); an adapted version of the Rochester Family Therapy Model (Landau-Stanton et al., 1993); structural (Gomez et al., 1995); Milan (Miller et al., 1994); integrative (Piercy, Trepper, & Jurich, 1993); narrative, systems, and collaborative (Walker, 1991); and ecosystemic (Walker, 1991) approaches. Particularly noteworthy is the narrative approach of Walker (1991), which builds positive narratives for families, and the multisystems approach of Boyd-Franklin and Boland (1995), which presents a family-focused, culturally sensitive, and systems-coordinated model. Family therapy for people living with AIDS and their families represents an excellent example of how the field has also not only adapted to a timely issue, but has found the inspiration, creativity, and strength to address it in a way that helps families, couples, and individuals live with dignity, respect, and hope.

Key Books, Chapters, and Articles

Therapist Issues: Attitudes and Knowledge of AIDS

Green, S., & Bobele, M. (1994). Family therapists response to AIDS: An examination of attitudes, knowledge, and contact. *Journal of Marital and Family Therapy, 20*(4), 349–367.

The authors discuss a survey of 457 clinical members of the American Association for Marriage and Family Therapy regarding their knowledge of AIDS, their attitudes toward people with AIDS, and their contact with gay men, lesbians, and people with AIDS. The authors discuss implications for clinical work and practice.

Family Therapy: Theories and Practice

Ackerman, F. (1989). Family systems therapy with a man with AIDS–related complex. *Family Systems Medicine, 7*(3), 292–304.

This article describes a case of 35–year–old man with AIDS–related complex in which Bowen Family Systems therapy was used.

Boyd–Franklin, N., Aleman, J., Steiner, G., Drelich, E., & Norford, B. (1995). Family systems interventions and family therapy. In N. Boyd–Franklin, G. L. Steiner, & M. G. Boland (Eds.), *Children, families, and HIV/AIDS: Psychosocial and therapeutic issues.* New York: Guilford Press.

The authors distinguish between family systems intervention, which provides direct, short–term care at critical junctures, and family therapy, which provides ongoing family treatment. The authors provide excellent case examples.

Boyd–Franklin, N., & Boland, M. (1995). A multisystems approach to service delivery for HIV/AIDS families. In N. Boyd–Franklin, G. L. Steiner, & M. G. Boland (Eds.), *Children, families, and HIV/AIDS: Psychosocial and therapeutic issues.* New York: Guilford Press.

The authors address the role of the therapist in supporting cooperative care for families of children with HIV/AIDS. These families may be dealing with a multitude of agencies, such as hospitals, clinics, schools, welfare services, child protective services, courts, juvenile justice, drug and alcohol treatment centers, visiting nurse programs, or foster care. The authors introduce a multisystems model to facilitate cooperative care. This model is family focused, culturally sensitive, and systems coordinated.

Britton, P., & Zarski, J. (1989). HIV spectrum disorders and the family: Selected interventions based on stylistic dimensions. *AIDS-Care, 1*(1), 85–92.

Centripetal and centrifugal family styles are used as a framework for presenting intervention strategies that allow the family to continue its developmental process. The authors discuss the life-cycle stage of the family and present a case example of a 28-year-old male.

Curtis, J. (1989). Treating AIDS: A family therapy perspective. In C. Kain (Ed.), *No longer immune: A counselor's guide to AIDS.* Virginia: American Association for Counseling and Development.

The author examines the use of a dynamic family approach for working with people with HIV infection and their significant others. Curtis emphasizes the importance of family involvement in the care of people with AIDS and discusses issues for family therapists.

Landau-Stanton, J., Clements, C. D., & Stanton, M. D. (1993). Psychotherapeutic intervention: From individual through group to extended network. In J. Landau-Stanton & C. Clements (Eds.), *AIDS health and mental health: A primary sourcebook.* New York: Brunner/Mazel.

The authors present therapeutic principles and techniques within an adapted version of the Rochester Family Therapy Model. The chapter provides an outstanding discussion of ways therapists may engage people affected by AIDS.

Maloney, B. (1988). The legacy of AIDS: Challenge for the next century. *Journal of Marital and Family Therapy, 14*(2), 143–150.

This article presents a 3-stage family therapy treatment method for working with people with AIDS and their families. The author discusses countertransference issues that threaten the therapeutic process.

Miller, R., Goldman, E., & Bor, R. (1994). Application of a family systems approach to working with people affected by HIV disease. In R. Bor & J. Elford (Eds.), *The family and HIV.* New York: Cassell.

The authors describe a family systems approach adapted from the Milan associates for counseling people with AIDS and their families, along with two case examples.

Piercy, F., Trepper, T., & Jurich, J. (1993). The role of family therapy in decreasing HIV high-risk behaviors among adolescents. *AIDS Education and Prevention, 5*(1), 71–86.

The authors identify HIV risk factors among adolescents and provide a rationale for using family therapy to prevent high risk for HIV behaviors among adolescents. They apply the integrative Purdue Brief Family Therapy Model to a family with a 15-year-old boy at risk for HIV infection.

Valentine, L., Bigner, J., Cook, A., & Guest, R. (1992). Assessment of the interpersonal themes in therapy of a person with AIDS. *Journal of Family Psychotherapy, 3*(2), 71–86.

The authors analyze the interpersonal themes at the beginning and end of therapy with a 37-year-old female with AIDS and suggest how the analysis of themes helps to evaluate the therapy process. The client underwent 10 sessions of individual therapy and 8 sessions of family therapy. Interpersonal themes included withholding, secrecy, self-erase, dependency, impatience, and frustration. The therapist transformed these themes to new responses of open communication, self-assertion, self-acceptance, and self-care.

Walker, G. (1991). *In the midst of winter: Systemic therapy with families, couples, and individuals with AIDS infection.* New York: Norton.

The author chronicles the challenges of persons with AIDS and their families, emphasizing that families facing death and stigmatization can often be a courageous source of strength and support. She employs both systems concepts and the narrative metaphor to frame the disease in a way that leaves room for living, dignity, and growth.

AIDS and Family Secrets

Black, L. (1993). AIDS and secrets. In E. Imber-Black (Ed.), *Secrets in families and family therapy.* New York: Norton.

The author discusses AIDS as a family secret, a secret in a marriage, a secret between a parent and child, and a secret from oneself. Black also presents powerful clinical case examples.

Walker, G. (1992). Family therapy in the context of AIDS. In T. Akamatsu, M. Stephenes, S. Hobfoll, & J. Crowther (Eds.), *Family health psychology.* Washington, DC: Hemisphere.

The author discusses critical issues for therapists working with people with AIDS and their families, and provides some principles for effective intervention. Walker describes key intervention tasks, including the need to empower families to identify caregiving resources, to construct positive narratives that counteract AIDS stigma, and to plan for the future.

Multiculturalism and AIDS

Boyd-Franklin, N., Aleman, J., Jean-Giles, M., & Lewis, S. (1995). Cultural sensitivity and competence: African-American, Latino, and Haitian families with HIV/AIDS. In N. Boyd-Franklin, G. L. Steiner, & M. G. Boland (Eds.), *Children, families, and HIV/AIDS: Psychosocial and therapeutic issues.* New York: Guilford Press.

This chapter discusses important issues in the lives of families and children from three cultural groups who are coping with HIV/AIDS. The authors stress the importance of recognizing diversity within each cultural group and present important information regarding the role of spirituality, reactions to therapy and health care, gender and language issues, perception of HIV, and family support.

Boyd-Franklin, N. (1993). Racism, secret-keeping, and African-American families. In E. Imber-Black (Ed.), *Secrets in family therapy.* New York: Norton.

The author addresses how secrets related to AIDS are kept in African American families and the response of African American families to family therapy (with case examples).

Parent–Child

Beckerman, N. (1994). Psychosocial tasks facing parents whose adult child has AIDS. *Family Therapy, 21*(3), 209–216.

This article examines the unique psychosocial tasks faced by parents of adult sons who have AIDS. The author outlines the role of the family therapist, with special attention to reducing isolation as parents move through the challenges of accepting and disclosing diagnosis to family and friends.

Dane, B. (1991). Anticipatory mourning of middle-aged parents of adult children with AIDS. *Families in Society, 72*(2), 108–115.

This article discusses a conceptual framework of anticipatory mourning for counseling parents of adult children with AIDS. The authors state that therapists should explore where the family is in its developmental life cycle and how the family has reacted to illness and loss in current and previous generations.

Shiga, N., Endo, Y., Tobe, S., & Yanagihara, S. (1992). Family counseling for HIV/AIDS patients. *Japanese Journal of Family Psychology, 6*(2), 121–132.

The authors present a case of family therapy in which the father had AIDS. The article emphasized counseling the man and his daughter. Counseling helped the daughter to anticipate mourning for her father without having to defend him from social prejudice against people with AIDS.

AIDS and Children

Gomez, K., Haiken, H., & Lewis, S. (1995). Support group for children with HIV/AIDS. In N. Boyd-Franklin, G. L. Steiner, & M. G. Boland (Eds.), *Children, families, and HIV/AIDS: Psychosocial and therapeutic issues.* New York: Guilford Press.

This chapter describes a support group for HIV-infected children held at a multidisciplinary treatment program that uses a structural family therapy model. Two cotherapists provide an environment that supports self-disclosure and peer bonds.

Krener, P., & Miller, F. (1991). Psychiatric response to HIV spectrum disease in children and adolescents. In S. Chess & M. Hertzig (Eds.), *Annual progress in child psychiatry and child development.* New York: Brunner/Mazel.

The authors use family therapy, as well as individual therapy, neuropsychological assessment, and psychopharmacological management. They also discuss the particular problems associated with each.

FAMILY SYSTEMS MEDICINE

Some have heralded family systems medicine as the "next frontier" of family therapy. The field of marriage and family therapy, which originally developed in opposition to the prevailing mechanistic medical model, has matured to the point at which therapists are willing to collaborate with physicians and other health-care providers. But what is family systems medicine and how was it established? What is the role of the medical family therapist? In this overview, we will answer these questions and suggest key publications and resources for those who wish to know more.

Family systems medicine grew from earlier attempts to understand the reciprocal influence of one's social context and health (see McDaniel, Hepworth, & Doherty, 1992, for a summary). The fields of family therapy and family medicine evolved simultaneously. In 1977, internist George Engel called for a new model of medicine, the biopsychosocial model, to supplant the prevailing model of biomedicine. He suggested a model in which one's biological, psychological, and social systems would be equally considered. The patient and the disease were considered in context.

The biopsychosocial model is one of the key theoretical tenets of family systems medicine, and the field of family medicine has adopted it as part of its theoretical core. With this model in mind, for example, the physician may understand the noncompliant diabetic child's behavior as playing some role in the family system. Similarly, the family therapist may take into account the impact of the course of a chronic illness on future life-cycle transitions.

Interest in family systems medicine burgeoned in the 1980s. The Society of Teachers of Family Medicine (STFM) sponsored a conference on the "Family in Family Medicine" in 1981. Initially attended primarily by family physicians, in recent years, annual conference attendance has been more evenly divided between family physicians and family therapists, and other related health and mental health professionals. In 1982, the Ackerman Institute sponsored a conference on "Therapy with Families of Physical Illness," which led to the creation of the journal *Family Systems Medicine*, edited by Don Bloch (1983). This journal, described in its subtitle as being "at the confluence of family therapy, systems theory and modern medicine" has been a major force in the field.

A number of key texts were published for family physicians and nurses that emphasized how families could be involved in medical care (Glenn, 1987; Wright & Leahey, 1987). Doherty and Baird (1983, 1987), a family therapist and a family physician, respectively, defined five levels of physician involvement with families: (1) minimal emphasis; (2) ongoing medical information and advice; (3) feelings and support; (4) systematic assessment and planned intervention; and (5) family therapy. They also identified the physician–patient–family triangle to conceptualize the interactions that can occur among these participants in the delivery of health care.

During the late 1980s and early 1990s, family systems medicine began to be embraced by the wider field of family therapy. Family therapists and family physicians delivered plenaries on the topic at the national American Association for Marriage and Family Therapy (AAMFT) conferences, and the AAMFT and STFM formed a joint task force. The Working Group for Family Therapists Practicing in Medical Settings was founded in 1991. With the title of their book, *Medical Family Therapy*, McDaniel et al. (1992) coined a new term. In this book, they describe in detail the role of the family therapist in family systems medicine.

Several prominent leaders in the field gathered in early 1994 to discuss family systems medicine in the rapidly changing arena of health care. This group established the Collaborative Family Health-Care Coalition, which advocates that, ideally, health care providers and mental health clinicians work under the same roof, share the biopsychosocial model, and provide holistic health care for families. The Coalition held its first national conference in July 1995, and has organized regional chapters throughout the United States and Europe.

Describing what is unique about medical family therapy, McDaniel et al. (1992) claim:

> It is distinguished by conscious attention to medical illness and its role in the personal life of the patient and the interpersonal life of the family. It combines biopsychosocial and family systems perspectives and uses them to work simultaneously with patients, families, health care professionals, and community groups and agencies. (p. 4)

Medical family therapists are trained to work with difficult cases in an intense and sometimes prolonged manner, beyond what is possible for other health care providers.

The family therapist has much to offer health-care providers in addressing some of the more difficult and frustrating aspects of their work. For example, as the therapist more fully understands the system and beliefs of a family, he or she may also more clearly understand issues of noncompliance with medical treatment or difficulties altering destructive health behaviors such as cigarette smoking or overeating. A medical family therapist might also help in other areas, including (1) chronic illness or disability; (2) childhood chronic or acute illness and its impact on marital and sibling relationships; (3) problematic relationships between health-care providers and patients or families; (4) treatment impasses and triangulation of the patient, family, and physician, or of the patient and competing multiple health-care providers; (5) somatic symptoms or chronic pain without clear physical etiology; (6) pregnancy loss or infertility; (7) death or unresolved loss; and (8) overutilization of health care services.

In addition to assisting with difficult cases, the family therapist practicing in a medical setting can enrich and be enriched by personal and professional interaction with colleagues from other disciplines. Health-care providers can benefit from ready access to a mental health clinician who understands the culture of medicine and is available to consult and support the health-care provider and to treat patients and families. The health-care team thus has multiple perspectives from which to devise effective treatment plans. Family therapists can also learn about the medical culture, various physical illnesses, and how to better appreciate the effect of biological processes on mental health and intimate relationships.

Although a large body of research demonstrates that the family has a powerful influence on physical health, the evidence for the effectiveness of *family* interventions in physical illness is less conclusive (Campbell & Patterson, 1995). There is an established literature on the cost-effectiveness of psychosocial interventions with physical health problems (see Katon & Gonzalez, 1994; Levenson, 1992; Mumford & Schlesinger, 1987; Mumford, Schlesinger, Glass, Patrick, & Cuerdon, 1984, for examples). Studies show that overall health-care expenditures can be offset in many cases when psychosocial interventions are applied and especially when hospital stays are shortened. More needs to be done to investigate the outcomes associated with medical family therapy, but initial clinical impressions and research findings are promising. It is particularly promising that some large managed care organizations are implementing collaborative approaches to care.

The ever-changing landscape of health care and mental health treatment demands cost-effective alternatives that emphasize quality of care and provider, and patient satisfaction. Collaborative family health care may be one such alternative. As Ransom (1984), one of the founders of family systems medicine recalls, "The family is the unit of illness, because it is the unit of living" (p. 110). Health care will continue to emphasize outpatient care and in-home treatment, which will automatically expand the role of the patient's family in treatment and prevention. Therefore, we will undoubtedly see more demand for those interested and trained in working at the confluence of families, systems, and health.

Key Resources

- Collaborative Family Health Care Coalition, 40 West 12th Street, New York, NY 10011-8604 (212-675-2477; E-mail: 72460.1142@compuserve.com; Fax: 212-727-1126). Sponsors annual conference, quarterly newsletter, and electronic mail network.
- *Families, Systems, and Health* (edited by Susan McDaniel, Ph.D., and Tom Campbell, M.D., of Rochester, New York). Primary journal of the field.

- Society for Teachers of Family Medicine (STFM), 8880 Ward Parkway, P.O. Box 8729, Kansas City, MO 64114. (1-800-274-2237). Group on Family in Family Medicine sponsors annual meeting in Amelia Island, Florida.

- Working Group for Family Therapists Practicing in Medical Settings. Contact: David Seaburn, University of Rochester, Department of Family Medicine, 885 South Avenue, Rochester, NY 14620. Publishes a directory and provides information on training opportunities.

Key Books and Articles[1]

Campbell, T. L., & Patterson, J. M. (1995). The effectiveness of family interventions in the treatment of physical illness. *Journal of Marital and Family Therapy, 21,* 545–583.

This excellent summary article appears in a special edition of the journal on the effectiveness of marital and family therapy. The authors present an exhaustive review of the literature in this area and display summaries of many of the studies they reviewed in user-friendly tables. They highlight those illnesses for which family interventions have been shown to be effective and recommend future areas of research. They conclude that the research supports the role of medical family therapy in the new health-care system.

Crane, D. D. (1986). The family therapist, the primary care physician, and the health maintenance organization: Pitfalls and possibilities. *Family Systems Medicine, 4,* 22–30.

Crane assists the therapist in making sense of the managed care medical context, while offering useful strategies for working effectively within HMOs.

Doherty, W. J. (1985). Family intervention in health care. *Family Relations, 34,* 129–137.

A good overview of the historical development and research on family interventions in health care is presented in this special issue on families and health care.

Doherty, W. J., & Baird, M. A. (1983). *Family therapy and family medicine: Toward the primary care of families.* New York: Guilford Press.

This book should be on the reading list of anyone interested in family health—physician or therapist. The authors describe five levels of physician involvement with families. These levels have been adopted as a fundamental framework for the field.

---

[1]Timothy F. Dwyer, Gary H. Bischof, Jacqueline L. Braeger, Carlos Leiro, and Philip J. Perez contributed to an earlier draft of this annotated bibliography as part of a Group Study on Family Systems Medicine in the Marriage and Family Therapy Doctoral Program at Purdue University.

Doherty, W. J., & Baird, M. A. (Eds.). (1987). *Family-centered medical care: A clinical casebook.* New York: Guilford Press.

The authors further clarify their five levels of physician involvement through numerous case examples of each level. Medical and mental health providers present cases, interspersed with comments from the editors, to illustrate family-centered medical care.

Doherty, W. J., & Campbell, T. (1988). *Families and health.* Newbury Park, CA: Sage.

This book contains an excellent summary of research on families and health. The authors also present a Family Health and Illness Cycle Model that defines the typical phases of a family's experience with illness and the health-care system.

Dym, B., & Berman, S. (1986). The primary health care team: Family physician and family therapy in joint practice. *Family Systems Medicine, 7,* 9–21.

This article presents an excellent example of family systems medicine in which primary care partnerships, consisting of a family physician and family therapist, see patients together in the same office. The authors view initial joint interviews as the cornerstone of accurate assessment and diagnosis of patients. They also claim that such collaboration will result in long-term cost-effectiveness.

Engel, G. L. (1977). The need for a new medical model: A challenge for biomedicine. *Science, 196,* 129–136.

In this landmark article, Engel proposes the biopsychosocial model of medicine, which serves as one of the theoretical foundations for the area of family systems medicine.

Engel, G. L. (1980). The clinical application of the biopsychosocial model. *American Journal of Psychiatry, 137,* 535–544.

Engel further explicates the clinical application of the biopsychosocial model in this important foundational work.

Illness in the family: Will systems thinking revolutionize medical treatment? *Family Therapy Networker* (1993, Vol. 17, January/February). Washington, DC: Family Therapy Networker.

This issue devotes several pages (pp. 18–43) to the role of family therapy in medicine and includes articles on medical family therapy and work with brain injury and cancer patients.

Glenn, M. (1985). Toward collaborative family-oriented health care. *Family Systems Medicine, 3,* 466–475.

Glenn provides a summary of the history of collaborative practice between physicians and several social science disciplines, particularly family therapy. He also gives a general overview of collaborative family health care, but does not address pragmatic practice issues.

Griffith, J. L., & Griffith, M. E. (1994). *The body speaks: Therapeutic dialogues for mind–body problems.* New York: Basic Books.

Replete with intriguing case examples, this book describes a narrative therapy for patients who present with somatic symptoms that arise at the complex mind–body interface. The authors also offer some creative ideas on the use of medication with these complex and often frustrating patients.

Hepworth, J., & Jackson, M. (1985). Health care for families: Models of collaboration between family therapists and family physicians. *Family Relations, 34,* 123–127.

This early article on models of collaboration between family therapists and family physicians uses the example of the death of a family member to describe several types of collaboration.

Hepworth, J., Gavazzi, S. M., Adlin, M. S., & Miller, W. L. (1988). Training and collaboration: Internships for family therapy students in a medical setting. *Family Systems Medicine, 6,* 69–79.

This article offers candid and personal perspectives (from a family therapy intern, family therapy supervisor, family medicine resident, and medical faculty member) of several persons involved in a family therapy internship in a medical setting.

Leahey, M., & Wright, L. M. (Eds.). (1987). *Families and life-threatening illness.* Springhouse, PA: Springhouse.

In this edited volume, the authors address nursing assessments and interventions of individuals and families with various life-threatening illnesses. Other titles in this family nursing series include *Families and Chronic Illness* (by the same editors) and *Families and Psychosocial Problems.*

McDaniel, S. H., Campbell, T. L., & Seaburn, D. B. (1990). *Family-oriented primary care: A manual for medical providers.* New York: Springer-Verlag.

Faculty in the University of Rochester's well-regarded Department of Family Medicine have compiled a practical manual for health-care providers interested in adopting a family-centered approach. This manual is a must for those teaching family systems to medical providers.

McDaniel, S. H., Hepworth, J., & Doherty, W. J. (1992). *Medical family therapy: A biopsychosocial approach to families with health problems.* New York: Basic Books.

Three pioneering family therapists in this area collaborate on what has become the bible for family therapists engaged in family systems medicine. Don't leave home as a medical family therapist without it.

Mauksch, L. B., & Leahy, D. (1993). Collaboration between primary care medicine and mental health in an HMO. *Family Systems Medicine, 11,* 121–135.

This article details how one large HMO has worked to dissolve inherent systemic barriers to collaboration. Data were collected from 15-person round-table interviews, followed by individual interviews with various medical, mental health, and business professionals of the HMO, yielding an uncommon insiders' view.

Ramsey, C. N. (Ed.). (1989). *Family systems in medicine.* New York: Guilford Press.

This academic volume brings together prominent scholars from the fields of family systems and medicine to address theoretical, research, and practice issues at the intersection of these fields.

Rolland, J. S. (1988). Family systems and chronic illness: A typological model. *Family Process, 27,* 143–168.

In this article, Rolland proposes a comprehensive conceptual typology of chronic illness that provides a framework whereby the relationship between individual and family dynamics, and chronic disease can be understood. He highlights onset, course, outcome, and degree of incapacitation as four significant dimensions of chronic illness.

Rolland, J. S. (1987). Chronic illness and the life cycle: A conceptual framework. *Family Process, 26,* 203–221.

Rolland provides a conceptual framework for thinking about the systems interface between chronic illness, individual development, and family life cycles. He also incorporates an analysis of the transgenerational aspects of illness, loss, and crisis. He uses clinical vignettes to elucidate this conceptual framework.

Rolland, J. S. (1994). *Families, illness, and disability: An integrative treatment model.* New York: Basic Books.

This is a natural extension of Rolland's two previous articles. In this book, Rolland distinguishes himself as a clear and comprehensive conceptual thinker in the area of family systems medicine. This is a must-read for those interested in helping families touched by chronic illness.

Saba, G., & Fink, D. (1985). Systems medicine and systems therapy: A call to a natural collaboration. *Journal of Strategic and Systemic Family Therapy, 4,* 15–31.

Saba and Fink offer a substantive overview of the "state of the art" in family systems medicine up to 1985. A particular strength of this article is the inclusion of historical information about the development of the family therapy field in relation to systems medicine. The authors also describe biological discoveries that influenced the development of systems theory.

Seaburn, D., Gawinski, B., Harp, J., McDaniel, S., Waxman, D., & Shields, C. (1993). Family systems therapy in a primary care medical setting: The Rochester experience. *Journal of Marital and Family Therapy, 19,* 177–190.

The authors explore physicians and patients' expectations of family therapists in their family practice residency setting. They also highlight other contextual factors that impinge on practice in this setting. This article provides an excellent insiders' view of one of the most prominent sites of collaborative family health care.

Seaburn, D., Lorenz, A., Gunn, W., Gawinski, B., & Mauksch, L. (1996). *Models of collaboration: A guide for mental health professionals working with health care practitioners.* New York: Basic Books.

This book describes several models of collaboration and illustrates these models through exemplary collaborative programs and settings. The authors include information from interviews they conducted with many of the leaders in the field. They also include chapters on the key ingredients of collaboration, outcome research, and training.

REFERENCES

Ackerman, F. (1989). Family systems therapy with a man with AIDS-related complex, *Family Systems Medicine, 7*(3), 292–304.

Adams-Westcott, J., & Isenbart, D. (1990). Using rituals to empower family members who have experienced child sexual abuse. In M. Durrant & C. White (Eds.), *Ideas for therapy with sexual abuse*. South Australia: Dulwich Centre Publications.

Anderson, H. (1991). Opening the door for change through continuing conversations. In T. Todd & M. Selekman (Eds.), *Family therapy approaches with adolescent substance abusers*. Boston: Allyn & Bacon.

Atwood, J. (1993). AIDS in African American and Hispanic adolescents: A multisystemic approach. *American Journal of Family Therapy, 21*(4), 333–351.

Beckerman, N. (1994). Psychosocial tasks facing parents whose adult child has AIDS. *Family Therapy, 21*(3), 209–216.

Berg, I., & Gallagher, D. (1991). Solution-focused brief treatment with adolescent substance abusers. In T. Todd & M. Selekman (Eds.), *Family therapy approaches with adolescent substance abusers*. Boston: Allyn & Bacon.

Berg, I. K., & Miller, S. D. (1992). Working with the problem drinker. New York: Norton.

Berson, N., & Herman-Giddens, M. (1994). Recognizing invasive genital care practices: A form of child sexual abuse. *The APSAC Advisor, 7*(1), 13–14.

Black, L. (1993). AIDS and secrets. In E. Imber-Black (Ed.), *Secrets in families and family therapy*. New York: Norton.

Bloch, D. (1983). Family systems medicine: The field and the journal. *Family Systems Medicine, 1*, 3–11.

Bor, R., & Elford, J. (1994). *The family and HIV*. London, UK: Redwood Books.

Boyd-Franklin, N. (1992). Racism, secret-keeping, and African-American families. In E. Imber-Black (Ed.), *Secrets in family therapy*. New York: Norton.

Boyd-Franklin, N., Aleman, J., Steiner, G., Drelich, E., & Norford, B. (1995). Family systems interventions and family therapy. In N. Boyd-Franklin, G. L. Steiner, & M. G. Boland (Eds.), *Children, families, and HIV/AIDS: Psychosocial and therapeutic issues*. New York: Guilford Press.

Boyd-Franklin, N., & Boland, M. (1995). A multisystems approach to service delivery for HIV/AIDS families. In N. Boyd-Franklin, G. L. Steiner, & M. G. Boland (Eds.), *Children, families, and HIV/AIDS: Psychosocial and therapeutic issues*. New York: Guilford Press.

Boyd-Franklin, N., Steiner, G. L., Boland, M. G. (1995). *Children, families, and HIV/AIDS: Psychosocial and therapeutic issues*. New York: Guilford Press.

Britton, P., & Zarski, J. (1989). HIV spectrum disorders and the family: Selected interventions based on stylistic dimensions. *AIDS-Care, 1*(1), 85–92.

Campbell, T. L., & Patterson, J. M. (1995). The effectiveness of family interventions in the treatment of physical illness. *Journal of Marital and Family Therapy, 21,* 545–583.

Cohan, N., & Atwood, J. (1994). Women and AIDS: The social construction of gender and disease. *Family Systems Medicine, 12*(1), 5–20.

Curtis, J. (1989). Treating AIDS: A family therapy perspective. In C. Kain (Ed.), *No longer immune: A counselor's guide to AIDS*. Alexandria, VA: American Association for Counseling and Development.

Dane, B. (1991). Anticipatory mourning of middle-aged parents of adult children with AIDS. *Families in Society, 72*(2), 108–115.

Davis, D. D. (1987). *Alcoholism treatment*. New York: Gardner.

Doherty, W. J., & Baird, M. A. (1983). *Family therapy and family medicine: Toward the primary care of families*. New York: Guilford Press.

Doherty, W. J., & Baird, M. A. (Eds.). (1987). *Family-centered medical care: A clinical casebook*. New York: Guilford Press.

Dolan, Y. M. (1989). "Only once if I really mean it": Brief treatment of a previously dissociated incest case. *Journal of Strategic and Systemic Therapies, 8*(4), 3–8.

Dolan, Y. M. (1991). *Resolving sexual abuse*. New York: Norton.

Donovan, D. M. (1988). Assessment of addictive behaviors: Implications of an emerging biopsychosocial model. In D. M. Donovan & G. A Marlatt (Eds.), *Assessment of addictive behaviors*. New York: Guilford Press.

Edwards, M. E., & Steinglass, P. (1995). Family therapy treatment outcomes for alcoholism. *Journal of Marital and Family Therapy, 21*(4), 475–510.

Elkin, M. (1984). *Families under the influence*. New York: Norton.

Engel, G. L. (1977). The need for a new medical model: A challenge for biomedicine. *Science, 196,* 129–136.

Fish, V., & Faynik, C. (1989). Treatment of incest families with the father temporarily removed: A structural approach. *Journal of Strategic and Systemic Therapies, 8*(4), 53–63.

Friedman, A., & Granick, S. (1990). *Family therapy for adolescent drug abuse*. Lexington, KY: Lexington Books.

Gelinas, D. J. (1983). The persisting negative effects of incest. *Psychiatry, 46,* 312–332.

Gilgun, J. F. (1991). Resilience and the intergenerational transmission of child sexual abuse. In M. Q. Patton (Ed.), *Family sexual abuse: Frontline research and evaluation*. Newbury Park, CA: Sage.

Glenn, M. (1987). *Collaborative health care: A family-oriented model*. New York: Praeger.

Glynn, T. (1981). From family to peer: A review of transitions of influence among drug using youth. *Journal of Youth and Adolescence, 10,* 363–384.

Glynn, T. (1984). Adolescent drug use and the family environment: A review. *Journal of Drug Issues, 14,* 271–295.

Gomez, K., Haiken, H., & Lewis, S. (1995). Support group for children with HIV/AIDS. In N. Boyd-Franklin, G. L. Steiner & M. G. Boland (Eds.), *Children, families, and HIV/AIDS: Psychosocial and therapeutic issues.* New York: Guilford Press.

Harbin, H., & Mazair, H. (1975). The families of drug abusers: A literature review. *Family Process, 14,* 411–431.

Henggeler, S., Borduin, C., Melton, G., Mann, B., Smith, L., Hall, J., Cone, L., & Fucci, B. (1991). Effects of multisystemic therapy on drug use and abuse in serious juvenile offenders: A progress report from two outcome studies. *Family Dynamics of Addiction Quarterly, 1,* 40–51.

Hindman, J. (1989). *Just before dawn.* Ontario, OR: Alexandria Associates.

Holder, H., Longabaugh, R., Miller, W. R., & Rubonis, A. V. (1991). The cost effectiveness of treatment for alcoholism: A first approximation. *Journal of Studies on Alcohol, 52,* 517–540.

James, B., & Nasjleti, M. (1983). *Treating sexually abused children and their families.* Palo Alto, CA: Consulting Psychologist Press.

Joanning, H., Thomas, F., Quinn, W., & Mullen, R. (1992). Treating adolescent drug abuse: A comparison of family systems therapy, group therapy, and family drug education. *Journal of Marital and Family Therapy, 18,* 345–356.

Katon, W., & Gonzales, J. (1994). A review of randomized trials of psychiatric consultation–liaison studies in primary care. *Psychosomatics, 35,* 268–278.

Landau-Stanton, T., Clements, C. D., & Associates. (1993). *AIDS health and mental health: A primary sourcebook.* New York: Brunner/Mazel.

Levenson, J. L. (1992). Psychosocial interventions in chronic medical illness: An overview of outcome research. *General Hospital Psychiatry, 14S,* 43S–49S.

Levine, C. (1994). AIDS and the changing concept of family. In R. Bor & J. Elford (Eds.), *The Family and HIV.* London: Redwood Books.

Lewis, R. A., Piercy, F. P., Sprenkle, D. H., & Trepper, T. S. (1990). The Purdue Brief Therapy Model for adolescent substance abusers. In T. Todd & M. Selekman (Eds.), *Family therapy approaches with adolescent substance abusers.* Boston: Allyn & Bacon.

Liddle, H. A., & Dakof, G. A. (1995). Efficacy of family therapy for drug abuse: Promising but not definitive. *Journal of Marital and Family Therapy, 21*(4), 511–544.

Liddle, H. A., Dakof, G. A., & Diamond, G. (1992). Adolescent substance abuse: Multidimensional family therapy in action. In E. Kaufman & P. Kaufmann (Eds.), *Family therapy of drug and alcohol abuse.* Boston: Allyn & Bacon.

Maddock, J. U., & Larson, N. R. (1995). *Incestuous families: An ecological approach to understanding and treatment.* New York: Norton.

Maloney, B. (1988). The legacy of AIDS: Challenge for the next century. *Journal of Marital and Family Therapy, 14*(2), 143–150.

Maltz, W. (1988). Identifying and healing the sexual repercussions of incest: A couples therapy approach. *Journal of Sex and Marital Therapy, 14*(2), 142–170.

McDaniel, S. H., Hepworth, J., & Doherty, W. J. (1992). *Medical family therapy: A biopsychosocial approach to families with health problems.* New York: Basic Books.

Miller, R., Goldman, E., & Bor, R. (1994). Application of family systems approach to working with people affected by HIV disease. In R. Bor & J. Elford (Eds.), *The family and HIV.* London: Redwood Books.

Mumford, E., & Schlesinger, H. J. (1987). Assessing consumer benefit: Cost offset as an incidental effect of psychotherapy. *General Hospital Psychiatry, 9,* 360–363.

Mumford, E., Schlesinger, H. J., Glass, G., Patrick, C., & Cuerdon, T. (1984). A new look at evidence about reduced cost of medical utilization following mental health treatment. *American Journal of Psychiatry, 141,* 1145–1158.

O'Farrell, T. J. (Ed.). (1993). *Treating alcohol problems: Marital and family interventions.* New York: Guilford Press.

Peters, S. D., Wyatt, G. E., & Finkelhor, D. (1986). Prevalence. In D. Finkelhor (Ed.), *Sourcebook on child sexual abuse.* Newbury Park, CA: Sage.

Piercy, F., & Frankel, B. (1986). *Training manual: Purdue brief family therapy.* West Lafayette, IN: Center for Instructional Services.

Piercy, F., & Frankel, B. (1989). The evolution of an integrative family therapy for substance abusing adolescents: Toward the mutual enhancement of research and practice. *Journal of Family Psychology, 3*(1), 5–25.

Piercy, F., Trepper, T., & Jurich, J. (1993). The role of family therapy in decreasing HIV high-risk behaviors among adolescents. *AIDS Education and Prevention, 5*(1), 71–86.

Ransom, D. (1984). Random notes: Patients have families. *Family Systems Medicine, 2,* 109–113.

Russell, D. E. H. (1986). *The secret of trauma: Incest influences of girls and women.* New York: Basic Books.

Schlossberger, E., & Hecker, L. (1996). HIV & family therapists' duty to warn: A legal and ethical analysis. *Journal of Marital and Family Therapy, 22,* 27–40.

Sheinberg, M., True, F., & Frankel, P. (1994). Treating the sexually abused child: A recursive, multimodal program. *Family Process, 33,* 263–276.

Shiga, N., Endo, Y., Tobe, S., & Yanagihara, S. (1992). Family counseling for HIV/AIDS patient. *Japanese Journal of Family Psychology, 6*(2), 121–132.

Stanton, M. D. (1978). The family and drug misuse: A bibliography. *American Journal of Drug and Alcohol Abuse, 5,* 151–170.

Stanton, M. D. (1979a). *Family structure and drug abuse: A review.* Report prepared for the Office of Program Development and Analysis, National Institute on Drug Abuse, Rockville, MD.

Stanton, M. D. (1979b). Family treatment approaches to drug abuse problems: A review. *Family Process, 18,* 251–280.

Stanton, M. D. (1981). An integrated structural/strategic approach to family therapy. *Journal of Marital and Family Therapy, 7,* 427–439.

Stanton, M. D., Todd, T., & Associates. (1982). *The family therapy of drug abuse and addiction.* New York: Guilford Press.

Szapocznik, J., Kurtines, W., Hervis, O., & Spencer, F. (1984). One person family therapy. In B. Lubin & W. A. O'Connor (Eds.), *Ecological approaches to clinical and community psychology.* New York: Wiley.

Szapocznik, J., Kurtines, W., & Contributors. (1989). *Breakthroughs in family therapy with drug abusing problem youth.* New York: Springer.

Szapocznik, J., Kurtines, W., Foote, F., Perez-Vidal, A., & Hervis, O. (1986). Conjoint versus one person family therapy: Further evidence for the effectiveness of conducting family therapy through one person. *Journal of Consulting and Clinical Psychology, 54,* 395–397.

Todd, T., & Selekman, M. (Eds.). (1991). *Principles of family therapy for adolescent substance abuse.* Boston: Allyn & Bacon.

Treadway, D. (1989). *Before it's too late: Working with substance abuse in the family.* New York: Norton.

Trepper, T. S., & Barrett, M. J. (1984). *Systemic treatment of incest: A therapeutic handbook.* New York: Brunner/Mazel.

Walker, G. (1991). *In the midst of winter: Systemic therapy with families, couples, and individuals with AIDS infection.* New York: Norton.

Walker, G. (1992). Family therapy in the context of AIDS. In T. Akamatsu, M. Stephenes, S. Hobfoll, & J. Crowther (Eds.), *Family health psychology.* Washington, DC: Hemisphere.

Wetchler, J. L., McCollum, E., Nelson, T., Trepper, T., & Lewis, R. (1993). Systemic couples therapy for alcohol-abusing women. In T. J. O'Farrell (Ed.), *Treating alcohol problems: Marital and family interventions.* New York: Guilford Press.

Wright, L. M., & Leahey, M. (1987). *Families and chronic illness.* Springhouse, PA: Springhouse.

Wyatt, G. E., & Peters, S. D. (1986). Issues in the definition of child sexual abuse in prevalence research. *Child Abuse and Neglect, 10,* 231–240.

13

Supervision and Training

DOUGLAS H. SPRENKLE
SUSAN G. WILKIE

STILL A RELATIVELY young field, marriage and family therapy seems to be emerging from its adolescence, and concomitantly, the subspecialty of supervision and training has experienced a childhood "growth spurt." The availability of literature on family therapy supervision and training has grown in the past two decades. There are now several books (Liddle, Breunlin, & Schwartz, 1988; Piercy, 1985; Todd & Storm, in press; Whiffen & Byng-Hall, 1982) on this topic. Particularly notable is the Liddle et al. (1988) *Handbook of Family Therapy Supervision and Training*, which attends to the teaching of particular models of supervision, the pragmatics of supervision, as well as contexts for training. The more recent Todd and Storm (in press), *The Complete Systemic Supervisor: Context, Philosophy, and Pragmatics* is a comprehensive look at the history and future of this emerging subdiscipline. Additionally, different perspectives on supervision and training have become available through a large number of published articles, book chapters and many workshops offered at regional and national conferences of the American Association for Marriage and Family Therapy (AAMFT).

In the last decade, social constructionism has greatly impacted the thinking of marriage and family therapists, and provides both challenges and opportunities for supervision (Bobele, Gardner, & Biever, 1995). Issues of power and authority have emerged to the forefront of training, supervision, and treatment.

The predominant approach in supervision theory building has been the extrapolation of family therapy approaches to the supervisory experience; unfortunately, this body of literature remains impressionistic and atheoretical. Furthermore, this literature continues to lack empirical verification, as attested in the research reviews by Kniskern and Gurman (1979), Avis and Sprenkle (1990), and Liddle (1991). These authors delineate important, researchable questions as a framework for the future of training and supervision research.

BASIC TERMS

Although the terms "therapy," "training," "supervision," and "consultation" are widely used in the literature, they are seldom defined and differentiated clearly.

Family "therapy," by definition, is the treatment of dysfunctional interpersonal systems of individuals who consider themselves to be "family." In most cases, the aim of therapy is to join the family in an effort to change, confront, or cope with present conflicts and problems. In this decade, the basic relationship of therapist to client has become more collaborative rather than complementary, with the therapist assuming a synergetic problem-solving role, avoiding taking the hierarchically superior position of "expert." This collaborative stance does not deny the inequities embedded in the therapeutic process. The therapist is more powerful by virtue of expertise, position, status, and being paid for therapy (Avis, 1991). The hierarchical nature of the relationship may be minimized or emphasized, depending on the therapeutic approach, but paramount is the therapist's ethical use of his or her position to empower individuals and families while engendering healthy functioning and psychological growth.

Family therapy is impacted by clients' expectations. Clients expect the therapist to support, guide, direct, or challenge them out of their difficulties. Unlike a decade ago, when the primary responsibility for the process and outcome of therapy was placed on the therapist, today, as Schwartz (1995) and many others recognize, the primary responsibility for creating change is shared between the therapist and the family. Along with the new collaborative attitudes and language of family therapy, issues of intimacy, authority, and gender have emerged as significant therapeutic categories.

"Training," is a process by which individuals learn to become therapists and acquire specific marriage and family therapy education. "Training" refers to the broad, comprehensive teaching of family therapy theories and techniques (such as in seminars, workshops, courses, and programs) that either precedes or occurs alongside the development of a trainee's clinical skills through supervised clinical practice (Saba & Liddle, 1986). Training involves both those learning to be therapists and experienced therapists who are trainers assisting in the learning process. Trainers are concerned with a general transmission of conceptual and clinical knowledge along with the promotion of personal awareness and growth of trainees. The trainer–trainee relationship, a form of teacher–student relationship, inherently involves degrees of complimentarity but, like the contemporary client–therapist relationship, today collaborative interaction is more valued. Informed by a postmodern philosophy, the learning process is becoming more collaborative and egalitarian. Anderson and Swim (1993) view the teacher's role as being an expert on process and the student's role as expert on "his or her problem, the expert on what he or she wants to learn and how the teacher can help him or her learn" (p. 151). In this view, "both are learners."

Sometimes the trainer's hierarchical position in relation to the trainee may be determined by institutional position. A professor, for example, has a more powerful position than students, even if the professor knows less than they do. Schwartz (1988) recommends that there be a wide enough discrepancy between trainer and trainee expertise to allow the trainee to trust that there is something to learn from the relationship. Typically, the trainer does have valuable expertise to share, and as training progresses, the experience of the trainer and trainees becomes less disparate, and the relationship naturally becomes more symmetrical.

"Supervision" refers to a continuous relationship, in a real-world work setting, which focuses on the specific development of a therapist's skills as he or she gains practical experience in treating client families (Saba & Liddle, 1986). It is the setting in which a less experienced therapist grapples with theory and case material to produce a unique and competent clinical style. Supervision is recognized as the part of the overall training of family therapists that deals with modifying their actual in-therapy behaviors (Lambert & Arnold, 1987). Focused attention on specific cases, therefore, is the hallmark of supervision. Although the supervision situation inherently possesses a power differential, the last 10 years have witnessed significant changes in the conceptualization of family therapy supervision.

The supervisory relationship involves the potential for considerable complementarity, since the settings in which supervisors operate (e.g., universities, social service agencies) confer authority on them in a variety of ways. For example, a supervisor has direct responsibility for the quality of work performed by the therapist being supervised. In actual practice, there is considerable variation in the supervisor–supervisee relationship, depending upon such factors as the skill level of the supervisee and the philosophy and approach of supervisor. Some models of supervision attempt to minimize the hierarchical nature of the relationship (e.g., functional family therapy, feminist approaches), whereas for other models, the supervisor maintains a clear position of authority (e.g., strategic approach, structural model; Kaiser, 1992). Additionally, at one extreme might be the supervision of beginners, involving close oversight and frequent suggestions; at the other extreme would be the supervision of experienced therapists for the purpose of fostering creativity and autonomy. Therefore, the relationship can range from one that is mostly complementary to one that is primarily symmetrical (Magee, 1985).

"Consultation" differs from supervision in that it is a short-term, symmetrical, peer-like relationship between a therapist and an invited expert. Consultation provides a setting to discuss difficult cases and get feedback, suggestions, and evaluation. The consultant's power is derived from his or her expertise and skill, as well as the therapist's invitation. The consultant has no formal stake in evaluating the therapist's progress in learning or job performance (Nielsen & Kaslow, 1980). Even highly experienced family therapists can benefit from the input of consultants for the purposes of overcoming therapeutic impasses, verifying diagnostic impressions, evaluating intervention strategies, and discussing clinical and ethical concerns. All therapists should be committed to an ongoing, lifelong quest for professional and personal growth, and consultations provide one avenue for fulfilling this commitment. Consultations can take place in a variety of forms, including discussion, observation through a one-way mirror, tape reviews, and cotherapy.

HISTORY AND OVERVIEW
OF THE STATE OF THE FIELD

Numbers and Types of Programs

Supervision and training take place in two major settings: (1) academic degree-granting programs, and (2) free-standing institutes. Programs may also be divided into (1) those that are accredited by the American Association for Marriage and Family Therapy (AAMFT) and (2) those that are not so accredited. The largest number of programs are freestanding and nonaccredited. Bloch and Weiss (1981) reported on the existence of over 175 training programs, only about 55 of which were degree granting. As of the winter of 1996, there were 75 commission-accredited programs, with the breakdown as follows: (1) 38 master's, plus 5 candidacy master's programs; (2) 11 doctoral, plus 1 candidacy doctoral program; and (3) 20 postdegree-level programs.

Brief History of Training Programs

Accredited and nonaccredited training programs vary in the degree to which their histories have been documented. In general, the histories on nonaccredited programs are less likely to have been written and disseminated. Like accredited programs, nonaccredited programs vary in quality;

however, because they are not standardized, their curricula may vary more than accredited programs. Because nonaccredited programs vary widely in course offerings, trainers, and physical facilities, these programs' merit must be evaluated on an individual basis. Accredited programs subject themselves to review by AAMFT's Commission on Accreditation for Marriage and Family Therapy Education (COAMFTE), which has been recognized by the U.S. Department of Education as the only official accrediting body for training programs in marriage and family therapy. The COAMFTE is also recognized by the Council on the Regulation of Post-Secondary Accreditation (CORPA). The COAMFTE periodically publishes rigorous requirements in terms of organizational guidelines, curriculum, faculty, physical facilities, and clinical training.

The early history of accredited programs is found in Nichols (1979), Smith and Nichols (1979), and Burman and Dixon-Murphy (1979). Briefly, although AAMFT (originally the American Association of Marriage Counselors, or AAMC) was founded in 1942, it did not publish standards on training centers in postgraduate professional marriage counseling until 1958. Standards for degree-granting programs were published in 1959. In its early years, AAMC was more concerned with establishing standards for marriage counselors (in 1949) and centers for marriage counseling (in 1953) than it was with training. It also assumed that marriage counseling was a professional activity that people entered after having earned a graduate degree in another discipline. Marriage counseling was typically learned through postgraduate internships (Nichols, 1979). This seemed reasonable, in that early practitioners considered marriage counseling supplemental to their primary occupations as psychologists, psychiatrists, social workers, ministers, and so forth (Broderick & Schrader, 1981).

By the time of the 1959 standards on graduate education in marriage counseling, certain universities had begun to develop graduate programs, which implied that marriage counseling was a separate area of graduate education and a professional field in its own right (Nichols, 1979). The early standards called for a 4-year-minimum doctoral program with internship. As the field developed, it was assumed that training would cease to be done primarily at the postdoctoral level and shift to doctoral programs in marriage counseling itself. During the 1950s, somewhat loosely defined doctoral programs could be found at Columbia University Teachers College, the University of Southern California, Florida State University, and Purdue University (Nichols, 1979).

The growth that subsequently occurred in graduate programs during the 1960s, 1970s, and 1980s has been primarily at the master's level. By 1971, AAMFT's standards concerning training centers in marriage and family counseling clearly designated the master's degree as the entry-level credential. By 1974, standards for degree programs were applicable to both master's and doctoral programs. The Commission on Accreditation for

Marriage and Family Therapy Education continually develops more stringent requirements for commission accredited programs, revising its standards about every 5 years. The most recently revised guidelines will be available in 1996.

Two of the oldest, accredited, freestanding programs are the Marriage Council of Philadelphia, which has offered training since 1947, and the Blanton–Peale Graduate Institute, which has offered training since 1956 (Burman & Dixon-Murphy, 1979). The freestanding programs have special appeal to those who already have advanced degrees and seek intensive training in marriage and family therapy, free of the constraints of a degree program, and lend themselves to the needs of part-time students.

Who Are the Supervisors?

There have been four studies of approved supervisors in AAMFT (Everett, 1980; McKenzie, Atkinson, Quinn, & Heath, 1986; Nichols, Nichols, & Hardy, 1990; Saba & Liddle, 1986). McKenzie et al. (1986) also included responses from half of the membership of the American Family Therapy Academy (AFTA). Nichols et al. (1990) conducted a 10-year replication study of Everett's (1980) survey of approved supervisors in AAMFT.

These studies indicate that demographic, educational, and supervisory work settings have changed in the 10 years preceding 1990. In the mid-1980s, about two-thirds of supervisors were men with an average age from mid- to late 40s. By 1990, there was a significant increase in the proportion of female supervisors and younger supervisors (under age 45; Nichols et al., 1990). The overwhelming majority were Caucasian, and over 50% had earned doctorates. McKenzie et al. reported a slight increase in master's-level supervisors over Everett's (1980; data gathered in 1976) figures. McKenzie et al. (1986) reported a significantly larger percentage who had less than 5 years of supervisory experience, whereas Nichols et al. (1990), found a mean MFT supervisory experience of 9.2 years. The largest group of supervisors, 42% in the McKenzie et al. study, supervise within their private practice. Although, Nichols et al. agree that private practice is the most common setting for supervising, their percentage was much smaller (27.6%), further stating that compared to the earlier study by Everett (1980) the supervisors were more likely to be supervising in formal settings such as private training institutes and less likely than their predecessors (39.4%) to be dealing with supervisees in private practice offices. McKenzie et al. (1986) also report a significantly smaller percentage (15.4%) of supervisors currently working within an educational setting than that reported in the earlier Everett study (26.3%). Saba and Liddle (1986), however, reported that AFTA subjects listed academic departments as their primary training–supervising site. Nichols et al. (1990) reported that 15% of their sample worked in accredited programs.

Interestingly, in the earlier three studies, none of the respondents listed "marriage and family therapist" as their primary professional identification. However, Nichols et al. (1990) found a greater number of supervisors identifying themselves as "marriage and family therapists," regardless of their education.

Methods Employed

Data on the actual use of the various supervisory modalities (see "Key Clinical Concepts" section for definitions) are found in studies by Henry (1983), McKenzie et al. (1986), Nichols et al. (1990), Saba and Liddle (1986), Sprenkle (1988), and Wetchler, Piercy, and Sprenkle (1989). The Saba and Liddle (1986) and Mckenzie et al. (1986) studies (of AAMFT-approved supervisors and AFTA members) suggested that even though supervisors believe that live supervision and videotape supervision are the most effective modalities, these were, in fact, used less frequently than such procedures as reviewing audiotapes and case notes. Studies of supervision in more formal training centers (Henry, 1983; Sprenkle, 1988) found that video and live supervision procedures predominate. In 1990, Nichols et al. reported that live supervision and process reports are used by approximately three out of five approved supervisors. The most dramatic change between 1980 and 1990 was the use of video recording, which nearly doubled (62.7% of approved supervisors). Wetchler et al. (1989) surveyed a randomly selected group of AAMFT-approved supervisors and their supervisees. Both groups rated videotape supervision as most effective, although individual case consultation was used most.

Theoretical Orientations

The earlier studies that examined theoretical orientations of supervisors–trainers indicated that the modal professional was not a "purist." The majority espoused an eclectic or integrative view. More recent findings indicate a decline in eclecticism as an orientation, with the major shift toward a systems orientation (Nichols et al., 1990). Additionally, Nichols et al. reported a decline in the popularity of personal therapy as part of training. With regard to training, the McKenzie et al. (1986), Sprenkle (1988), and Henry (1983) studies all found that the structural and strategic models were taught most frequently. Also relatively popular were experiential (Whitaker), communication/humanistic (Satir), and intergenerational (Bowen, Framo) approaches. No doubt, contemporary preferences would include a large percentage of trainers with orientations influenced by social construction-ism, including narrative, solution-focused and collaborative language system models.

KEY CONCEPTS AND CLINICAL SKILLS

Supervisory Modalities

Live Supervision

Live supervision entails the supervisor observing the therapy as it actually occurs. Eight different forms of live supervision (see Figure 13.1) can be delineated by using (1) temporal, (2) spatial, and (3) personnel dimensions. With regard to timing, live supervision can be "immediate" or "delayed." With regard to space, it can occur from within the therapy room or outside it. With regard to personnel, it can include one supervisor or a team of two or more persons.

The Temporal Dimension. Regarding timing, delayed feedback (given after the session is completed) is less popular than immediate feedback, since it offers no opportunity to engender during-therapy change. One advantage of delayed feedback is that it gives the therapist the opportunity to work "solo" (perhaps to increase his or her confidence). It also may serve as a "bridging modality" for therapists who will be moving on to settings where live supervision is not feasible.

Immediate feedback can occur through a variety of mechanisms. Two of the most popular are the telephone and the "bug in the ear." The latter entails the supervisor speaking to the therapist through a hearing-aid-type device, which may be either wireless or connected to the trainee by wire. Essentially, it is a one-way form of communication that, from the family's

	Individual supervision		Team supervision	
	Within room	Outside room	Within room	Outside room
Immediate				
Delayed				

FIGURE 13.1. Supervisory modalities for live supervision.

point of view, is unobtrusive. Earphone interventions are typically brief and direct, and if done skillfully, can be carried out as though the therapist originated them. Disadvantages include the inability to clarify messages and the potential for the therapist to become dependent on the supervisor (Byng-Hall, 1982).

A characteristic of the telephone that may be seen as either an advantage or a disadvantage is the fact that it interrupts the interaction of the session. As such, it serves as an intervention in and of itself, apart from the message being sent. This may be useful, for example, if the supervisor wants to stop an inappropriate or destructive family interaction. Also, there is the opportunity to clarify and/or amplify interventions, and communication is potentially two way. On the other hand, the telephone lacks the immediacy and unobtrusiveness of the earphone. A recent exploratory study by Frankel and Piercy (1990) examined the immediate effects of family therapy live supervision phone-ins on therapist and client behaviors, as well as the parallel process between live supervision and therapy. Findings suggest that effective use of "teaching" and "support" behaviors by the supervisor during phone-ins predicted change in parallel trainee behaviors, which seem to result in more cooperative behaviors from the family. Many creative ways in which to use the telephone in live supervision are described by Coppersmith (1980).

Other ways in which a supervisor may intervene immediately include coming into the room and giving directives either to the supervisee or directly to the family (a procedure used often by Salvador Minuchin). Or the supervisor may request that the therapist come out for a midsession conference. This request can be made by telephone, by earphone, or by knocking on the door. Of course, the therapist may come out on his or her own initiative. Finally, the supervisor (or team) may send the therapist written messages. Examples of the framing of such messages and their impact are described in Breunlin and Cade (1981). Smith, Smith, and Salts (1991) studied the impact of supervisor interruptions on participants of therapy. Their findings support the position that the probable benefits of live supervision outweigh the immediate and transitory costs of disruption to the therapy process; however, they do emphasize the need to familiarize clients with the process and advise paying close attention to possible effects of interruptions for the clients. Two general guidelines are offered: (1) keep interruptions to a minimum, and (2) avoid interrupting during emotionally intense moments.

The Spatial Dimension. Concerning the spatial dimension of live supervision, supervisory input is much more likely to come from outside the room than from within it. Since one-way mirrors are not always available, however, the supervisor (or team) may stay in the same room as the therapist and family. One article has called this "direct open supervision" (Olson & Pegg, 1979).

We also know of several centers in which behind-the-glass observation is possible, but direct open supervision is often the method of choice (Hoffman, 1993; Landau & Stanton, 1983). One potential advantage of the "open" method is that the family may benefit from hearing what the supervisor says. Another advantage is that the supervisor can better detect the emotional climate of the family from within the room. Disadvantages include loss of a different perspective that may come from spatial distance, the loss of leverage made possible by feedback outside of the family's awareness (including a markedly reduced potential for indirect interventions), and a reduced ability to use technical language. The supervisor may also be overly protective of the therapy, avoid conflict (and/or disagreement), or usurp the therapist's authority (Carter, 1982). Although the one-way mirror has been very useful in the history of marriage and family therapy, some current advances in the field contemplate its problematic nature. Young (1989/1990), in "A Critical Look at the One-Way Screen," raises some clinical, political, and ethical concerns. The author questions the value of seeing the mirror as a barrier distinguishing the "objective" from the "subjective." Young suggests viewing the mirror as "two-way" rather than one-way, recognizing that both in-front and behind-mirror positions offer different but valid views, and appreciating the constraints and strengths of each. Denying this poses danger regarding issues of power and hierarchy.

The Personnel Dimension. Concerning the personnel dimension, the field has witnessed an explosion in the use of team supervision approaches, probably due to the enormous influence of the Milan and Ackerman groups. Although there are no data on the matter, team supervision may be the norm rather than the exception in training settings where live supervision is practiced. Teams differ in a variety of ways, including the extent to which they are composed of peers (as opposed to being formed around a senior supervisor) and participate in the formulation of interventions. Team supervision has the advantages of facilitating brainstorming (and hence of enhancing creativity), of developing camaraderie among team members, and of enhancing learning among team members as well as therapists (Heath, 1983). Indeed, Roberts (1983) considers the team an important "third tier" (alongside the therapist and supervisor) that needs to be nurtured every bit as much as the therapist. Roberts offers guidelines for the development of effective collaborative therapy teams.

Anderson (1987), Coppersmith (1980), DeShazer and Molnar (1984), Landau and Stanton (1983), Papp (1980), and Roberts et al. (1989) offer rich illustrations of ways in which teams can be used in highly creative ways to affect the therapy process. For example, the team can be used as "Greek chorus" to support, confront, provoke, confuse, or challenge the family. The therapist can side with or oppose the chorus. In the latter case, this "split" highlights the family's ambivalence about change and gives the therapist leverage to capitalize on resistance (e.g., "The team is convinced you can't make this change, but I believe you've got the stuff to do it"). Roberts et al. (1989) offer a type of dual supervision in which both an observing team and a treatment team work behind the mirror at the same time. Anderson and his colleagues (1987), influenced by constructivism, developed the reflecting team concept. The reflecting team is a team behind the one-way mirror that watches a session with a family. The family and the therapist then go behind the mirror and watch the team, now in the therapy room, discuss their perceptions of the interview. Alternately, the reflection team remains in the observation room, but the lighting and sound are reversed. In yet another variation, the reflecting team comes into the therapy room.

Recognizing the major implications of the reflecting team as well as the "new epistemology" for supervision in marriage and family therapy, Prest, Darden, and Keller (1990) adapted the reflecting team concept for use in group supervision. This adaptation offers a supervision group and a reflecting team at two different levels. The reflecting team observes the group supervision process from behind a one-way mirror, and after about 45 minutes, the two groups switch rooms, and the reflecting team discusses their observations regarding the supervision process. Among other things, this affords the supervisee the opportunity to be a "fly on the wall" (metalevel) to his or her own process.

Whatever the form of live supervision, it is clear that the basic modality has advantages. Any other method is ex post facto, in that there is no opportunity to influence therapeutic interventions (live supervision with delayed feedback is also ex post facto). Like videotape review (to be discussed), live supervision provides reliable information about the therapist's nonverbal as well as verbal skills, but, unlike video review, it gives the supervisor some sense of the emotional climate of the session. If this immediacy is buffered by a one-way mirror, the method also provides a metaperspective on the therapy that is quite advantageous (Aradi, 1985). The supervisor is freer to concentrate upon patterns and to detect ways the therapist might be participating in dysfunctional transactions (Berger & Dammann, 1982). Moreover, family members generally like live supervision procedures (Piercy, Sprenkle, & Constantine, 1986). The most obvious disadvantages of live supervision are the physical and mechanical requirements. In addition, as Beroza (1983) notes, the modality has the potential for undermining therapists confidence. Postmodern thinking, in addition to current theoretical approaches, has shed some critical light on how we view and practice live supervision of marital and family therapy (Liddle & Halpin, 1978; Young, 1989/1990).

Ex Post Facto Methods of Supervision

The Case Presentation. The case presentation entails the therapist giving a verbal report of a session or case to the supervisor or supervisory group.

As noted earlier, the method is used quite frequently and is often a supplement to other more expensive forms such as live supervision or video review. In addition to low cost and convenience, the method has the advantage of disciplining the therapist to integrate data and present them as a coherent whole. Case supervision helps train the memory to review and think about cases; it invites the therapist to learn to trust his or her memory. A therapist who is unable to condense the relevant aspects of a session and does not communicate well with supervisors will usually have similar difficulty carrying this out in therapy. Moreover, the emotional distance from the actual therapy experience may allow a more relaxed learning and planning environment. In addition, this is also a good method for reviewing one's metagoals and progress, as opposed to focusing on a single case. Finally, in a group context, the method lends itself well to role playing and other forms of behavior rehearsal. McCollum and Wetchler (1995) present a compelling case for the use of case consultation, even when live and video modalities are readily available.

Other than its ex post facto nature, the obvious other major disadvantage is the supervisor's inability to determine what actually occurred in sessions, and hence his or her inability to truly assess and monitor therapist performance (Aradi, 1985). However, overreliance on live and video supervision and "exact material" seems to foster the expert position of the supervisor as an authority who knows the best way to conduct therapy. Case supervision is the distillation of the themes the therapist has heard. Because that the therapist is the person who actually sat and talked with the clients, he or she is the "expert" on that experience. We agree with McCollum and Wetchler (1995) that this form of supervision should be revived and reevaluated by marriage and family therapists.

The Review of Case Notes. Review of the case entails rereading the supervisee's written accounts of the therapy session, most typically, but not necessarily, in the absence of the supervisee (Aradi, 1985). The primary advantage of this method is that it encourages the therapist to describe behaviors, hypotheses, interventions, goals, and so on, in an organized manner, especially if a structured form for case notes is utilized. The report can also serve as a stimulus for discussion during supervision. As with the case presentation, a possible disadvantage is that this modality may provide highly unreliable information. An example of a useful form for case notes is found in Fisher and Sprenkle (1980).

Audiotape Review. Audiotape review entails the supervisor listening to all or part of the audiotape of a session (either with or in the absence of the therapist). The advantage of this over the case presentation and review of case notes is that the supervisor does have accurate information concerning at least the auditory dimensions of the therapist–family interaction.

Even though important nonverbal information is lost, the supervisor is better able to assess the therapist's progress and give useful feedback. The audiotape review method is also cheaper and more convenient than video or live supervision.

Disadvantages of the audiotape review method include its ex post facto nature, the loss of nonverbal communication, and the fact that the process is often considered boring. For best results, the supervisor should encourage the therapist to edit his or her audiotape into short sequences that highlight crucial incidents or areas in which the therapist is "stuck" or desires input from the supervisor.

The advantages of each of the ex post facto methods may be maximized by using several such methods in concert. For example, a therapist–supervisor audiotape review may precede or be used in conjunction with a case presentation, where interventions and family dynamics heard on the tape are discussed in more depth.

Videotape Review. The visual component makes videotape review the most advantageous of the ex post facto methods. Most importantly, the supervisor has the opportunity to observe and evaluate the supervisee's perceptual, conceptual, and executive skills, rather than having to rely solely on the trainee's reports. In addition, as Whiffen (1982) notes, videotape provides three unique opportunities: (1) It freezes time so that a crucial sequence can be studied; (2) the therapist sees him- or herself subjectively as one of the contributors to the system; and (3) the effect of the intervention can be observed and assessed. The videotape review even has certain advantages over live supervision. It can be done at a convenient time and at a leisurely pace. Subtle gestures and mannerisms are often lost in live supervision. The fact that key segments may be played and relayed can be of enormous pedagogical significance. Selekman and Todd (1990) describe a didactic exercise they call "searching for strengths," in line with supervision of the solution-focused model. The exercise involves the trainee watching a short segment of videotape and generating two or more descriptions of the family. The opportunity afforded the therapist by videotape supervision to directly observe his or her own appearance, style, mannerisms, and interventions cannot be underestimated. In our opinion, even when live supervision is readily available, it should be supplemented with videotape review. Videotape review is one of the most powerful self-teaching tools in the therapist's training experience. For interesting reading on the theoretical basis for this modality, consult Breunlin, Karrer, McGuire, and Cimmarusti (1988).

Videotape review has most of the same disadvantages as the other ex post facto methods. One potential, unique disadvantage is that it is a rather cool medium. Poignant moments often appear to be toned down on video, and they seem less powerful or may even go unnoticed (Aradi, 1985).

Cotherapy

Cotherapy, although typically a therapeutic modality, is sometimes utilized as a form of supervision. This is the method of choice in the experiential school (Whitaker & Keith, 1981). It typically combines elements of both live and ex post facto supervision. The supervisor is with the trainee in the room and can intervene as the case progresses; however, the bulk of the feedback to the trainee (cotherapist) is typically given outside the therapy hour. The therapeutic advantages of cotherapy have been described elsewhere (Whitaker & Keith, 1981). As a supervisory modality, it allows the trainee to observe his or her mentor, enables him or her to balance interacting with the family with watching for patterns, and often reduces the anxiety over being solely responsible for the session. Potential disadvantages include trainee dependency on the supervisor, the trainee's lack of awareness of the supervisor's goals or intentions, lack of clarity with regard to responsibility for the case, competition or conflicting strategies, and the potential for the supervisor to adopt the "expert" role, thereby devaluing and disempowering the training therapist.

Other Clinical Concepts

Conceptual, Perceptual, and Executive Skills

Three types of skills have been described in an influential article by Cleghorn and Levin (1973), and this description has influenced others who have delineated and categorized therapeutic skills (e.g., Falicov, Constantine, & Breunlin, 1981; Tomm & Wright, 1979). "Conceptual skills" relate to the trainee's ability to look at the raw data of the session through the lens of family therapy. "Perceptual skills" are required to see and describe accurately the behavioral data of a therapy session. "Executive skills" include all therapeutic interventions, as well as activities necessary to prepare for therapy (e.g., effective telephone contacts) and case management (e.g., making referrals).

Isomorphism

The isomorphism of therapy and supervision has been strongly emphasized in writings by Howard Liddle (Liddle, 1982b; Liddle & Saba, 1984; Liddle & Schwartz, 1983). Basically, Liddle argues that although therapy and training–supervision are different, they are nonetheless parallel processes. What one does in supervision–training is guided by what one believes are the central tasks of therapy. For example, for the structural–strategic professional, both therapy and supervision–training include the processes of joining and restructuring. Furthermore, what happens between the supervisor and trainee tends to be paralleled in the relationship between the therapist and clients (Schwartz et al., 1988; Frankel & Piercy, 1990).

Presession, Midsession, and Postsession Meetings

"Presession," "midsession," and "postsession" are terms used widely in the literature on live supervision to describe interactions at different points between supervisor and trainee. In the presession meeting, the supervisor and trainee review goals and plans for the session. Midsession meetings typically occur behind the mirror, in a different office or, at times, in the therapy room. They serve as midway processing for what is occurring in the session, as an opportunity to plan interventions or homework, and as a "breather" from the intensity of the therapy. In a postsession meeting, the therapist and supervisor debrief. Typically, the therapist's thoughts and feelings about the session are processed, along with feedback and ideas from team members and the supervisor, and plans for the subsequent session are discussed.

Structuring and Relationship Skills

Described by Alexander and his colleagues (e.g., Alexander, Barton, Schiavo, & Parsons, 1976), structuring and relationship skills are generic family therapy skills that cut across theoretical orientations. "Structuring skills" are the abilities necessary to structure a session, such as being direct, being clear, and modeling good communication. "Relationship skills" are those necessary to create an interpersonal climate where change can take place. They include humor, warmth, and the ability to connect feelings with behaviors. Alexander et al. (1976), in their influential study, found that these two sets of skills accounted for 60% of the variance in treatment outcome. Relationship skills alone accounted for 45% of the outcome variance.

Relationships are essential instruments of therapy. Just as vital as the therapeutic relationship is the supervisory relationship. Kaiser (1992) identified the following salient elements of the supervisory relationship: (1) accountability, (2) personal awareness, (3) trust, (4) power and authority; and introduced a theoretical framework for understanding these elements based on principles of ethical relationships. Anderson and Swim (1995) reflect a postmodern philosophy in their discussion of supervision "as collaborative conversation," emphasizing the role of language, conversation, self, and story. They view the supervisor as more of a mentor in a partnership with the supervisee in which both individuals create knowledge together. The supervisor's stance is one of "not knowing," such that he or she does not have access to privileged information, accepts the randomness of unique human experience, is receptive to being informed by the supervisee, and gives primary importance to the supervisee's voice.

MAJOR ISSUES IN THE FIELD

In an important review article, Liddle (1982a) identified five generic training issues that form the outline for this section.

Who Should Teach and Be Taught Family Therapy?

It remains unclear today which are the most relevant and salient variables for the selection of both family therapy trainees and trainers. It is not known whether previous psychotherapy experience, significant life experience, or other factors help to determine the effectiveness of a family therapist. To what extent are family therapists "made" or "born"? AAMFT's Commission on Supervision is the first group to grapple seriously with qualifications for supervisors, although the majority of persons supervising family therapy in this country are not credentialed by this organization.

What Should Be Taught?

The issue of the content of supervision is controversial because of the aforementioned isomorphism between therapy and supervision. Because there are a variety of schools of therapy, it is not surprising that there are a variety of schools of training–supervision. Liddle et al. (1988) as well as McDaniel, Weber, and McKeever (1983) show how several therapy models have been translated into supervisory modalities consistent with the theories of change, including structural, strategic, and family-of-origin, and experiential, brief, integrative, and functional family therapies. Reflecting more current therapeutic approaches, Selekman and Todd (1990) offer a collaborative supervisory model based on solution-focused therapy, whereas White (1989/1990) presents ideas about a structure for training and supervision that is informed by ideas derived from narrative therapy. Breunlin, Rampage, and Eovaldi (1994) advocate supervision of family therapy from an integrative perspective, affording bridges between pure systems and psychoanalytic family therapy models, as well as between family therapy and other forms of therapy. Other examples of models of supervision based on therapy theories are found in Connell (1984) and Keller and Protinsky (1984).

Another issue related to the content of training is whether trainees should be schooled in one pure approach and whether eclectic training models lead to confusion or contradiction (Liddle, 1982b). Liddle et al. (1988) offer approaches to training in various "pure" family therapy models. Others present integrative models of training, such as structural–strategic and Bowen approaches (McCollum, 1990), and structural–strategic and symbolic–experiential (Todd & Greenberg, 1987). Breunlin et al. (1994) offer an integrated perspective based on the metaframeworks perspective (Breunlin, Schwartz, & Mac Kune-Karrer, 1992).

The extent to which a trainee's personal life should be examined in training is also controversial. Some curricula are designed with the purpose of integrating theory and skills training with the trainee's own family-of-origin or person-of-the-therapist issues either simultaneously (Aponte, 1992; McDaniel & Landau-Stanton, 1991) or sequentially (McCollum, 1990). Aponte (1994) recognizes that training programs that integrate personal work on the self with clinical practice will struggle with issues of boundaries and dual relationships, as well as the line between training and therapy. However, given that the therapist's personal characteristics may be the most powerful determinants of treatment effectiveness, it seems only ethical that training programs aim at producing personal growth in trainees as they learn the art and skill of marriage and family therapy.

AAMFT guidelines for training program accreditation stress that special emphasis should be given to the impact on sexism and gender role stereotyping on the individual and the family (COAMFTE, 1994). Gender issues have become a relatively new focus in family therapy training in the past decade. A survey of the role of gender in family therapy training programs conducted by the Womens Task Force of the American Family Therapy Academy (AFTA) discovered that few programs identify with a feminist model or have a clearly defined sense of gender awareness (Coleman, Avis, & Turin, 1990). The authors interpret the results to suggest that the subject of gender is absent in most family therapy training and is least likely to be taught through a regularly scheduled course; rather, gender is addressed primarily when issues emerge in class or supervision (Coleman et al., 1990). Several feminist family therapists have criticized systems theory and called for training and supervision that is feminist informed. Wheeler, Avis, Miller, and Chaney (1986) give many detailed suggestions for developing a training program and supervision experience that embodies feminist content, values, and behavior. More recently, Storm (1991) describes a master's level course with the goal of developing a gender-sensitive systemic view in evaluating theory and participating in clinical work. Roberts (1991) presents four experiential exercises to help address gender issues in either therapy or training. Given the preponderance of male leadership in the history of our field, along with the increasing number of women obtaining professional degrees and moving into more leadership roles, attention to the impact of gender on supervision and training can no longer be ignored.

Finally, trainers are being challenged to identify and differentiate specific clusters of skills that are associated with the various approaches to supervision. An attempt to specify supervisory skills for the structural–strategic approach is offered by Liddle and Schwartz (1983). More recently, Liddle et al. (1988) devoted an entire section of their book to conceptual, behavioral, and technical aspects of family therapy supervision. Five chapters explicitly provide "skill-focused explorations of various aspects of the mechanics of supervising family therapists" (p. xv). Skills associated with specific models are also delineated in Todd and Storm (in press). Although there are no research data guiding how to supervise, Haley (1988), viewing various supervision approaches, identifies three major areas of focus: (1) the client's problem situation; (2) the therapist's personality; and (3) therapy skills; and discusses some consequences of each training focus.

How Should the Content and Skills Be Taught?

Many family therapies rely heavily on right-brain activities, such as meta-phor, pattern recognition, and humor. Frequently, however, trainers try to teach such right-hemispheric operations through left-hemispheric methods, such as reading and writing. There is little consensus as to how one should teach such nondigital processes. Also, certain theoretical models, such as Whitaker's experiential therapy, do not lend themselves well to goal-specific objectives. Liddle's (1982c) article on using mental imagery to create therapeutic and supervisory realities and Prosky's (1982) chapter on the use of analogic and digital communication in training are among the first publications in the literature to address this issue.

Another promising method, adapted from individual therapy training, is microtraining. Its application to family therapy is described in Street and Treacher (1980). Specific family therapy skills are described and demon-strated to students with video examples. Students are then challenged to demonstrate the skills while being taped. They observe their own work and receive feedback. Tools can often provide useful vehicles for training. Two recent developments for training include the Calgary Family Intervention Model (Wright & Leahey, 1994), an organizing framework for conceptu-alizing a fit between interventions and a domain of family functioning, and the Systemic Therapy Sessions Summary Form (Bernstein & Burge, 1988), a tool for enhancing training in systemic therapy.

The *Handbook of Family Therapy Training and Supervision* (Liddle et al., 1988) explores various models of family therapy and how differences in therapy models reflect differences in training. Furthermore, the contribution of several authors (Storm; Anderson & Swim; Bobele, Gardner, & Biever; Amundson; Cantwell & Holmes; Merl; Turner & Fine; and Stewart & Amundson) celebrating collaborative, postmodern supervision is compiled in the *Journal of Systemic Therapies* (Vol. 14, Summer 1995).

How Does the Setting Influence Training, and How Does Training Influence the Setting?

As anyone who has tried to teach family therapy in a non-family-therapy setting knows, the discipline has considerable political ramifications (Framo, 1976; Haley, 1975; Liddle, 1978). Some systems resist family therapy yet are operating according to systemic theory. For this reason, Liddle (1982a) believes that we need the ability to make interactional–structural assessments of the training systems and the ecosystem in which it functions, and to prepare students and organizations for the personal and political consequences of adopting a systemic view. Liddle et al. (1988) offer seven chapters discussing different forms and settings for training and the unique challenges of each context.

How Should Training Be Assessed?

A traditional marker of a field's growth is a coherent body of research offering support for the efficacy of the field's positions or perspectives. The issue of research on training–supervision is explored later in more detail. Suffice it to say here that it is a grossly neglected area, ready for exploration. If the "bottom line" of training is to produce effective therapists, it is a sad commentary that there is only one training–supervision study Stolk and Perlesz (1990) in which the therapeutic outcome is the dependent variable.

TEACHING TOOLS AND TECHNIQUES

As noted at the outset of this chapter, training is a generic term that encompasses all aspects of family therapy education. As such, the topic is too broad to be covered here. In fact, this entire book can be seen only as a partial answer to the question "What is training?" Beyond the model curriculum of the Commission on Accreditation for Marriage and Family Therapy Education (1991) and the revision now in process, readers are referred to several useful resources. For example, Liddle and Saba (1982) have describes an introductory family therapy course that demonstrated the isomorphic relationship between teaching and therapy. Nichols (1979) has written a general article on doctoral programs in family therapy, and Everett (1979) has written a similar article about master's programs. There are also several articles describing the curricula of particular programs (e.g., Garfield, 1979; L'Abate, Berger, Wright, & O'Shea, 1979; Liddle et al., 1988; McCollum, 1990; McDaniel & Landau-Stanton, 1991). Wheeler et al. (1986) and Storm (1991) describe guidelines for incorporating feminist-informed content and process in family therapy training. More recently, articles have been published describing the content and teaching methods for courses in ethical, legal, and professional issues in family therapy (Piercy & Sprenkle, 1983) and family therapy outcome research (Sprenkle & Piercy, 1984). Additionally, a general article on the process of family therapy classroom education, which delineates basic educational assumptions and the variety of techniques applicable to many courses, has been prepared (Piercy & Sprenkle, 1984). Finally, Piercy and Sprenkle (1985) have written a chapter on the process of helping students develop their own integrative theories of family intervention.

The remainder of this section offers suggestions for a course specifically on family therapy supervision. Such a course might entail both a content track and a clinical track. The content track is fulfilled through a seminar that meets for several hours each week. Activities (from Sprenkle, 1988) include the following:

1. Students are asked to prepare outlines and critiques of the major readings on supervision published in the past 5 years.
2. They write brief papers in response to a series of questions about supervision; this helps them to articulate their personal therapy of supervision. Here are some example questions:
   a. What is the relationship between your theory of therapy and your theory of supervision?
   b. What are the implications of operating from a specific framework versus an eclectic approach?
   c. What are the relative advantages and disadvantages of live supervision, case conferences, audiotaping, videotaping, and the other modes of supervision?
   d. Develop a plan for the assessment of your supervision. This should include methods for assessing your supervisory strengths as well as limitations.
3. Students are asked to observe the faculty supervisors for several weeks. Then they are required to make an oral presentation on the theory and practice of the supervision of the faculty members.
4. They present their own goals as supervisors, using the Goal Attainment Scaling format. These goals, developed early in the course, are used to evaluate progress at the end of the term.
5. Class members prepare a worksheet that a supervisor could use to help a therapist increase his or her supervisory skills.

One published model is by Schwartz (1981). For example, a student might develop a worksheet to facilitate learning circular diagramming. Another might prepare one to teach positive connotation (Constantine, Stone Fish, & Piercy, 1984). Alternatively, students may develop forms for supervisory note taking, such as the one published by Heath (1983). Williams (1994) developed a useful tool called the supervision Feedback Form for training family therapy supervisors. Originally, the form was developed for supervisees to provide constructive and concrete feedback to the supervisor; however, the author identifies several other uses for the form in training supervisors.

The clinical track focuses on supervision of supervision, a process described in articles by Constantine, Piercy, and Sprenkle (1984) and by

Liddle, Breunlin, Schwartz, and Constantine (1984). At Purdue University, for example, several supervisors in training are assigned to a supervisor of supervisors (a faculty member). The supervisors in training are assigned to one of the practica in the on-campus Marriage and Family Therapy Clinic, which typically meets from 2:00 to 9:00 P.M. The supervisors in training and the supervisor of supervisors meet at the beginning and end of this time to discuss progress of therapists, specific issues that have arisen during the process of supervision, and the group process (Constantine et al., 1984). During the balance of the time, the supervisors in training conduct presession meetings with the therapists, do live supervision of cases, and conduct posttherapy feedback sessions. In addition, they typically meet with the therapist before supervision begins in order to establish a relationship, to discuss the therapists' overall goals for supervision, and to ascertain how the supervisors in training can be helpful. The supervisor of supervisors keeps his or her contact with the therapist to a minimum and works through the supervisors in training. The supervisor of supervisors is not in the therapy room during the pre- or postsession meetings but remains in the observation booth to monitor the work of the supervisors in training. A supervisor of supervisors, may, however, call in to make suggestions and/or provide support for the supervisors in training. The supervisors in training answer all such calls to ensure that there is little direct contact between therapist and the supervisor of supervisors (Constantine et al., 1984; Sprenkle, 1988).

RESEARCH ISSUES

In an empirical evaluation of the training program of the Family Institute of Chicago, Tucker and Pinsof (1984) assert that most positive reports of training outcome

> have been based primarily on clinical impressions . . . or training self reports post training. . . . Unfortunately, these positive conclusions rest on the tacit and untested assumption that a self-reported, positive training experience is associated with change in actual practice or outcome with patients. In fact, no research evidence exists to show that training in marital and family therapy increases clinical effectiveness. Consequently, family therapy training has been planned and conducted without the benefit of a scientific foundation. (p. 437)

Unfortunately, this quotation accurately reflects the state of research in the field. Avis and Sprenkle (1990) report a lack of research on family therapy supervision and training, identifying minimal research on (1) evaluating training programs, (2) studying effectiveness of specific live supervision techniques, and (3) examining the process of live supervision. As noted earlier in this chapter, there is only one study that directly connects training and family therapy client outcome. Stolk and Perlesz (1990) offer the first attempt in the field to study the effects of training on family therapy outcome. Their findings suggest families seen by second-year trainees tended to be actually less satisfied with therapy than families seen by first-year trainees.

Fortunately, however, in recent years there have been some studies that indirectly (inferentially) assess the degree to which a particular program teaches its trainees those skills believed to be associated with positive therapy outcome (Avis & Sprenkle, 1990). In the first major review on research in training in marriage and family therapy, Kniskern and Gurman (1979) noted that training can be evaluated by several other criteria: (1) Does the training increase the trainee's conceptual knowledge about family functions? (2) Does the training have an impact on the trainee's personal life?

Description of Recent Studies

Avis and Sprenkle (1990) located 15 studies on family therapy training that were not discussed in the Kniskern and Gurman (1979) review. They fell into two major categories: (1) Six described the development of instruments for measuring the outcome of training/supervision; and (2) nine actually evaluated training programs. The latter assessed the impact of a variety of training–learning experiences on the trainees' skills and behavior.

Evaluation Instruments

Although evaluation of trainees' performances is a multifaceted, multiphasic task requiring integration of information from various sources, behavioral measures of trainee performance have been developed. The Allred Interaction Analysis for counselors (Allred & Kersey, 1977) was developed to provide family therapy trainees with "a method for acquiring meaningful, objective feedback about counseling behaviors" (p. 17). It has seven categories for therapist behaviors and three categories for client behaviors. Pinsof (1979) developed the Family Therapist Behavioral Scale to specify clinically relevant verbal behaviors of family therapists. It comprises 19 mutually exclusive code categories, based theoretically on the executive skills identified by Cleghorn and Levin (1973). Pinsof (1981) has used this system to devise his more complex Family Therapist Coding System, which was designed to be totally "reconstructive" (i.e., the therapist can reconstruct what happened in the session by examining the codes). Additionally, Tucker and Pinsof (1984) developed the Family Concept Assessment Task and Rating Scale for measuring the degree to which therapists conceptualize clinical material from a family systems perspective. Piercy, Laird, and Mohammed (1983) developed the Family Therapist Rating Scale as a measure of in-therapy skills. It consists of 10 items within each of five skill categories (Structuring, Relationship, Historical, Structural/Process, and Experiential). It is the first coding system to describe nonverbal behaviors and is more global than Allred and Pinsof's scale. Breunlin, Schwartz, Krause, and Selby (1983) developed a training evaluation instrument that consists of a 30-minute videotape of a simulated family therapy session, followed by a series of multiple-choice questions about the session. It was designed to be easily quantifiable and does not require the laborious task of coding or rating actual therapy sessions or tapes.

Evaluation of Family Therapy Training

Studies that have actually evaluated training programs are noted here. Tomm and Leahey (1980) compared three methods of teaching basic family therapy assessment to beginning medical students. Churven and McKinnon (1982) investigated the impact of a 3-day intensive workshop in basic therapy on the cognitive and intervention skills of 24 trainees. Byles, Bishop, and Horn (1983) investigated the results of a training program designed to teach family therapy skills to 24 master's-level social workers who were employed at a family service agency. Kolevzon and Green (1983) examined the differential effect of three types of family therapy training on therapists' therapeutic assumptions and in-therapy behavior. Mohammed and Piercy (1983) examined the differential effect of two training methods on the acquisition of structuring and relationship skills. Tucker and Pinsof (1984) completed a comprehensive evaluation of 19 family therapy trainees who had completed the first year of a training program at the Family Institute of Chicago. Fenell, Hovestadt, and Harvey (1986) compared the effect of two types of supervision on trainees' acquisition of family therapy skills as measured by the Family Therapy Rating Scale (FTRS) (Piercy et al., 1983). Pulleybank and Shapiro (1986) evaluated a 9-month structural family therapy training program at Eastfield Children's Center in Campbell, California. Finally, Zaken-Greenberg and Neimeyer (1986) examined changes in the conceptual and executive skills of 44 subjects (22 family trainees and 22 comparisons) over a 16-week semester.

Conclusions and Recommendations

On the basis of these 15 studies, Avis and Sprenkle (1990) reached the following conclusions:

1. There are now several instruments with some degree of reliability and validity that appear able to distinguish beginning and advanced

therapists, to measure the acquisition of conceptual and/or intervention skills, and to offer feedback to therapists on their in-therapy behavior.

2. There is evidence that various types of family therapy training produce an increase in trainees' cognitive and intervention skills.
3. In-service family therapy training programs for agency staff members may be an effective way to increase agency services.
4. Beginning assessment skills may be as effectively taught by using traditional classroom methods as by using more expensive experiential methods.
5. Sequencing of training activities may be a significant variable in the acquisition of family therapy skills.
6. Cognitive and intervention skills may develop independently of each other.

Avis and Sprenkle (1990) also made the following recommendations:

1. There is a need for controlled research on both training and supervision. Only four of the studies noted previously used some type of comparison group, and only one (Tomm & Leahey, 1980) used random assignment and had an adequate sample size.
2. There is a need for replications of existing studies in order to confirm or disconfirm what have to be considered tentative findings. Such replications will require much more specification of teaching–supervisory methods used, context of training, and conditions under which training occurs.
3. There is an urgent need for more valid and reliable instruments to measure change in trainee skills. The instruments developed thus far, although promising, either have problems with reliability and validity or are so complex that they use overwhelming amounts of information and are too cumbersome and time consuming for the average person to administer.
4. There remains a need for research that directly assesses the impact of training upon therapeutic outcome.
5. Various design improvements are necessary to make research in this area methodologically adequate. These include specifying and controlling trainer–supervisor-in-training variables, including more follow-ups to determine the stability of training effects, using more adequate samples, and assuring trainer–investigator nonequivalence.
6. Comparative studies will be increasingly necessary to answer the specificity question; that is, what training is effective, when, for whom, under what conditions, and for what type of clinical situation?

Additional research recommendations are found in Liddle's (1991) comprehensive review of the field. He concludes his section on research and evaluation:

> Surely, this represents what is perhaps the most important future area of development in training and supervision. Producing the next generation of family therapists, given the complexities of our world and the field, will not be easy. We need to know what is effective and why. Questions about criteria and methods to determine effectiveness are now being asked and answered. A small revolution is happening in which practical instruments are being developed that can help us assess our work. This growing literature is becoming one of the most exciting areas of our field. (p. 685)

KEY BOOKS, CHAPTERS, AND ARTICLES

Overviews

Postmodern supervision. (1995). *Journal of Systemic Therapies, 14*(2).

This entire issue of the journal is dedicated to postmodern supervision. Cheryl Storm opens the issue with a discussion of the implications of social constructivism for supervision, followed by an outstanding article by Harlene Anderson and Susan Swim, in which they describe supervision as a "collaborative conversation." The remaining six articles cover various topics, such as supervisory approaches deriving from social construction theory (Bobele, Gardner, & Biever; Cantwell & Holmes; Turner & Fine), postmodern and narrative supervision (Amundson); dilemmas presented by social constructionism in supervision (Bobele, Gardner, & Biever); reflecting supervision derived from the reflecting team model (Merl); and professional ethics and postmodern supervision (Stewart & Amundson). This is an intriguing and informative issue that is very useful to supervisors, trainers, and those learning to supervise.

Liddle, H. A. (1982). Family therapy training: Current issues, future trends. *International Journal of Family Therapy, 4*, 31–47.

This article extrapolated five realms of focus from previous literature on family therapy training: (1) personal, (2) content, (3) methodology, (4) context, and (5) evaluation. Corresponding to each domain, the following questions are raised: (1) Who should teach or be taught family therapy? (2) What should be taught? (3) How should the content be taught? (4) How do the training system and training methods influence each other? and (5) How should training be assessed? The article thoroughly examines controversial issues in training that have yet to be resolved. Although the author shows some bias for learning from a particular theory as opposed to eclecticism, he otherwise attempts to present both sides of the issues.

Liddle, H. A. (1991). Training and supervision in family therapy: A comprehensive and critical analyses. In A. Gurman & D. Kniskern (Eds.), *Handbook of family therapy* (Vol. 2). New York: Brunner/Mazel.

In probably the most comprehensive chapter-length treatment available, Liddle covers the history of supervision, the seminal writings in the field, major conceptual and theoretical issues, methods of training and supervision, schools and approach specific models, and descriptions of training programs. His section on research and evaluation is particularly noteworthy as he covers a number of studies (both published and unpublished) that are not treated in the Avis and Sprenkle (1990) review of research in this area.

Liddle, H. A., Breunlin, D. C., & Schwartz, R. C. (Eds.). (1988). *Handbook of family therapy training and supervision*. New York: Guilford Press.

This superior book provides a comprehensive examination of family therapy training and supervision. The book is organized into six sections, including (1) an overview; (2) various models and approaches to training; (3) pragmatics of supervision; (4) contexts for training; (5) special issues and topics in family therapy training and supervision; and (6) an extensive appendix of the family therapy training and supervision literature. This is one of the most comprehensive books on supervision and training, and it incorporates various perspectives and contributions from leaders in the field of marriage and family therapy.

Piercy, F. P. (Ed.). (1985). *Family therapy education and supervision*. Binghamton, NY: Haworth. (Also published as Vol. 1, No. 4, of the *Journal of Psychotherapy and the Family*.)

This volume includes some excellent articles on topics such as family therapy theory building, feminist training, training implications of family therapy as a profession or a professional specialty, and an introduction and consumer's guide to family therapy supervision. Many of the contributors are leaders in the area of family therapy training, and many of the articles provide a firsthand view of training approaches that the reader may use as either a trainer or a participant.

Nichols, W. C., Nichols, D. P., & Hardy, K. V. (1990). Supervision in family therapy: A decade restudy. *Journal of Marital and Family Therapy, 16*(3), 275–285.

These authors conducted a 10-year replication study of Everett's (1980) survey of AAMFT supervisors. This broad and informative article found several interesting and significant differences from the earlier survey of supervisors. It is useful in obtaining a general grasp of AAMFT-approved supervisors and supervision, as well as identifying researchable questions in the area of supervision.

Simon, R., & Brewster, F. (1983). What is training? *Family Therapy Networker, 7*(2), 25–29, 66.

The authors of this article take a "human interest" approach to the topic of training. They identify five phases a student in any training program might encounter, emphasizing the feelings that such a process might arouse. This article is peppered with interesting quotes from leaders in the field that reveal their dilemmas with family therapy and supervision. The article is not intended to be a rigorous discourse on training but rather an evocative experience with the subject matter, putting the reader in touch with the emotional issues involved from either side of the one-way mirror.

Todd, T., & Storm, C. (in press). *The complete systemic supervisor: Context, philosophy and pragmatics.* Needham Heights, MA: Allyn & Bacon.

This cutting edge book coves the area of systemic supervision with much breadth and depth. The book is divided into six sections: (1) history and future of MFT supervision; (2) ethical and contextual issues; (3) ideas, values, and beliefs underlying models of supervision; (4) issues of power and collaboration within the supervisory relationship; (5) methods and interventions; and (6) training supervisors. This book is a valuable contribution to the growing literature in MFT supervision.

White, M. B., & Russell, C. S. (1985). The essential elements of supervisory systems: A modified Delphi study. *Journal of Marital and Family Therapy, 21*(1), 33–53.

This study identifies the essential elements, generated by a panel of AAMFT Approved Supervisors, important to the outcome of marriage and family therapy supervision. Variables identified by the expert panel are organized into five categories: (1) supervisor variables; (2) supervisee variables; (3) supervisor–supervisee relationship variables; (4) supervisory interaction variables; and (5) contextual variables. This article begins to lay the foundation for a comprehensive model of MFT supervision. This article could facilitate training as well as research in the area of supervision.

Live Supervision

Berger, M., & Dammann, C. (1982). Live supervision as context, treatment, and training. *Family Process, 21,* 337–344.

The uniqueness of this contribution lies in the willingness of the authors to examine not only the advantages of live supervision, but also the potential pitfalls. The article addresses the inevitable struggle between the perceptions of therapist and supervisor that originate from opposite sides of the one-way screen. In addition, the value of varying perspectives is lauded, and the synthesis of multiple views is recommended for enhanced treatment and training.

Byng-Hall, J. (1982). The use of the earphone in supervision. In R. Whiffen & J. Byng-Hall (Eds.), *Family therapy supervision: Recent developments in practice.* New York: Grune & Stratton.

The author describes the main uses of the "bug in the ear," its advantages and disadvantages, and ways to utilize the modality most effectively. The importance of the supervisor being sensitive to the trainee's position is stressed, because the method is potentially intimidating as well as helpful.

Roberts, J., Matthews, W., Bodin, N., Cohen, D., Lewandowski, L., Novo, J., Pumilia, J., & Willis, C. (1989). Training with O (observing) and T (treatment) teams in live supervision: Reflections in the looking glass. *Journal of Marital and Family Therapy, 15*(4), 397–410.

This article discusses ways to work with both a treatment and observing team behind the mirror simultaneously. This group, consisting of two supervisors and six trainees, used the T and O format to (1) look at their group process, (2) integrate the Milan model and Ericksonian hypnotherapy, and (3) provide a structure for the two supervisors to work without getting in each other's way. This article could be very useful for training in that it provides a clear and interesting description of using T and O teams, illustrated by clinical examples. This technique allows for creativity and flexibility in its use.

Coppersmith, E. I. (1980). Expanding uses of the telephone in family therapy. *Family Process, 19,* 411–417.

Creative uses of the telephone in family therapy are described. The author gives examples of calls to the therapist, calls from the team to specific family members, and calls between family members. These case examples demonstrate the impact of the format on recalcitrant families. The author additionally shows how she simultaneously capitalized on use of the team for both therapeutic and training purposes.

Olson, U., & Pegg, P. F. (1979). Direct open supervision: A team approach. *Family Process, 18,* 463–469.

This article describes the model utilized by the Family Therapy Training Institute of London. Here, "direct" refers to supervisory intervention that are made directly and immediately to the therapists during a family session. "Open" means that the supervisor and other team members are present in the same room as the family during sessions. The functions of the team in this model include combining expertise and support, serving as actors or models for behaviors for the family, and providing feedback about the session to both the therapist and the family. Four forms of direct supervision are discussed: authoritarian, supportive, explorative, and collaborative. The problems as well as the benefits of such a supervisory approach are discussed.

Papp, P. (1980). The Greek chorus and other techniques of paradoxical therapy. *Family Process, 19,* 45–57.

This important article describes the process of paradoxical family therapy, including the indications, principles, and limitations of such techniques as reframing, prescription, and reversals. The "Greek chorus" (the supervisory team) is highlighted as useful to several paradoxical interventions appropriate for a family resistant to change. This article is rich in examples and is a prime source for a family resistant to change. This article is rich in examples and is a prime source for family therapists interested in live supervision and/or paradoxical intervention strategies.

Supervisory Skills and Techniques

Breunlin, D. C., & Cade, B. (1981). Intervening in family systems with observer messages. *Journal of Marital and Family Therapy, 7,* 453–460.

The authors describe an approach to family therapy in which observers become part of the therapeutic team by sending messages in to the session. Five components of observer messages are discussed: function, target, timing, content, and delivery. Guidelines for effective team functioning and implications for training are also considered. In addition to presenting practical suggestions for implementing this mode of therapy, the article includes a thoughtful discussion of the evolution of the role of observers from passive to active participants in the therapeutic process.

Heath, T. (1983). The live supervision form: Structure and theory for assessment in live supervision. In J. C. Hansen & B. P. Keeney (Eds.), *Diagnosis and assessment in family therapy.* Rockville, MD: Aspen Systems.

The author uses a live supervision instrument as a vehicle to present his theory and practice of supervision. The instrument is isomorphic to the activity for which it is designed. It is structured, goal specific, and theory based. The purpose of the instrument (supervision) is described, followed by a clear and thorough analysis of its components.

Liddle, H. A. (1982). Using mental imagery to create therapeutic and supervisory realities. *American Journal of Family Therapy, 10,* 68–72.

This is a short but potent article that reminds supervisors to create experiential bridges for their supervisees through the use of visual and auditory imagery. The thoughts presented are innovative and provocative and set the mind spinning in new directions. This is an unusually analogic style for the author, and the content will probably be a refreshing addition to a supervisor's repertoire.

Liddle, H. A., & Schwartz, R. C. (1983). Live supervision/consultation: Conceptual and pragmatic guidelines for family therapy trainers. *Family Process, 22,* 477–490.

In this article, the authors provide a rather thorough list of live supervision skills. These skills could be useful to supervisors in developing learning objectives and/or evaluation tools for live supervision.

Nielsen, E., & Kaslow, F. (1980). Consultation in family therapy. *American Journal of Family Therapy, 8,* 35–42.

The authors advocate the regular use of consultants (either peers of visiting experts) by experienced family therapists for the purposes of overcoming therapeutic impasses, verifying diagnostic impressions, confirming intervention strategies, and stimulating professional and personal development. Consultations can take place in several forms, including discussion, tape reviews, observation through a one-way mirror, and participation in a session as cotherapist. Concrete recommendations are made for the careful preparation for and carrying out of consultant-conducted interviews, with special emphasis on the way that such interviews can best by integrated into the continuing process of therapy.

Roberts, J. (1983). The third tier: The overlooked dimension in family therapy training. *Family Therapy Networker, 7*(2), 30–31, 60–61.

The case is made that the field of family therapy should begin to "appreciate the importance of the larger therapeutic–educational system that includes the supervisor, therapist, family, and the group of trainees behind the mirror" (p. 30).

The author identifies supervisory responsibilities in developing a "collaborative team" that will expand the potential of the training group. Some of the training techniques suggested are likely to be controversial, in that team trainees may be left unsupervised to rise to the occasion on their own.

Family Therapy Education and Training

Aponte, H. J. (1992). Training the person of the therapist in structural family therapy. *Journal of Marital and Family Therapy, 18*(3), 269–281.

This article offers a model for training therapists in the use of self, grounded in structural family therapy. Case examples illustrate the personal training in a clinical context. This article could be valuable to those who value self-of-the-therapist issues in the training and practice of marriage and family therapy.

Aponte, H. J. (1994). How personal can training get? *Journal of Marital and Family Therapy, 20*(1), 3–15.

This article acknowledges that person of the therapist training is essential to becoming a effective therapist. However, dealing with one's own personal issues in training raises concerns about dual relationships. The author offers a distinction between dual qualities and dual relationships, and provides an illustration of clinical training. Guidelines are provided for trainers and trainees using this "person–practice model" to protect against violations and promote a constructive association between the two qualities of the training program.

Breunlin, D. D., Karrer, B. M., McGuire, D. E., & Cimmarusti, R. A. (1988). Cybernetics of videotape supervision. In H. A. Liddle, D. C. Breunlin, & R. C. Schwartz (Eds.), *Handbook of family therapy training and supervision.* New York: Guilford Press.

The authors offer a model of videotape supervision organized by second-order cybernetics. Additionally, in this chapter, videotape supervision based on psychodynamic, first- and second-order cybernetics are compared, and a set of guidelines is proposed for effective videotape supervision. This chapter is an important contribution to an underdeveloped area in the literature on marriage and family therapy supervision.

Coleman, S., Avis, J., & Turin, M. (1990). A study of the role of gender in family therapy training. *Family Process, 29,* 365–374.

This article reports on a survey conducted by the Women's Task Force of the American Family Therapy Association on the extent gender issues were included in family therapy training programs. Overall, results suggest that the subject of gender is absent in most family therapy training and is usually addressed only when issues arise in class or in supervision. This is an extremely important article with rather startling findings. We hope it will serve to inform and motivate educators and trainees about the need for attention to the role of gender in training programs.

Keller, J. F., & Protinsky, H. (1984). A self-management model for supervision. *Journal of Marital and Family Therapy, 10,* 281–288.

This article presents the model of supervision used in the family therapy program at Virginia Polytechnic Institute and State University at the time the article was written. It is based on the assumption that as supervisees develop an understanding of their own family-of-origin issues and patterns, they will be better able to interrupt those patterns as they are reenacted in the therapeutic context. Self-understanding is emphasized as an essential ingredient in the therapist's management of self in the clinical setting. The article's main value lies in its elaboration of how psychodynamic and family-of-origin concepts may be applied to the process of supervision, and it will undoubtedly be of greatest interest to those working from these orientations.

Lebow, J. L. (1987). Developing a personal integration in family therapy: Principles for model construction and practice. *Journal of Marital and Family Therapy, 13*(1), 1–14.

This article offers guidelines for therapists to help in building their own personal integrative method of family therapy. The author suggests that clinicians organize their own efforts at integration around a number of principles allied around five foci: (1) the need for a personal paradigm, (2) the assimilation of aspects of scholastic approaches, (3) the role of the person of the therapist, (4) the adaptation of the model to specific cases, and (5) the pathways toward the development of a personal integrative model. This can serve as a useful model for therapists in developing their own theories of change and approaches to therapy.

McCollum, E., & Wetchler, J. (1995). In defense of case consultation: Maybe "dead" supervision isn't dead after all. *Journal of Marital and Family Therapy, 21,* 155–166.

This article presents a compelling case for the use of case consultation, even when live and video modalities are readily available. The authors propose four "tasks" to be accomplished in case consultations to provide organization to the process and facilitate the examination of broader contextual issues. This is an interesting and exciting contribution to a field that is famous for supervision based on "raw data"—such as live and video supervision.

McDaniel, S., & Landau-Stanton, J. (1991). Family-of-origin work and family therapy skills training: Both–and. *Family Process, 30,* 459–471.

This article presents a family-of-origin curriculum designed to integrate the trainee's own family-of-origin work with live supervision and skills training. Traditionally, training programs have advocated one position. These authors make an important contribution to the field by offering a model for training that includes a focus on *both* clinical skills *and* the self of the-therapist.

McDaniel, S. H., Weber, T., & McKeever, J. (1983). Multiple theoretical approaches to supervision: Choices in family therapy training. *Family Process, 22,* 491–500.

This article chooses several family therapy orientations to illustrate how supervision may be used to further the training of a family therapist in ways consistent with the orientations' respective theories of human behavior and change. Structural, strategic, experiential, and family-of-origin approaches to supervision are described, along with an exploration of the similarities and differences in these particular approaches. This article includes a discussion of the relative merits of multiple versus single theoretical orientations in family therapy training programs. Recommendations are offered with regard to training and supervision as it relates to the developmental level of the trainee.

Piercy, F. P., & Sprenkle, D. H. (1983). Ethical, legal, and professional issues in family therapy: A graduate level course. *Journal of Marital and Family Therapy, 9*(4), 393–401.

This presentation of a 16-week academic course in ethical, legal, and professional issues facing family therapists may be used as a model for training clinicians in real-life dilemmas typically not described in texts. In addition, students are offered assignments and experiential activities geared to promote their own professional development. Although it is conceded that the topics covered are not comprehensive, the course is global enough in focus that the sources introduced provide a solid foundation and launching pad for exploring related considerations.

Piercy, F. P., & Sprenkle, D. H. (1984). The process of family therapy education. *Journal of Marital and Family Therapy, 10*(4), 399–407.

Suggestions for the process of graduate family therapy education are prefaced with theoretical assumptions promoting student involvement and critical evaluation of the works in the field. Examples of course assignments intended to combine theory, research, and practice are included, along with multiple assessment methods for capitalizing upon student strengths. This is a prime source for family therapy trainers seeking to expand their existing models of instruction.

Roberts, J. (1991). Sugar and spice, toads and mice: Gender issues in family therapy training. *Journal of Marital and Family Therapy, 17*(2), 121–132.

Roberts offers four experiential exercises that can be used in training to help trainees address gender issues. These activities could also be adopted to be used with clients. These exercises address what we have learned about gender in our families growing up, through our culture, and through various therapy models. These activities can be very helpful in attending to person-of-the-therapist, supervision, clinical, and classroom issues relating to gender.

Stolk, Y., & Perlesz, A. (1990). Do better trainees make worse family therapists? A followup study of client families. *Family Process, 29*, 45–58.

This is the first empirical study evaluating the effects of training on family therapy outcome. The purpose of this study was to evaluate the effectiveness of the training course in preparing trainees for successful work with families. The findings suggest that families seen by second-year trainees tended to be less satisfied with therapy then families seen by first-year trainees. Although the findings are constrained by the methodological limitations of the study, this groundbreaking study is very thought provoking for both trainers and trainees of family therapy.

Tomm, K. M., & Wright, L. M. (1982). Multilevel training and supervision in an outpatient service program. In R. Whiffen & J. Byng-Hall (Eds.), *Family therapy supervision: Recent developments in practice.* New York: Grune & Stratton.

This chapter articulates many of the policies and procedures adopted at the family therapy program at the University of Calgary. Training facilities, content of training, levels of training, methods of training, and evaluation methods are covered. The hallmark of this piece is the author's discussion of circular pattern diagramming as a teaching tool.

Wheeler, D., Avis, J., Miller, L., & Chaney, S. (1986). Rethinking family therapy education and supervision: A feminist model. *Journal of Psychotherapy and the Family, 1*(4), 53–72.

These authors provide a feminist approach to family therapy. The model proposed describes perceptual, conceptual, and executive skills in relations to three phases of therapy: (1) developing and maintaining a working alliance between the family and the therapist, (2) defining the problem, and (3) facilitating change. Issues of training and supervision in a feminist model are discussed. This is an excellent article that is very useful for both trainers and learners incorporating a feminist lens in their work.

Whiffen, R. (1982). The use of videotape in supervision. In R. Whiffen & J. Byng-Hall (Eds.), *Family therapy supervision: Recent developments in practice.* New York: Grune & Stratton.

The excellent, brief chapter discusses the various uses of videotape in the process of family therapy supervision. Addressed are its contributions to teaching circular functioning in systems, increasing the therapist's awareness of his or her own contribution to the system, encouraging skill development, and offering useful feedback to the family, along with helpful examples of each. A format is suggested for using videotapes within supervisory sessions in such a way as to maximize learning and minimize boredom. Finally, administrative considerations and issues related to the actual process of filming and using the camera are discussed.

Supervision of Supervision

Liddle, H. A., Breunlin, D. C., Schwartz, R. C., & Constantine, J. A. (1984). Training family therapy supervisors: Issues of content, form, and context. *Journal of Marital and Family Therapy, 10*(2), 139–150.

This article elaborates on the form, structure, and process of a program to train family therapy supervisors in the live supervision of structural–strategic therapy. The program includes a small-group supervision seminar, individual supervision-of-supervision meetings, and a supervision group that involves the direct observation–supervision of the work of a supervisor in training. This article would be quite useful for anyone involved in supervision of supervision.

Family Therapy Skills

Cleghorn, J. M., & Levin, S. (1973). Training family therapists by setting learning objectives. *American Journal of Orthopsychiatry, 43,* 439–446.

The authors of this classic article exhibit considerable clarity in distinguishing behavioral objectives for basic-level, advanced, and experienced family therapists. Distinctions among the proposed categories of perceptual, conceptual, and executive skills are less clear, although the classification is cited widely in the family therapy training literature. Therapists who are making the transition from individual therapy to systemic modalities will find this source particularly valuable, as will their trainers.

Falicov, C. J., Constantine, J. A., & Breunlin, D. C. (1981). Teaching family therapy: A program based on training objectives. *Journal of Marital and Family Therapy, 7,* 497–505.

This article represents an initial step in identifying family therapy training objectives toward the goal of training evaluation. Observational, conceptual, and therapeutic skills are delineated for a direct, problem-solving, family therapy approach. The authors concede that the curriculum components in their training program probably overlap and should be more integrated in practice than their list of objectives would suggest.

Wright, L., & Leahey, M. (1994). Calgary Family Intervention Model: One way to think about change. *Journal of Marital and Family Therapy, 20,* 381–396.

This article presents a framework for conceptualizing a fit between family functioning and clinical interventions. The model is called the Calgary Family Intervention Model, and it offers specific ideas for interventions in cognitive, affective, or behavioral domains of family functioning. This article and the framework described could be very useful for trainees as well as for more experienced clinicians.

Tomm, K. M., & Wright, L. M. (1979). Training in family therapy: Perceptual, conceptual, and executive skills. *Family Process, 18*(3), 227–250.

A rather thorough linkup between perceptual/conceptual skills and corresponding executive skills is presented with numerous examples for family therapists' use in sessions. The model delineates therapist functions, competencies, and skills to be displayed over the course of therapy, and provides a handy reference for trainers who wish to underscore the strengths of their trainees as well as areas needing improvement. The bulk of this article is in outline form and may be difficult to absorb in one sitting.

Evaluation

Avis, J., & Sprenkle, D. (1990). Outcome research on family therapy training: A substantive and methodological review. *Journal of Marital and Family Therapy, 16*(3), 241–264.

This article examines developments in empirical research in family therapy training from 1979 to 1986. The article assesses present knowledge concerning training outcomes in marital and family therapy, evaluates research methodologies, and makes recommendations for future research. This is an extremely important article for trainers, supervisors, therapists, and researchers in the field of marriage and family therapy.

Everett, C. A., & Koerpel, B. J. (1986). Family therapy supervision: A review and critique of the literature. *Contemporary Family Therapy, 8,* 62–74.

This article critically reviews 5 years of supervision literature, from 1980 to 1985. The authors address several key points: (1) Supervision is a crucial aspect in the growth of our field; (2) there has not been a careful enough examination of the process of supervision; (3) the supervision literature remains atheoretical and underresearched, and questions pertaining to research and theory have not been articulated; (4) MFT supervision is isolated from related fields; and (5) there is a need for more conceptual and theoretical clarity.

Frankel, B. R., & Piercy, F. P. (1990). The relationship among selected supervisor, therapist, and client behaviors. *Journal of Marital and Family Therapy, 16*(4), 407–421.

This study examined the immediate effects of family therapy live supervision phone-ins on therapist and client behaviors as well as the parallel process between live supervision and therapy. This study is one of the few in the field of marriage and family therapy that researches the important concept of isomorphism in training and therapy.

Kniskern, D. P., & Gurman, A. S. (1979). Research on training in marriage and family therapy: Status, issues, and directions. *Journal of Marital and Family Therapy, 5,* 83–92.

This overview of the evaluative literature for family therapy training raises many important research questions. The article exposes the "empirical ignorance" associated with gaps in the profession's knowledge base regarding training and is thorough in raising issues for clinicians, supervisors, and researchers alike. The authors pinpoint a variety of uncharted areas ripe for investigation.

Wetchler, J. L., Piercy, F. P., & Sprenkle, D. H. (1989). Supervisors' and supervisees' perceptions of the effectiveness of family therapy supervisory techniques. *The American Journal of Family Therapy, 17,* 35–47.

This survey on the perceptions of the effectiveness of supervisory techniques of AAMFT-approved supervisors and their supervisees found that although both rated videotape supervision the most effective, they utilized individual case consultation most frequently. This study offers an important perspective by providing information on the perceptions and use of supervisory techniques from both supervisors' and supervisees' perspectives. This type of exploration is vital in understanding and fostering more collaborative supervisory relationships.

REFERENCES

Alexander, J., Barton, C., Schiavo, R., & Parsons, B. (1976). Systems-behavioral interventions with families of delinquents: Therapist characteristics, family behavior, and outcome. *Journal of Consulting and Clinical Psychology, 44,* 656–664.

Allred, G., & Kersey, F. (1977). The AIAC, a design of systemically analyzing marriage and family counseling: A progress report. *Journal of Marriage and Family Counseling, 3,* 17–26.

Anderson, H., & Swim, S. (1993). Learning as collaborative conversation: Combining the student's and teacher's expertise. *Human Systems, 4,* 145–160.

Anderson, H., & Swim, S. (1995). Supervision as collaborative conversation: Connecting the voices of supervisor and supervisee. *Journal of Systemic Therapy, 14,* 1–13.

Anderson, T. (1987). The reflecting team: Dialogue and metadialogue in clinical work. *Family Process, 26*(4), 415–428.

Aponte, H. (1992). Training the person of the therapist in structural family therapy. *Journal of Marital and Family Therapy, 18,* 269–282.

Aponte, H. (1994). How personal can training get? *Journal of Marital and Family Therapy, 20,* 1–16.

Aradi, N. (1985). *Advantages and disadvantages of the major forms of family therapy supervision.* Unpublished manuscript prepared for a seminar on supervision, Purdue University, West Lafayette, IN.

Avis, J. (1991). Power politics in therapy with women. In T. J. Goodrich (Ed.), *Women and power: Perspectives for family therapy.* New York: Norton.

Avis, J., & Sprenkle, D. H. (1990). A review on outcome research on family therapy training: A substantive and methodological review. *Journal of Marital and Family Therapy, 16*(3), 241–264.

Berger, M., & Dammann, C. (1982). Live supervision as context, treatment, and training. *Family Process, 21,* 337–344.

Bernstein, R., & Burge, S. (1988). A record-keeping format for training systemic therapists. *Family Process, 27*(3), 339–349.

Beroza, R. (1983). The shoemaker's children. *Family Therapy Networker, 7*(2), 31–33.

Bloch, D., & Weiss, H. (1981). Training facilities in marital and family therapy. *Family Process, 20,* 133–146.

Bobele, M., Gardner, G., & Biever, J. (1995). Supervision as social construction. *Journal of Systemic Therapies, 14*(2), 14–25.

386 FAMILY THERAPY SOURCEBOOK

Breunlin, D. C., & Cade, B. (1981). Intervening in family systems with observer messages. *Journal of Marital and Family Therapy, 7*, 453–460.

Breunlin, D. C., Karrer, B. M., McGuire, D. E., & Cimmarusti, R. A. (1988). Cybernetics of videotape supervision. In H. A. Liddle, D. C. Breunlin, & R. C. Schwartz (Eds.), *Handbook of family therapy training and supervision*. New York: Guilford Press.

Breunlin, D., Rampage, C., & Eovaldi, M. (1994). Family therapy supervision: Toward an integrative perspective. In R. Mikesell, D. D. Lusterman, & S. McDaniel (Eds.), *Family psychology and systems therapy: A handbook*. Washington, DC: American Psychological Association.

Breunlin, D. C., Schwartz, R. C., Krause, M. S., & Selby, L. M. (1983). Evaluating family therapy training: The development of an instrument. *Journal of Marital and Family Therapy, 9*(1), 37–47.

Breunlin, D., Schwartz, R., & Mac Kune-Karrer, B. (1992). *Metaframeworks: Transcending the models of family therapy*. San Francisco: Jossey-Bass.

Broderick, C. B., & Schrader, S. S. (1981). The history of professional marriage and family therapy. In A. S. Gurman & D. P. Kniskern (Eds.), *Handbook of family therapy*. New York: Brunner/Mazel.

Burman, E., & Dixon-Murphy, T. (1979). Training in marital and family therapy at free standing institutes. *Journal of Marital and Family Therapy, 5*, 29–42.

Byles, J., Bishop, D., & Horn, D. (1983). Evaluation of a family therapy training program. *Journal of Marital and Family Therapy, 9*, 299–304.

Byng-Hall, J. (1982). The use of the earphone in supervision. In R. Whiffen & J. Byng-Hall (Eds.), *Family therapy supervision: Recent developments in practice*. New York: Grune & Stratton.

Carter, E. (1982). Supervisory discussion in the presence of the family. In R. Whiffen & J. Byng-Hall (Eds.), *Family therapy supervision: Recent developments in practice*. New York: Grune & Stratton.

Churven, P., & McKinnon, T. (1982). Family therapy training: An evaluation of a workshop. *Family Process, 21*, 345–352.

Cleghorn, J. M., & Levin, S. (1973). Training family therapists by setting instructional objectives. *American Journal of Orthopsychiatry, 43*, 439–446.

Coleman, S., Avis, J., & Turin, M. (1990). A study of the role of gender in family therapy training. *Family Process, 29*(4), 365–374.

Commission on Accreditation for Marriage and Family Therapy Education. (1994). *Manual on accreditation*. Washington, DC: American Association for Marriage and Family Therapy.

Connell, G. M. (1984). An approach to supervision of symbolic–experiential psychotherapy. *Journal of Marital and Family Therapy, 10*, 273–280.

Constantine, J. A., Piercy, F. P., & Sprenkle, D. H. (1984). Live supervision in family therapy. *Journal of Marital and Family Therapy, 10*, 95–97.

Constantine, J. A., Stone Fish, L. S., & Piercy, F. P. (1984). A systematic procedure for teaching positive connotation. *Journal of Marital and Family Therapy, 10*(3), 313–316.

Coppersmith, E. I. (1980). Expanding uses of the telephone in family therapy. *Family Process, 19,* 411–417.

DeShazer, S., & Molnar, A. (1984). Changing teams/changing families. *Family Process, 22,* 481–486.

Everett, C. (1979). The masters degree in marriage and family therapy. *Journal of Marital and Family Therapy, 5,* 7–13.

Everett, C. (1980). An analysis of AAMFT supervisors: Their identities, roles, and resources. *Journal of Marital and Family Therapy, 6,* 215–226.

Falicov, C. J., Constantine, J. A., & Breunlin, D. C. (1981). Teaching family therapy: A program based on training objectives. *Journal of Marital and Family Therapy, 7,* 497–505.

Fenell, D. L., Hovestadt, A. J., & Harvey, S. J. (1986). A comparison of delayed feedback and live supervision models of marriage and family therapist clinical training. *Journal of Marital and Family, 12,* 181–186.

Fisher, B. L., & Sprenkle, D. H. (1980). Family therapy conceptualization and use of "case notes." *Family Therapy, 2,* 177–184.

Framo, J. (1976). Chronicle of a struggle to establish a family unit within a community mental health center. In P. J. Guerin (Ed.), *Family therapy: Theory and practice.* New York: Gardner.

Frankel, B. R., & Piercy, F. P. (1990). The relationship among selected supervisor, therapist, and client behaviors. *Journal of Marital and Family Therapy, 16*(4), 407–421.

Garfield, R. (1979). An integrative training model for family therapists: The Hahnemann Master of Family Therapy program. *Journal of Marital and Family Therapy, 5,* 15–22.

Haley, J. (1975). Why a mental health clinic should avoid family therapy. *Journal of Marriage and Family Counseling, 1,* 3–14.

Haley, J. (1988). Reflections on supervision. In H. A. Liddle, D. C. Breunlin, & R. C. Schwartz (Eds.), *Handbook of family therapy training and supervision.* New York: Guilford Press.

Heath, T. (1983). The live supervision form: Structure and theory for assessment in live supervision. In J. C. Hansen & B. P. Keeney (Eds.), *Diagnosis and assessment in family therapy.* Rockville, MD: Aspen Systems.

Henry, P. W. (1983). *The family therapy profession: University and institute perspectives.* Unpublished doctoral dissertation, Purdue University, West Lafayette, IN.

Hoffman, L. (1993). *Exchanging voices.* London: Karnac Books.

Kaiser, T. (1992). The supervisory relationship: An identification of the primary elements in the relationship and an application of two theories of ethical relationships. *Journal of Marital and Family Therapy, 18,* 283–296.

Keller, J. F., & Protinsky, H. (1984). A self-management model for supervision. *Journal of Marital and Family Therapy, 10,* 281–288.

Kolevzon, M. S., & Green, R. G. (1983). Practice and training in family therapy: A known group study. *Family Process, 22,* 179–190.

Kniskern, D. P., & Gurman, A. S. (1979). Research on training in marriage and family: Status, issues and directions. *Journal of Marital and Family Therapy, 5,* 83–92.

L'Abate, L., Berger, M., Wright, L., & O'Shea, M. (1979). Training family psychologists: The family studies program at Georgia State University. *Professional Psychology, 10,* 58–65.

Lambert, M. J., & Arnold, R. C. (1987). Research and the supervisory process. *Professional Psychology: Research and Practice, 18*(3), 217–224.

Landau, J., & Stanton, M. D. (1983). Aspects of supervision with the "Pick-A-Dali Circus" model. *Journal of Strategic and Systemic Therapies, 2*(2), 31–39.

Liddle, H. A. (1978). The emotional and political hazards of teaching and learning family therapy. *Family Therapy, 5,* 1–12.

Liddle, H. A. (1982a). Family therapy training: Current issues, future trends. *International Journal of Family Therapy, 4,* 31–47.

Liddle, H. A. (1982b). On the problems of eclecticism: A call for epistemologic clarification and human scale theories. *Family Process, 21,* 243–250.

Liddle, H. A. (1982c). Using mental imagery to create therapeutic and supervisory realities. *American Journal of Family Therapy, 10,* 68–72.

Liddle, H. A. (1991). Training and supervision in family therapy: A comprehensive and critical analysis. In A. Gurman and D. Kniskern (Eds.), *Handbook of family therapy* (Vol. 2). New York: Brunner/Mazel.

Liddle, H. A., Breunlin, D. C., & Schwartz, R. C. (Eds.). (1988). *Handbook of family therapy training and supervision.* New York: Guilford Press.

Liddle, H. A., Breunlin, D. C., Schwartz, R. C., & Constantine, H. A. (1984). Training family therapy supervisors: Issues of content, form, and context. *Journal of Marital and Family Therapy, 10*(2), 139–150.

Liddle, H. A., & Halpin, R. J. (1978). Family therapy training and supervision literature: A comparative review. *Journal of Marriage and Family Counseling, 4,* 77–98.

Liddle, H. A., & Saba, G. W. (1982). Teaching family therapy at the introductory level: A conceptual model emphasizing a pattern which connects training and therapy. *Journal of Marital and Family Therapy, 8,* 63–72.

Liddle, H. A., & Saba, G. (1984). The isomorphic nature of training and therapy: Epistemological foundation for a structural–strategic training program. In J. Schwartzman (Ed.), *Families and other systems: The macrosystemic context of family therapy.* New York: Guilford Press.

Liddle, H. A., & Schwartz, R. C. (1983). Live supervision/consultation: Conceptual and pragmatic guidelines for family therapy trainers. *Family Process, 22,* 477–490.

Magee, R. (1985). *Advantages and disadvantages of various forms of family therapy supervision.* Unpublished manuscript prepared for a seminar on supervision, Purdue University, West Lafayette, IN.

McCollum, E. (1990). Integrating structural, strategic, and Bowen approaches to family therapy supervision. *Contemporary Family Therapy, 12*(1), 23–34.

McCollum, E., & Wetchler, J. (1995). In defense of case consultation: Maybe "dead" supervision isn't dead after all. *Journal of Marital and Family Therapy*, *21*, 155–166.

McDaniel, S., & Landau-Stanton, J. (1991). Family-of-origin work and family therapy skills training: Both–and. *Family Process, 30*, 459–471.

McDaniel, S. H., Weber, T., & McKeever, J. (1983). Multiple theoretical approaches to supervision: Choices in family therapy training. *Family Process, 22*, 491–500.

McKenzie, P. N., Atkinson, B. J., Quinn, W. H., & Heath, A. (1986). Training and supervision in marriage and family therapy. *The American Journal of Family Therapy, 14*, 293–303.

Mohammed, Z., & Piercy, F. P. (1983) The effects of two methods of training and sequencing on structuring and relationship skills of family therapists. *American Journal of Family Therapy, 4*, 64–71.

Nichols, W. C. (1979). Doctoral programs in marital and family therapy. *Journal of Marital and Family Therapy, 5*, 23–28.

Nichols, W. C., Nichols, D. P., & Hardy, K. V. (1990). Supervision in family therapy: A decade restudy. *Journal of Marital and Family Therapy, 16*(3), 275–285.

Nielsen, E., & Kaslow, F. (1980). Consultation in family therapy. *American Journal of Family Therapy, 8*, 35–42.

Olson, U., & Pegg, P. F. (1979). Direct open supervision: A team approach. *Family Process, 18*, 463–469.

Papp, P. (1980). The Greek chorus and other techniques of paradoxical therapy. *Family Process, 19*, 45–57.

Piercy, F. P. (Ed.). (1985). *Family therapy education and supervision*. Binghamton, NY: Haworth. (Also published as Vol. 1, No. 4, of the *Journal of Psychotherapy and the Family*)

Piercy, F. P., Laird, R. A., & Mohammed, Z. (1983). A family therapist rating scale. *Journal of Marital and Family Therapy, 9*, 49–60.

Piercy, F. P., & Sprenkle, D. H. (1983). Ethical, legal, and professional issues in family therapy: A graduate level course. *Journal of Marital and Family Therapy, 9*(4), 393–401.

Piercy, F. P., & Sprenkle, D. H. (1984). The process of family therapy education. *Journal of Marital and Family Therapy, 10*(4), 399–407.

Piercy, F. P., & Sprenkle, D. H. (1985). Family therapy theory development: An integrated training approach. In F. P. Piercy (Ed.), *Family therapy education and supervision*. Binghamton, NY: Haworth.

Piercy, F. P., & Sprenkle, D. H., & Constantine, J. A. (1986). Family members' perceptions of live observation/supervision: An exploratory study. *Contemporary Family Therapy: An International Journal, 8*(3), 171–187.

Pinsof, W. M. (1979). The Family Therapist Behavior Scale (FTBS): Development and evaluation of a coding system. *Family Process, 18*, 451–461.

Pinsof, W. M. (1981). Family therapy process research. In A. S. Gurman & D. P. Kniskern (Eds.), *Handbook of family therapy*. New York: Brunner/Mazel.

Prest, L., Darden, E., & Keller, J. (1990). "The fly on the wall" reflecting team supervision. *Journal of Marital and Family Therapy, 16*(3), 256–273.

Prosky, P. (1982). The use of analogic and digital communication in training systems perception and intervention. In R. Whiffen & J. Byng-Hall (Eds.), *Family therapy supervision: Recent developments in practice*. New York: Grune & Stratton.

Pullet Blank, E., & Shapiro, R. J. (1986). Evaluation of family therapy trainings. *Family Process, 25,* 591–598.

Roberts, J. (1983). The third tier: The overlooked dimension in family therapy training. *Family Therapy Networker, 72*(2), 30–31, 60–61.

Roberts, J. (1991). Sugar and spice, toads and mice: Gender issues in family therapy training. *Journal of Marital and Family Therapy, 17*(2), 121–132.

Roberts, J., Matthews, W., Bodin, N., Cohen, D., Lewandowski, L., Novo, J., Pumilia, J., & Willis, C. (1989). Training with O (observing) and T (treatment) teams in live supervision: Reflections in the looking glass. *Journal of Marital and Family Therapy, 15,* 397–410.

Saba, G. W., & Liddle, H. A. (1986). Perceptions of professional needs, practice patterns, and initial issues facing family therapy trainers and supervisors. *American Journal of Family Therapy, 14,* 109–122.

Schwartz, R. C. (1981). The conceptual development of family therapy trainees. *American Journal of Family Therapy, 9,* 89–90.

Schwartz, R. C. (1988). The trainer–trainee relationship in family therapy training. In H. A. Liddle, D. C. Breunlin, & R. C. Schwartz (Eds.), *Handbook of family therapy training and supervision*. New York: Guilford Press.

Schwartz, R. C. (1995). *Internal family systems therapy*. New York: Guilford Press.

Schwartz, R. C., Liddle, H. A., & Breunlin, D. C. (1988). Muddles in live supervision. In H. A. Liddle, D. C. Breunlin, & R. C. Schwartz (Eds.), *Handbook of family therapy training and supervision*. New York: Guilford Press.

Selekman, M., & Todd, T. (1990). *Co-creating a context for change in supervision: Application of the solution-focused model*. Unpublished manuscript.

Smith, C. W., Smith, T. A., & Salts, C. J. (1991). The effects of supervisory interruptions on therapists and clients. *American Journal of Family Therapy, 19*(3), 250–256.

Smith, V. G., & Nichols, W. C. (1979). Accreditation in marital and family therapy. *Journal of Marital and Family Therapy, 5,* 95–100.

Sprenkle, D. H. (1988). Training and supervision in degree-granting graduate programs in family therapy. In H. A. Liddle, D. C. Breunlin, & R. C. Schwartz (Eds.), *Handbook of family therapy training and supervision*. New York: Guilford Press.

Sprenkle, D. H., & Piercy, F. P. (1984). Research in family therapy: A graduate level course. *Journal of Marital and Family Therapy, 10*(3), 225–240.

Stolk, Y., & Perlesz, A. (1990). Do better trainees make worse family therapists? A follow-up study of client families. *Family Process, 29,* 45–58.

Storm, C. (1991). Placing gender in the heart of MFT masters programs: Teaching a gender sensitive systemic view. *Journal of Marital and Family Therapy, 17*(1), 45–52.

Street, E., & Treacher, A. (1980). Microtraining and family therapy skills. *Journal of Family Therapy, 2,* 243–257.

Todd, T., & Greenberg, A. (1987). No question has a single answer: Integrating discrepant models in family therapy training. *Contemporary Family Therapy, 9,* 116–137.

Todd, T., & Storm, C. (in press). *The complete systemic supervisor: Context, philosophy and pragmatics.* Needham Heights, MA: Allyn & Bacon.

Tomm, K. M., & Leahey, M. (1980). Training in family assessment: A comparison of three teaching methods. *Journal of Marital and Family Therapy, 6,* 453–457.

Tomm, K. M., & Wright, L. M. (1979). Training in family therapy: Perceptual, conceptual, and executive skills. *Family Process, 18,* 227–250.

Tucker, S. J., & Pinsof, W. M. (1984). The empirical evaluation of family therapy training. *Family Process, 23,* 437–456.

Wetchler, J. L., Piercy, F. P., & Sprenkle, D. H. (1989). Supervisors' and supervisees' perceptions of the effectiveness of family therapy supervisory techniques. *American Journal of Family Therapy, 17,* 35–47.

Wheeler, D., Avis, J., Miller, L., & Chaney, S. (1986). Rethinking family therapy education and supervision: A feminist model. In F. Piercy (Ed.), *Family therapy education and supervision.* Binghamton, NY: Haworth.

Whiffen, R. (1982). The use of videotape in supervision. In R. Whiffen & J. Byng-Hall (Eds.), *Family therapy supervision: Recent developments in practice.* New York: Grune & Stratton.

Whiffen, R., & Byng-Hall, J. (Eds.). (1982). *Family therapy supervision: Recent developments in practice.* New York: Grune & Stratton.

Whitaker, C. A., & Keith, D. V. (1981). Symbolic–experiential family therapy. In A. S. Gurman & D. P. Kniskern (Eds.), *Handbook of family therapy.* New York: Brunner/Mazel.

White, M. (1989/1990, Summer). Family therapy training and supervision in a world of experience and narrative. *Dulwich Centre Newsletter,* pp. 27–38.

Williams, L. (1994). A tool for training supervisors: Using the Supervision Feedback Form (SFF). *Journal of Marital and Family Therapy, 20,* 311–315.

Wright, L., & Leahey, M. (1994). Calgary Family Intervention Model: One way to think about change. *Journal of Marital and Family Therapy, 20,* 381–396.

Young, J. (1989/1990, Summer). A critical look at the one-way screen. *Dulwich Centre Newsletter,* pp. 5–11.

Zaken-Greenberg, F., & Neimeyer, G. J. (1986). *The impact of structural family therapy training on conceptual and executive skills. Family Process, 25,* 599–608.

14

~

Research in Family Therapy

DOUGLAS H. SPRENKLE
DEREK BALL

FOR FAMILY therapy to mature as a discipline and become respectable in the mental health field, it must be able to authenticate its efficacy through high-quality research (Pinsof & Wynne, 1995). Moreover, there should be a synergistic interplay among research, theory, and practice (Olson, 1976; Sprenkle, 1976). It is certainly no secret that theory (often "armchair" theory) has far outstripped the field's ability to authenticate it. Our practice, sad to say, is too often a grab bag of techniques, few of which have been proven superior to others in reasonably controlled investigations. This is ironic, since, as Wynne (1983) states, our field began with a strong bond between research and practice. It is too often true that clinicians and researchers tend to be two different types of people who do not understand each other's language and concerns, and seldom talk to each other (Olson, 1981; Schwartz & Breunlin, 1983). Our field remains too often dominated by charismatic clinician/teachers whose ideas have rarely been empirically tested with anything approaching scientific rigor (Sprenkle & Bischoff, 1995).

NEED FOR SPECIFIC TRAINING
IN FAMILY THERAPY RESEARCH

Because family therapy is a unique discipline, training in family therapy research cannot be adequately completed by simply taking traditional research methods courses. Most courses and books on research are developed by people with little understanding of family therapy. Sociologists tend to emphasize large-scale survey research and design, and sampling and analysis techniques that are of marginal relevance to family therapy researchers. Traditional psychologists often emphasize experimental designs that cannot be easily replicated in family therapy settings. Research examples infrequently focus on intervention, and if they do, they often are not sensitive to the special problems of measuring family interaction and change. Other issues of interest to family therapy researchers (e.g., the cost-effectiveness of interventions, attention to process as well as outcome variables) are seldom understood by most methodologists. Sprenkle and Moon (1996) edited the first book written specifically about family therapy research methodology. Because of the aforementioned concerns, the editors of this volume required chapter authors to utilize family therapy examples in their presentations of quantitative, qualitative, and mixed research methodologies.

This chapter opens with a glossary of basic terms related to family therapy research. Then, a number of basic content areas and relevant resources and teaching strategies are described. The chapter concludes with an annotated bibliography of key resources on family therapy research.

KEY CONCEPTS

Although quantitative methods have dominated the field of marriage and family therapy research, there is a growing awareness that qualitative measures are also important for the field's growth (Piercy & Sprenkle, 1990). Qualitative methods are seen as a means for expanding and enhancing quantitative research and giving a contextual understanding of quantitative data (Moon, Dillon, & Sprenkle, 1990). Due to their distinctive differences, we have separated qualitative and quantitative concepts; but we have included concepts from both areas to emphasize the impact both have on marriage and family therapy research.

Qualitative Concepts

Critical theory. An approach to theory, critical theory states that humans interact with what they "know" and that their values and beliefs play a large part in how they "know" (Rediger, 1996). Similar to social constructionists, critical theorists avoid the positivist notion of a neutral approach to research. Instead, they emphasize an active interaction with one's values, both chosen and unchosen, that they believe pervade one's research approach.

Ethnography. A study in which the researcher closely observes and possibly participates in, the daily lives of the research participants, ethnographic research could study the lives of therapists or observe and record the experiences of being a family therapy client (Newfield, Sells, & Smith, 1996).

Focus group. In this qualitative approach to data collection, a moderator facilitates a group discussion on a prescribed topic (Piercy & Nickerson, 1996). The moderator can open up a free discussion or choose to probe for specific examples from the group participants. The moderator then writes down themes of the discussion and analyzes the transcript of the focus-group session.

Grounded theory. A methodology in which theory development arises out of data that is collected and analyzed systematically (Rafuls & Moon, 1996), grounded theory is a process in which data is collected and analyzed for emergent themes and theoretical categories. These categories are then used to inform further data collection, and the loop continues building.

Phenomenology. This methodology is one in which the researcher does not assume an a priori definition of the experience under study. Instead, the researcher learns about the subject by experiencing it (Rahilly, 1993). This methodology is primarily an inductive approach and fits nicely into the social constructionist framework.

Social construction. The philosophy that knowledge does not exist apart from the knower and, rather, emerges from the social interaction between people, and therefore is not an objective entity but a relativistic result of social relationships (Boss, Dahl, & Kaplan, 1996) is called social construction. Important concepts to the social constructionist researcher are meaning, language, and experience of the participants. There is also a distinction made between constructionism and constructivism. Although often used interchangeably, constructivism, a term with roots in biology, is a scientific metaphor that views reality as a product of individually unique human processes. In contrast, constructionism is based in a philosophy of community processing and views reality as a result of interaction (Mills & Sprenkle, 1995).

Triangulation. As a means of establishing validity in qualitative research, in triangulation, data is collected from more than one source and, if possible, by more than one method (Moon et al., 1990). The purpose of this multiple data collection is to check on the validity of the initial observation and rule out any alternative hypotheses.

Quantitative Concepts

Clinical versus statistical significance. Clinical significance is obtained when a previously dysfunctional person scores in the functional range after treatment. This measure differs from statistical significance, which simply evaluates group means. Although differences between two treatment groups may be significantly different statistically, those who have statistically improved may not have become functional as a result of treatment. Clinical significance offers such information (Sprenkle & Bischoff, 1995).

Comparative studies of outcome. In the marriage and family therapy field, studies that compare different types of marital and family therapy with each other and with other therapies (Gurman & Kniskern, 1978) are called comparative studies of outcome. An example of the former would be Shadish, Ragsdale, Glaser, and Montgomery's (1995) investigation of various marital treatment modalities. An example of the latter would be Joanning, Thomas, Quinn, and Mullen's (1992) comparisons of family versus individual treatment. Pinsof and Wynne (1995) caution about comparisons between family and individual treatment, because frequency of treatment may be a mediating factor in outcome differences.

Controlled studies of outcome. These studies include random assignment by the investigator to at least one experimental treatment group and one control group. The latter could be a no-treatment and/or an alternative treatment group. Most controlled studies in marriage and family therapy have been published in the last two decades. Although Kniskern (1985) is amenable to noncontrolled exploratory research, Pinsof and Wynne (1995) call for more methodologically rigorous studies, including random assignment and control groups.

Core battery. Marital and family therapists, like individual therapists, have argued the relative merits of a core or common battery of assessment instruments. The clear advantage would be comparability across studies. It appears, however, that there is not sufficient consensus in the field concerning what dependent variables should be utilized to reach agreement on a core battery (Gurman & Kniskern, 1981). Pinsof and Wynne (1995) call for a combination of a standard core battery used in all studies and then a context-specific battery that captures the unique aspects of the individual study.

Cost-effectiveness analysis and cost–benefit analysis. These two sets of procedures can help decision makers determine the value of psychotherapy. In cost-effectiveness analysis (CEA), the investigator determines what the costs of therapy (personnel, facilities and equipment, patient's time, etc.) are in dollar terms. The effects can be in any unit (e.g., increase in marital satisfaction scores). A CEA study in marriage and family therapy might examine the relative cost of conjoint versus conjoint group treatment in reducing marital distress. Cost–benefit analysis (CBA) is more difficult, because it requires that the effects of outcomes must also be in dollar terms (e.g., money saved from reduced worker absenteeism due to marital therapy for chemically dependent couples). CBA leads to a ratio whereby total benefits are divided by total costs. This ratio must be greater than one if the intervention is to be deemed worthwhile (Pike, MacKinnon, & Piercy, 1996). Cost-effectiveness measures are seen as increasingly important variables in marriage and family research (Pinsof & Wynne, 1995).

Design criteria. In their classic review article on research in marriage and family therapy, Gurman and Kniskern (1978, pp. 820–821) gave the field an influential list of 14 criteria by which the adequacy of outcome studies may be evaluated. Points are assigned for each criterion (e.g., "controlled assignment of treatment condition," 5 points). Point totals enable one to classify the design of a study on a continuum from "poor" to "very good."

Deterioration effects. Research in marriage and family therapy that focuses on whether some clients get worse or are harmed by intervention is called deterioration effects. Gurman and Kniskern (1978) estimate that 5–10% of clients or relationships get worse in marriage and family therapy using a large number of uncontrolled studies of nonbehavioral therapy. A recent review by Pinsof and Wynne (1995) has shown that there has not been a replicated or controlled study of marriage and family therapy in which marriage and family therapy clients had poorer outcomes than those receiving no therapy.

Discovery versus verification. Uncontrolled or descriptive studies may be argued to be of value if they are viewed to be operating in the context of discovery (discovering or exploring new relationships, generating hypotheses, etc.). Qualitative research can also be a means for discovery (Sprenkle & Moon, 1996). Experimentally controlled studies are done in a context of verifying theoretically or empirically derived hypotheses. Pinsof and Wynne (1995) call for more experimentally controlled studies in the field of marriage and family therapy.

Effect size. This is the most typical dependent variable in meta-analysis (to be discussed). In its most common expression, it is the difference between two means divided by a standard deviation. In most cases, researchers employing meta-analysis subtract the mean of the control group from the mean of the experimental group and divide by the standard deviation of the control group (Shadish et al., 1995).

Efficacy versus effectiveness. These two terms are measures of helpfulness of a particular treatment that are defined somewhat differently. Efficacy is a measure of whether a treatment works in a controlled, experimental, research setting. Effectiveness is a measure of whether a treatment works in nonexperimental, "normal therapy" conditions (Pinsof & Wynne, 1995).

Exhaustiveness (of a coding system). Defined as the degree to which the instrument codes every possible therapist and/or client behavior, Pinsof's (1981) Family Therapy Coding System is an example of an exhaustive coding system.

Experimental research. This is a study in which an investigator manipulates (has control over) at least one independent variable (see also Ex post facto research). In marriage and family therapy research, this independent variable is typically the treatment. Experimental research in this field typically involves the random assignment of subjects to groups and the random assignment of treatment to groups (Lyness & Sprenkle, 1996). Some authors (e.g., Todd &

Stanton, 1983) do not believe that random assignment of therapists to treatment is advisable, because this means that a therapist must try to utilize a method to which he or she may not be committed. Good experimental designs are reviewed in Kerlinger (1986, Chap. 18).

Ex post facto research. Literally, this is research "from what is done afterward." There can be no random assignment of subjects or treatment, because the independent variables have already occurred. The investigator begins with observations of dependent variables and retrospectively studies the independent variables (Kerlinger, 1986). Beck and Jones's (1973) study of the effectiveness of family service agency therapy is a good example of ex post facto research.

History. One of the major threats to validity in poorly controlled research, history specifically refers to extraneous variables that occur during a study that might affect outcome and could inadvertently be attributed to the intervention under study (Kerlinger, 1986). For example, if subjects in a Couples Communication Program (CCP) outcome study attended a Marriage Encounter (ME) weekend, the latter might contribute to the observed change during this time period (see also Maturation).

Maturation. Another threat to validity in uncontrolled research, maturation is similar to history, except that extraneous variables are not specific. It refers more to general change or growth as a result of passage of time or daily living (Kerlinger, 1986). The fact that most untreated people recover from divorce with the passage of time might threaten an uncontrolled (no "no-treatment" control group) study of the effectiveness of a divorce recovery versus intervention program.

Mediating versus ultimate goals. When measuring outcome in marriage and family therapy, researchers need to distinguish between goals that represent enabling or intermediate (mediating) conditions and those that represent the final or broader (ultimate) goals of therapy. For example, if getting Sally to attend school is an ultimate goal, a mediating goal might be to increase the parents' authority with their children. Shadish (1992) emphasizes the importance of including both in studies of outcome and criticizes the overemphasis on ultimate goals.

Meta-analysis, narrative report, and box score. Terms that relate to procedures for reviewing and summarizing research results. In its most generic sense, meta-analysis is any literature review that uses a quantitative approach to summarize results across studies. A common metric is identified and then used to standardize studies in order to combine results (Wampler, 1982). The most common metric is the "effect size" (see above), which typically transforms results into standard deviation units. A good example of meta-analysis is the Shadish et al. (1995) analysis of the efficacy and effectiveness of marital and family therapy. The more typical qualitative literature review is the narrative report, in which the researcher makes his or her own subjective integration of the data. The box score approach to reviewing the literature typically tallies studies on the basis of statistically significant results. For example, "non-behavioral family therapy has yielded results superior to those of no treatment in 8 out of 13 comparisons, with five finding no differences" (Gurman & Kniskern, 1978, p. 845). Meta-analysts assert that relying on statistical significance ignores subtle but meaningful change and does not often measure the magnitude of change.

 Process research. This research focuses on the attempt to operationally and/or reliably describe the actual events within the therapy process (Gurman, Kniskern, & Pinsof, 1986). Process researchers believe their endeavors are essential to answer the specificity question of what treatment (intervention) by what therapist works best for what clients under what circumstances (Paul, 1967). Process research is still somewhat new, but Gurman et al. (1986) offer the field some research strategies that may elucidate the relationship between process and outcome variables. They advocate for a "new process perspective" that looks not at the relationship between the therapy process and some final, distant outcome, but rather envisions "outcome" as a series of smaller "episodes" in therapy in which some kind of theoretically significant event occurs (Piercy & Sprenkle, 1990).

 Reactive measures. The act of measuring subjects often changes them. A measurement is reactive when the subject is directly involved in the study and he or she reacts to the measurement process itself. A nonreactive measure is an unobtrusive or passive measure and does not itself change the subject's behavior (Lambert & Hill, 1994). In family therapy research, measures of weight gain following anorexia or recidivism (as measured by arrests) following family therapy for delinquency are considered nonreactive measures.

 Reconstructivity (of a coding system). The ability of a coding system to permit clinically meaningful reconstruction of the specific behaviors or experiences denoted by the codes is called reconstructivity. Pinsof's (1981) Family Therapy Coding System is high on reconstructivity.

 Regression effects. Another threat to validity, this term refers to the fact that very high and low scores on a test are often due to chance factors; upon a second testing, they are likely to regress toward the mean (Kerlinger, 1986). For example, high pretest scores for some individuals will yield lower posttest scores and vice versa. These changes will often occur independently of treatment.

 Reliability. Essentially, this is the stability and consistency of measurement by an instrument. Like "validity" (see below), reliability cannot be dealt with comprehensively here.

 "Test–retest reliability" is ascertained by having subjects take an instrument on several occasions and then correlating these scores. Developers of coding systems for behavioral measures report measures of "interrater reliability," which is the degree to which two or more raters agree when coding the same data. "Intrarater reliability," on the other hand, is the degree to which a single rater agrees with him- or herself when coding the same data at two different time periods. Adequate intrarater reliability shows that a coding system can be learned and applied consistently, whereas interrater reliability shows that different raters have the same understanding and are consistent. Researchers in marriage and family therapy are also concerned with the "internal consistency reliability" of their instruments. Items within a subscale, for example, are analyzed to make sure that they correlate positively with other subscale items (or a hypothesized universe for such items, as in Cronbach's alpha).

Single-case designs. In marriage and family therapy research, designs that measure a single couple, family or individual are called single-case designs. Typically, a baseline is established by repeated measures of a dependent variable in the absence of intervention. Then an independent (usually treatment) variable is introduced, with the effect noted in the dependent variable. Finally, the process of withdrawing and introducing treatment is repeated several times (Dickey, 1996). The results may then be replicated across different subjects, behaviors, or settings (Kazdin, 1994). Although the method has been touted as promising for research in the field (Kazdin, 1992), several important issues related to single-case designs have not been adequately addressed (Kazdin, 1994).

Stimulus heterogeneity. When researching the effect of different therapeutic behaviors, the researcher must control for the fact that families (and hence the degree of difficulty of cases) differ. Stimulus heterogeneity across treatment groups may be maximized through (1) random assignment of families and therapists, or (2) standardization of the in-therapy behavior of the family members through the use of actors or a simulated therapy situation in which the therapist responds to a family or videotape (Pinsof, 1981).

Triple threat. A term coined by David Olson (1976), triple threat refers to the ideal synergistic interplay among theory, research, and practice in the family field. A therapist will be a better clinician, for example, if his or her practice is guided by theory and is tested empirically. Each of the three domains enriches the other two.

Treatment on demand (TOD). This method was devised as an alternative to no-treatment control groups due to ethical concerns about not treating clients. Each control family has access to a therapist "on demand" (if necessary), but such visits are severely limited in number (Gurman & Kniskern, 1981). Todd and Stanton (1983) criticize the TOD design because there is self-selection among those clients who do not use TOD sessions, those who do but do not exceed the limits, and those who exceed the cutoff number of sessions.

Validity. A complex topic, validity can only be dealt with in broad strokes here. In marriage and family therapy research, "internal validity" would ask the question of whether the treatment being studied really made a significant difference. The major threats to internal validity are such aforementioned issues as history, maturation, regression, and reactive measurement effects (Kerlinger, 1986). Researchers in marriage and family therapy are also frequently interested in several other types of validity, as follows: The "content validity" of an instrument reflects the extent to which it samples the universe of content about the particular construct being measured. Most typically, instrument developers utilize a panel of experts to help determine whether the instrument sufficiently represents the content of what it purports to represent. For example, the content related to intergenerational family process should be included in the items of a family differentiation scale (Bray, Williamson, & Malone, 1984). "Discriminant validity" represents the ability of an instrument to distinguish between individuals or groups that are assumed to differ on the variable being measured (e.g., beginning and experienced therapists have been shown to differ on the Family Therapist Rating Scale; see Piercy, Laird, & Mohammed, 1983). "Predictive validity" refers to the ability of an instrument to predict future behaviors or outcomes on another variable. Alexander, Barton, Schiavo, and Parsons's (1976) measure of structuring and relationship skills has been shown, for example, to predict therapy outcome.

"Construct validity" is concerned with the degree to which the instrument, in fact, measures the theoretical construct it was designed to measure. Allred's research with the Allred Interaction Analysis for Counselors (Allred & Kersey, 1977) represents one of the few attempts within family therapy research to formally test the construct validity of an instrument (Pinsof, 1981, p. 736).

FOUNDATIONS FOR FAMILY THERAPY RESEARCH: CONTENT AREAS AND LEARNING ACTIVITIES

Review of Basic Experimental Designs

Comments on the Area

Although most family therapists have had some training in methodology and statistics, an excellent review of research design can be found in Kerlinger (1986). These chapters review the typical faulty designs and explain carefully the components of good designs. They deal well with such threats to validity as history, maturation, reactivity, and regression effects, and they discuss major forms of reliability and validity.

Learning Activity

Students are given a hypothetical situation and then asked, in small groups, to develop a study utilizing the various designs. Here is one example: "You are a family therapist who has devised what you consider to be an effective program of mediating child custody disputes. Your local court system has given you funding to test your model. Describe your study utilizing a matched-subjects experimental design. Also, make a list of the strengths and limitations of this design." Different small groups are assigned different designs.

Lessons from Psychotherapy Research

Comments on the Area

It is instructive to review the history of psychotherapy research, beginning with Eysenck's (1952) challenge that nonbehavioral psychotherapy is ineffective. There are many lessons to be learned from this rich history, and psychotherapy research forms an excellent foundation for the study of family therapy research. Parloff (1980) is an excellent single resource. His monograph describes the basic research designs used in psychotherapy research, delineates the difficulties in conducting research, and critically evaluates the various methods of integrating findings such as box-score analysis and meta-analysis. Parloff also devotes several chapters to a topic that has (until recently) never been adequately discussed in the family therapy research literature, namely, methods for conducting cost-effectiveness research in MFT (Pike, MacKinnon, & Piercy, 1996).

Learning Activity

Students (individually or in teams) are assigned to play the roles of the various protagonists in a debate on the effectiveness of psychotherapy. For example, one student, playing the role of "Eysenck," throws down the gauntlet to the psychotherapy profession and offers a rationale for his or her challenge. Another student, playing the role of "Bergin," disputes Eysenck's findings by telling how he or she recomputed Eysenck's treatment remission rates using different assumptions and procedures. Depending on time and the number of students, the debate can continue through the most recent challenge to psychotherapy.

Learning Activity 2

The most comprehensive sourcebook about psychotherapy research is by Garfield and Bergin (1994). One can pursue the ideas noted previously in more depth by assigning key chapters in this handbook.

Learning Activity 3

In small groups, students are asked to design a CEA or CBA of some aspect of family therapy.

Key Review Articles

Comments on the Area

The review articles on family therapy research constitute the "forest" in which are set the "trees" of the individual investigations that follow. There have been many review articles, and these are catalogued by Alexander, Holtzworth-Munroe, and Jameson (1994). In our judgment, although there is some value in all these articles, the most comprehensive and indispensable reviews are those by Alexander et al. (1994), Gurman and Kniskern (1978, 1981), Gurman et al. (1986), Sprenkle and Bischoff (1995), and Pinsof and Wynne (1995). They offer "state-of-the-art" information that addresses such important topics as the following: (1) How effective are the family therapies? (2) Which family therapies are the most effective? (3) What therapist factors, client factors, and treatment factors influence the effectiveness of family therapies? (4) What are the major measurement problems in family therapy outcome research? and (5) What are the key directions for future research?

The Alexander et al. (1994) review first examines the impact of various forms of marital therapy such as behavioral, emotion-focused, and insight-oriented therapies. Research on specific disorders such as depression and alcoholism are also discussed. Certain limitations to the current research are listed, including longitudinal, developmental, contextual, and measurement issues. Qualitative research and meta-analysis are also discussed. The Alexander et al. (1994) chapter may be the most comprehensive coverage to date of methodological issues. The Pinsof and Wynne (1995) work will probably remain the benchmark volume on the substantive results of family therapy research for years to come.

Learning Activities

The review articles refer to a series of debates that students can pursue further using original source materials. For example, several authors (Jacobson, 1978; Wells & Dezen, 1978a, 1978b) have challenged Gurman and Kniskern's (1978) use of uncontrolled or otherwise weak studies in accumulating knowledge about the effectiveness of marital and family therapy. Another potential debate concerns the relative merits of various approaches to control groups. Jacobson (1978) considers the no-treatment control group to be the essential ingredient in adequate design. Gurman and Kniskern (1981) note considerable difficulties with the design and offer the TOD approach as an alternative. Todd and Stanton (1983), in turn, criticize the TOD approach and offer several varieties of parallel treatment groups as more productive alternatives. As another example, Sprenkle and Bischoff's (1995) chapter details the controversy surrounding the merits of qualitative versus quantitative approaches to family therapy research.

Students are asked to play the role of the various protagonists in these debates, which can become quite heated.

Instrumentation

Comments on the Area

There are many important issues in the assessment of change in marital and family therapy. A few important principles discussed in the literature include the following:

1. The measurement of family therapy outcome requires multiple perspectives. We agree wholeheartedly with Pinsof and Wynne (1995) that variance in outcome is greatly affected by who is asked (client, therapist, friend) and how the data are collected. A helpful table (Gurman & Kniskern, 1981, p. 770) illustrates a variety of perspectives and shows how they vary in the degree of inference involved in making an evaluative judgment about a family. For example, a therapist's rating of a family as "enmeshed" is a high-inference judgment, relative to a researcher's examining hospital records to determine whether rehospitalization occurred following therapy. Several books are available that are compendia of family therapy measurement instruments. These include Fischer and Corcoran (1994), Fredman and Sherman (1987), L'Abate and Bagarozzi (1993), and Touliatos, Perlmutter, and Straus (1990).

2. An instrument package should include both standardized forms and measures tailor-made to specific cases (Pinsof & Wynne, 1995). Standardized instruments allow for increased confidence concerning reliability and validity as well as comparisons across studies. Conversely, ideographic measures enable the researcher to address the presenting problem as well as the therapist's unique goals for the case. We agree with Todd and Stanton (1983) that measures of the family's primary complaints should be the sine qua non of outcome research.

3. There should be attention to both ultimate and mediating goals. Pinsof and Wynne (1995) stress the importance of distinguishing between goals that represent the end toward which one hopes to move a family and the means or subgoals one employs to achieve this end.

4. The units to be assessed, at a minimum, include the identified patient, the marriage, and the total system.

Learning Activity 1: An Exercise in Multiple Research Perspectives

Students are presented with a case vignette of a family whose principle complaint its the poor school performance and truancy of a teenage son. The parents also make reference to communication difficulties in the marital dyad and the wife's lack of sexual desire. Students are divided into small groups and are challenged to formulate as many research perspectives as possible. In keeping with Gurman and Kniskern (1981), each perspective must include a statement of the type of information sought (e.g., performance on clinically relevant, nonfamilial objective criteria); an illustration of this type of information (e.g., school grades); and an opinion about the best judge or source of this information (e.g., school records). Students are also asked to note several disadvantages of using this criterion as the sole measure of outcome in family therapy. Alternatively, students are asked to brainstorm a variety of family therapy research questions. Utilizing the chapters in Sprenkle and Moon (1996), which describe qualitative, quantitative, and mixed methods for doing family therapy research, students are challenged to note which methods are most appropriate for answering these questions and why.

Learning Activity 2: Assessment Workup

Students perform a comprehensive family assessment on a volunteer family. The literature offers several suggestions for comprehensive family assessment (Sprenkle & Bischoff, 1995). Students are encouraged to use tools and techniques that tap the individual, couple, and family units, and to employ several of the research perspectives discussed earlier.

Implications of the New Epistemologies for Family Therapy Research

Comments on the Area

Assigning Colapinto (1979) or Doherty (1995) as a reading sensitizes the students to the fact that research paradigms are not neutral or value free, but rather reflect one's epistemology. Colapinto (1979) shows how different epistemologies lead to significant differences in such key concepts as "problems" and "solutions." Therefore, what may be deemed "therapeutic success" in one framework may become "therapeutic failure" in another. Fisher (1982) discusses the frequent discrepancy between transactional theories and individual assessment methods. Many of our assessment methods focus exclusively on the individual, assume that one can know a family perspective by summing the total of individual viewpoints, and reflect linear causality. Russell, Olson, Sprenkle, and Atilano (1983) stress that there is often no clear correspondence between presenting individual symptoms (e.g., alcoholism) and type of family system. Keeney (1983) writes persuasively that any attempt to describe a phenomenon (e.g., a family) is itself an intervention and alters the thing described, just as statements about the stock market ("It is going up") create the very phenomenon being "described." Tomm (1983, 1986) also attacks the myth of objective observation and asserts that we need to give more attention to the process of investigation itself. In addition, he discusses how the traditional scientific method of dividing phenomena into smaller segments more amenable to objectification frequently kills the beast in an attempt to understand it. Holistic patterns are reduced to contrived causal explanations that do not fit clinical realities. These so-called "new-wavers" (Gurman, 1983b) also call for a greater appreciation of the roles of intuition and creativity in research. They also favor qualitative methods and believe that research should be evaluated by the community of "stakeholders" (most notably the therapists who use the methods being tested) rather than by artificial "scientific" standards (Atkinson, Heath, & Chenail, 1991). Since the context of discovery is deemed as important as the context of verification, descriptive research should be accorded more prestige, and hypothesis testing should no longer be considered the only royal road to the researcher's kingdom. In a spirited defense of traditional research methodology, "old hatters" Cavell and Snyder (1991), Gurman (1983a, 1983b), Kniskern (1983), and Shields (1986) point out that it is the only current ethical and responsible way to address the kinds of questions about efficacy of our treatments that are being raised by consumers, government agencies, and third-party payers, as well as by therapists. Although the total context of family interaction is circular, important therapeutic subprocesses are linear. Families pay therapists on the premise that therapy (cause) produces change (effect). These writers also catalogue the impressive gains already made by family therapy research and caution us not to throw out the baby with the bathwater until and unless some better way is found. Indeed, they assert, responsible traditional researchers have always been aware of the subjectivity of their underlying assumptions and the fallacy of truly objective and value-free inquiry. Careful traditional researchers are also very much aware of contextual variables and frequently employ statistical techniques (e.g., correlational analysis) that are consistent with circular causality.

Learning Activity

The class is divided into two groups ("old hatters" vs. "new wavers"). Each designates a spokesperson to begin debate, and the protagonists are seated in opposing chairs in the front of the room. At any time other members of either group can stand behind the spokesperson and act as an "alter ego" for him or her in the debate. The initial stimulus question is this: "Resolved, that traditional research methods are the only ethically responsible means presently available by which we can assess the efficacy of our work and study the facts influencing therapeutic outcomes" (Gurman, 1983a, p. 229).

Qualitative Research

Learning Activity 1

After reviewing some of the important components of qualitative research from readings such as Moon et al. (1990), have the students construct a research question and design a qualitative research project including methodology, data collection, data analysis, and discussion that matches the question. The qualitative chapters in Sprenkle and Moon (1996) are also helpful here.

Learning Activity 2

Taking an existing quantitative study and, maintaining the research question and theoretical underpinnings as much as possible, students design a qualitative study in place of the current quantitative approach. Questions considered include how the measurement, data collection, data analysis, write-up, results, discussion, and conclusions would differ from or resemble the existing quantitative study. The qualitative and quantitative chapters in Sprenkle and Moon (1996) are useful here.

KEY BOOKS, CHAPTERS, AND ARTICLES

Many annotated citations of important research studies are given in the other topical chapters of this volume and hence are not included here. The works summarized here are either of a general nature or are not pertinent for the other chapters.

Alexander, J., Holtzworth-Munroe, A., & Jameson, P. (1994). The process and outcome of marital and family therapy: Research review and evaluation. In A. Bergin & S. Garfield (Eds.), *Handbook of psychotherapy and behavior change* (4th ed.). New York: Wiley.

This chapter first examines the impact of various forms of marital therapy such as behavioral, emotion-focused, and insight-oriented therapies. Research on specific disorders such as depression and alcoholism are also discussed. Certain limitations to the current research are listed, including longitudinal, developmental, contextual, and measurement issues. Qualitative research and meta-analysis are also discussed.

Beck, D. F., & Jones, M. A. (1973). *Progress on family problems: A nationwide study of clients and counselors' views on family agency services.* New York: Family Service Association of America.

This publication reports on a large-sample study of 3,956 cases seen at Family Service Association agencies throughout the United States. Among the hundreds of findings was the fact that the strongest predictors of outcome were the relationship between the client and therapist and the agreement on the agenda for therapy. The study is significant because of the unique method of statistical control, made possible by the huge sample. This nonexperimental study is one of the few sources of information about such variables as the race of the therapist and the effect of client fees.

Beck, D. F., & Jones, M. A. (1976). *How to conduct a client follow-up study.* New York: Family Service Association of America.

This is a primer for agencies that wish to carry out an evaluation of therapy services along the lines of the Beck and Jones (1973) Family Service Association study. Almost every detail from questionnaires to computation procedures to record keeping is discussed.

Bergin, A., & Lambert, M. (1994). The evaluation of therapeutic outcomes. In A. Bergin & S. Garfield (Eds.), *Handbook of psychotherapy and behavior change* (4th ed.). New York: Wiley.

This review extends and broadens Bergin's coverage of the therapeutic outcome literature in the earlier edition of this volume. The authors give detailed summaries of major comparative studies and consider therapeutic modalities as well. Psychotherapists should be encouraged by the authors' assessment of the evidence for the positive effects of psychotherapy, but perhaps humbled by their conclusion that client characteristics and therapist personal factors still contribute more to outcome variance than therapeutic technique. Although not a chapter on family therapy research, this is an excellent resource on psychotherapy outcome research.

Bray, J., & Jouriles, E. (1995). Treatment of marital conflict and prevention of divorce. *Journal of Marital and Family Therapy, 21,* 461–474.

This article reviews the literature on the effectiveness of marital therapy in preventing marital separation and divorce. The results suggest that marital therapy reduces marital conflict and increases marital satisfaction. Most of the research is short term, and long-term results are rare. The long-term results that exist are positive, but the authors suggest that further long-term research is needed. Predictors of positive outcome, clinical significance, and cost-effectiveness are also discussed.

Campbell, T., & Patterson, J. (1995). The effectiveness of family interventions in the treatment of physical illness. *Journal of Marital and Family Therapy, 21,* 545–584.

This article reviews the literature on the effectiveness of family therapy treatment of physical illness. Results, for the most part, are inconclusive but are positive in some areas. Family therapy seems to be effective in dealing with childhood illnesses such as diabetes and asthma. Other areas of effectiveness, although not as strong, are dealing with cardiovascular and neurologic problems, and anorexia nervosa. Recommendations for future research are also discussed.

Chamberlain, P., & Rosicky, J. (1995). The effectiveness of family therapy in the treatment of adolescents with conduct disorders and delinquency. *Journal of Marital and Family Therapy, 21,* 441–460.

This article reviews the literature on recent (1988–1994) studies done on the treatment of conduct disorders of adolescents. In general, family-based treatments were effective. Barriers to successful treatment include attrition, family stress, lack of social support, and specific child variables. They suggest that results from research-based studies may overestimate the effectiveness of a treatment, because clinic-based studies consistently showed lower results.

Cookerly, J. (1976). Evaluating different approaches to marriage counseling. In D. Olson (Ed.), *Treating relationships.* Lake Mills, IA: Graphic.

This chapter reviews four studies (completed in a private-practice setting) designed to test the relative effectiveness of six types of marriage counseling: individual, individual group, concurrent, concurrent group, conjoint, and conjoint group. Overall, the conjoint approach produced the best results except for those couples who went on to divorce. The conjoint group modality was almost as good and was decidedly better for those who went on to divorce.

Cookerly, J. (1980). Does marital therapy do any lasting good? *Journal of Marital and Family Therapy, 10,* 393–396.

This is the report of a 5-year longitudinal investigation comparing couples in a private practice who received conjoint as opposed to nonconjoint treatment. Conjoint couples were more likely to remain married and to have much higher "good" outcomes, higher "moderate" outcomes, and lower "poor" outcomes than nonconjoint couples. The results also suggest that conjoint therapy may facilitate somewhat earlier and healthier divorces.

Doherty, W., & Simmons, D. (1996). Clinical practice of marriage and family therapists: A national survey of therapists and their clients. *Journal of Marital and Family Therapy, 22,* 9–25.

This article presents the first national data on the mental health services provided by marriage and family therapists. The survey was based, in part, on the questionnaire developed by the National Institute of Mental Health, meaning that for the first time, marriage and family therapists were asked questions comparable to other federally recognized mental health providers. The results suggest that marriage and family therapists treat a wide range of mental health problems and that the length of treatment is relatively short in comparison to individual treatment. Client satisfaction and functional improvement are also reported to be high.

Edwards, M., & Steinglass, P. (1995). Family therapy treatment outcomes for alcoholism. *Journal of Marital and Family Therapy, 21,* 475–510.

This article is a meta-analysis of 21 studies of family therapy treatment of alcoholism. Family therapy was effective at motivating alcoholics to enter treatment, and it was marginally more effective at enhancing outcome of treatment over individual treatment alone. Gender, investment in the relationship, and perceived support from the spouse were all mediating factors in the outcome. Recommendations for future research are also made.

Estrada, A., & Pinsof, W. (1995). The effectiveness of family therapies for selected behavioral disorders of childhood. *Journal of Marital and Family Therapy, 21,* 403–440.

This article reviews the research done on the effectiveness of family therapy with certain behavioral disorders of childhood. The results are strong for family-centered and child-centered family therapy with children presenting conduct disorders and autism, even at long-term follow-up. Although family therapy can affect noncompliance and aggression in children with attention-deficit/hyperactivity disorder, it does not seem to help with the core symptoms any more than the medication helps. Other tentative results are discussed regarding the family-based treatment of childhood phobias and anxieties. Limitations and suggestions for future research are also mentioned.

Fischer, J., & Corcoran, K. (1994). *Measures for clinical practice: A sourcebook. Volume 1: Couples, families and children*. New York: Free Press.

This book begins by reviewing some of the basic principles of measurement and then moves on to discuss different types of measurement tools, the advantages and disadvantages of rapid assessment instruments, and how to select measures for ones practice. The majority of the book is devoted to presenting different assessment instruments. The instruments are divided into three sections focused on instruments for couples, instruments for families, and instruments for children.

Fisher, L. (1982). Transactional theories but individual assessment: A frequent discrepancy in family research. *Family Process, 21,* 313–320.

The author contends that although most family therapy theories are transactional, the assessment tools most often used in outcome studies assess, at best, relational-level variables. Fisher offers a number of suggestions regarding how to use many of the present assessment tools and also calls for the development of new research tools to assess marriage and family change on a more comprehensive transactional level.

Giblin, P., Sprenkle, D., & Sheehan, R. (1985). Enrichment outcome research: A meta-analysis of premarital, marital and family findings. *Journal of Marital and Family Therapy, 11,* 257–272.

This article presents the findings of a meta-analysis of 85 studies of premarital, marital, and family enrichment. Findings are presented in terms of overall effectiveness as well as relevant program, subject, design, measurement, and analysis characteristics. An average overall effect size of .44 was found, indicating that the average person who participates in an enrichment program is better off than 67% of those who do not. Measurement variables (rather than those related to program content, leadership, or participants) proved to be the most powerful predictors of outcome. This article provides an interesting overview of what is known and unknown in enrichment research, as well as a useful discussion of the process of doing a meta-analysis.

Goldstein, M., & Miklowitz, D. (1995). The effectiveness of psychoeducational family therapy in the treatment of schizophrenic disorders. *Journal of Marital and Family Therapy, 21,* 361–376.

This review of the literature on family psychoeducational interventions with schizophrenia divides the literature into two "generations." The first generation focused on comparing family-oriented approaches with medication to medication treatments alone. The results were strongly in favor of the family-oriented treatment plus medication. The second generation focused on more complex study designs. These results suggested that the efficacy of family intervention when added to medication is mediated by a number of other variables.

Greenberg, L., and Pinsof, W. (1986). Process research: Current trends and future prospects. In L. S. Greenberg & W. Pinsof (Eds.), *The psychotherapeutic process: A research handbook*. New York: Guilford Press.

This chapter, as an introduction to the authors' book on process research, discusses major trends in process research and future directions of process research in the field of marriage and family therapy. Among the trends discussed are integrating process and outcome research, conceptualizing process research in a smaller way, investigating the therapeutic alliance, and involving clients' feedback in process research. Among the future directions suggested are viewing the psychotherapeutic process systemically, moving toward a multilevel perspective, and coordinating research programs.

Gurman, A. (1983). Family therapy research and the "new epistemology." *Journal of Marital and Family Therapy, 9*, 227–234.

This article provides a convincing counterargument to the position of the "new epistemology" family therapists who challenge the value of traditional research designs and methods. The author argues that conventional research methodology presents the only ethically responsible and practical approach for evaluating the effectiveness of marriage and family therapy. Several issues are presented that strongly support the compatibility of traditional research strategies with a systemic theoretical perspective. The author proposes that research questions should be posed in a way that acknowledges the multidimensionality of the therapeutic process.

Gurman, A., & Kniskern, D. (1978). Research on marital and family therapy: Progress, perspective and prospect. In S. Garfield & A. Bergin (Eds.), *Handbook of psychotherapy and behavior change* (2nd ed.). New York: Wiley.

This is the first of Gurman and Kniskern's classic reviews of outcome research. Although the chapter has historical significance, the information is available in more up-to-date form (Gurman & Kniskern, 1981; Gurman, Kniskern, & Pinsof, 1986). The authors' influential design criteria (see the "Key Concepts" section) are included.

Gurman A., & Kniskern, D. (1981). Family therapy outcome research: Knowns and unknowns. In A. Guram & D. Kniskern (Eds.), *Handbook of family therapy*. New York: Brunner/Mazel.

This key chapter summarizes the state of outcome research in the field of family therapy at the time of the book's publication. The authors present an overview of what is known and not known regarding the relative effectiveness of different marriage and family therapies for specific clinical populations and problems, as well as factors that contribute to therapeutic effectiveness regardless of method (treatment factors, patient–family factors, and therapist factors). The authors also address a number of crucial issues in doing outcome research in family therapy. The chapter is comprehensive, in that it includes an excellent discussion of both the current state of knowledge and important questions and directions for the future. It is essential reading for clinicians and researchers alike.

Gurman, A., Kniskern, D., & Pinsof, W. (1986). Research on the process and outcome of marital and family therapy. In S. Garfield & A. Bergin (Eds.), *Handbook of psychotherapy and behavior change* (3rd ed.). New York: Wiley.

The authors diverge from their previous reviews (Gurman & Kniskern, 1978, 1981) in that there are few tables; the material is organized primarily around research relative to specific clinical disorders and clinical populations (child and adolescent disorders, psychosomatic disorders, divorce therapy, etc.). The chapter also includes an enlightening history of research in the field and a discussion of the new epistemological challenge to traditional research. William Pinsof had a major influence on the large section of the chapter devoted to process research. A variety of recommendations about design and measurement issues are also included.

Hazelrigg, M., Cooper, H., & Borduin, C. (1987). Evaluating the effectiveness of family therapies: An integrative review and analysis. *Psychological Bulletin, 101,* 428–442.

This article is the first attempt to statistically integrate family therapy effectiveness research. The results showed that family therapy had positive effects in comparison to no-treatment and alternative treatment controls using family interactions and behavior ratings as measures. Follow-up data showed continued, although diminished, positive effects. Suggestions are made for future outcome research in family therapy.

Henggeler, S., Borduin, C., & Mann, B. (1993). Advances in family therapy: Empirical foundations. In T. Ollendick & R. Prinz (Eds.), *Advances in clinical child psychology* (Vol. 15). New York: Plenum Press.

This review offers the contention that family therapy, especially those schools with a behavioral focus, can be an empirically effective way in which to treat problems of childhood and adolescence. Family therapy approaches to externalizing problems, such as antisocial behavior and delinquency, and internalizing behaviors, such as schizophrenia and affective disorders, are discussed in terms of their effectiveness. Finally, suggestions for the future direction of family therapy research are made.

Hill, C. (1992). An overview of four measures developed to test the Hill Process Model: Therapist intentions, therapist response modes, client reactions, and client behaviors. *Journal of Counseling and Development, 70,* 728–739.

This article first presents a brief history of process research. This historical perspective then leads into a discussion of the Hill Process Model. Four measures of the model, including therapist intentions, therapist response modes, client reactions, and client behaviors, are presented. Future directions of methodological issues, measurement development, and research areas are also discussed.

Jacobson, N. (1991). Behavioral versus insight-oriented marital therapy: Labels can be misleading. *Journal of Consulting and Clinical Psychology, 59,* 142–145.

Jacobson, N. (1985). Family therapy outcome research: Potential pitfalls and prospects. *Journal of Marital and Family Therapy, 11,* 149–158.

The author proposes a series of design recommendations for family therapy outcome research: (1) The proportion of clients who improve should become a standard descriptive statistic; (2) between-model outcome studies should deemphasize statistically significant differences between treatments and should focus more on clinical significance, relative effect size, and demonstrable replicability; (3) the use of random assignment and a control group should be compromised only under specified conditions; (4) there is a need to compare results in research-structured and clinically flexible conditions; (5) more research is need on the optimal level of therapist experience and the extent to which therapists should be treated as an independent variable in the overall design; and (6) the primary outcome measure should be the most direct possible research of the presenting problem. A response to this article by Kniskern and a brief rejoinder by Jacobson follow in the same issue of the journal.

Johnson, S., & Greenberg, L. (1988). Relating process to outcome in marital therapy. *Journal of Marital and Family Therapy, 14,* 175–183.

This article, noting a serious lack of process research in comparison to the outcome research at the time it was written, attempts to analyze the process of change in emotionally focused marital therapy. Results indicated conformation of the theoretical assumptions of the model. This is a classic process research study and a good model for doing process research.

Kniskern, D. (1983). The new wave is all wet. *Family Therapy Networker,* 7(4), 38, 60–62.

In response to the claims of the new epistemologists that traditional methods of scientific research are inappropriate, Kniskern offers a "plea for caution and conservatism." He points out that the traditional research methods have served the cause of family therapy well by demonstrating its effectiveness in many areas of clinical practice. He suggests that, although the linear and analytic approaches of typical outcome studies may be epistemologically limited, they nevertheless will continue to be of great interest to several consumer groups, namely, prospective clients, third-party payers, and mental health professionals in other fields. So far, says Kniskern, the "new wave" has not produced any serious alternatives to existing research strategies.

Liddle, H., & Dakof, G. (1995). Efficacy of family therapy for drug abuse: Promising but not definitive. *Journal of Marital and Family Therapy, 21,* 511–544.

This article reviews the research done on family therapy approaches to treatment of drug abuse. Many studies confirm the effectiveness of family therapy at engaging and retaining drug users in treatment and significantly reducing drug use and other problem behaviors. The authors caution a blanket endorsement of a family therapy approach, as there is not a large enough number of studies and those studies that do exist have some methodological limitations. Suggestions are made for continued research in this area.

Moon, S., Dillon, D., & Sprenkle, D. (1990). Family therapy and qualitative research. *Journal of Marital and Family Therapy, 16,* 357–373.

This article introduces the qualitative research paradigm and encourages its further application to family therapy research. It introduces some characteristics of qualitative research, including the role of the researcher, sampling techniques, data collection and analysis, and reporting results. Possible benefits and pitfalls for family therapy research are also discussed.

Parloff, M. (1980). *The efficacy and cost-effectiveness of psychotherapy* (Office of Technical Assessment, Document 052-003-00783-5). Washington, DC: U.S. Government Printing Office.

This report provides a review of four issues centrally related to the evaluation of psychotherapy: (1) the definition and complexity of psychotherapy; (2) the degree to which psychotherapy is amenable to scientific analysis and the availability of appropriate methods for studying psychotherapy; (3) the evidence as to psychotherapy's efficacy, including the results of analyses that synthesize findings across studies; and (4) the appropriateness of CEA and CBA of psychotherapy and the results of their application.

Piercy, F., & Sprenkle, D. (1990). Marriage and family therapy: A decade review. *Journal of Marriage and the Family, 52,* 1116–1126.

This review summarizes the trends in theory construction and research methodology from 1980 to 1989. Standard theories such as strategic and Milan systemic therapy are discussed, in addition to current theoretical trends such as the new epistemology and feminist critiques of family therapy. Trends in research such as doing within-school comparisons, moving from outcome alone to process and outcome, and adding qualitative research to the established quantitative paradigm are discussed. Recommendations for research are also made.

Pinsof, W. (1981). Family therapy process research. In A. Gurman & D. Kniskern (Eds.), *Handbook of family therapy.* New York: Brunner/Mazel.

This is an essential chapter for methodologists and researchers in the family therapy field. Pinsof explicates the vital function of process research, which is to operationalize and/or reliably describe the in-therapy events that may suggest the effectiveness of a therapy. Furthermore, process research can test clinical theories about the nature and relative effects of different techniques and treatment strategies. The chapter includes a comprehensive literature review of process research, describes the methodological issues involved, and provides a framework for the conduct of process research within the family therapy field.

Pinsof, W., & Wynne, L. (1995). The efficacy of marital and family therapy: An empirical overview, conclusions, and recommendations. *Journal of Marital and Family Therapy, 21,* 585–613.

Based on the other articles in the special issue on the effectiveness of MFT, the authors draw some general conclusions. Research has supported the efficacy of broadly defined marital and family therapy for the treatment of many disorders. Recommendations are made for methodology and conceptualization of effectiveness. Methodological recommendations include having clear definitions and dealing with attention effects. Conceptualization recommendations include developing a set of core outcome batteries, guiding research with theory, and including more cost-effectiveness measures in research done in marriage and family therapy.

Prince, S., & Jacobson, N. (1995). A review and evaluation of marital and family therapies for affective disorders. *Journal of Marital and Family Therapy, 21,* 377–402.

This review looks at the effectiveness of marital and family therapy in the treatment of affective disorders. This review not only reports the research findings but also evaluates the available treatment outcome data, with special emphasis on predictors of treatment success and cost-effectiveness issues. They then suggest priorities for future research, including dealing with gender issues, preventive measures, and more rigorous research designs.

Russell, C., Olson, D., Sprenkle, D., & Atilano, R. (1983). From family symptom to family system: Review of family therapy research. *American Journal of Family Therapy, 11,* 3–14.

Effective outcomes are linked to the interaction between symptom reduction and healthy family dynamics. The authors demonstrate the fallacy of the assumption that all families presenting with the same symptom (e.g., alcoholism) have similar family system organizations. A research design linking symptom to system is introduced.

Schwartz, R., & Breunlin, D. (1983). Why clinicians should bother with research. *Family Therapy Networker, 7*(4), 22–27.

The authors point out the gap between researchers and clinicians, and the steps necessary to bridge it. The authors make three good recommendations for presenting research findings to clinicians: (1) The paper should be readable and understandable; (2) the treatment itself should be described and explained in a precise and thorough manner; and (3) results should be presented in terms of their clinical as well as statistical significance.

Shadish, W., Montgomery, L., Wilson, P., Wilson, M., Bright, I., & Okwumabua, T. (1993). *Journal of Consulting and Clinical Psychology, 61,* 992–1002.

This article is a meta-analysis of 163 randomized studies on the effectiveness of marriage and family therapy. Results suggest that marital and family clients have a more improved outcome than control clients. Findings also focused on differences between family therapy and other orientations and differences within marital and family therapy. A review of methodological issues including internal validity, external validity, and construct validity is also presented.

Shadish, W., Ragsdale, K., Glaser, R., & Montgomery, L. (1995). The efficacy and effectiveness of marital and family therapy: A perspective from meta-analysis. *Journal of Marital and Family Therapy, 21*, 345–360.

This article reports major findings from a multiproject meta-analysis of the effectiveness of marriage and family therapy. Their results showed that no orientation is superior to another, and MFT is neither superior nor inferior to individual therapy but is sometimes more cost-effective. Questions and concerns about the way in which MFT is studied are indicated, and suggestions are made for improving research done in this area. Questions are also raised about the generalizability of research to actual clinical practice.

Simmons, D., & Doherty, W. (1995). Defining who we are and what we do: Clinical practice patterns of marriage and family therapists in Minnesota. *Journal of Marital and Family Therapy, 21*, 3–16.

This article is based on a survey of AAMFT clinical members in the state of Minnesota. Results showed that MFT practice is relatively short term and that therapy with families and couples is shorter than therapy with individuals. Results also showed that MFTs treat a wide range of serious problems and that MFT clinical practice was comparable to other established mental health professions.

Snyder, D., Wills, R., & Grady-Fletcher, A. (1991). Long-term effectiveness of behavioral versus insight-oriented marital therapy: A 4-year follow-up study. *Journal of Consulting and Clinical Psychology, 59*, 138–141.

Snyder, D., Wills, R., & Grady-Fletcher, A. (1991). Risks and challenges of long-term psychotherapy outcome research: Reply to Jacobson. *Journal of Consulting and Clinical Psychology, 59*, 146–149.

This series of articles focuses on the comparison of long-term effects of behavioral (BMT) and insight-oriented (IOMT) marital therapies. The original Snyder et al. article found that in a long-term, 4-year follow-up, a significantly higher percentage of BMT couples experienced divorce. Jacobson responded that the treatment manual used in this study for BMT inadequately represented BMT as it was currently conceived and points out that many clinical skills present in the IOMT approach were integral to current BMT. Snyder et al. responded by disputing Jacobson's characterization of BMT and IOMT and pointed out that BMT still fails to address affective and unconscious conflictual themes in marital interaction.

Sprenkle, D., & Bischoff, R. (1995). Research in family therapy: Trends, issues, and recommendations. In M. Nichols & R. Schwartz (Eds.), *Family therapy: Concepts and methods* (3rd ed.). Needham Heights, MA: Allyn & Bacon.

This chapter begins with issues in family therapy research. Among the issues discussed are legitimization of family therapy, a gap between research and practice and between qualitative and quantitative measurement, statistical versus clinical significance, and cost-effectiveness research. The next section focuses on outcome results in a number of substantive areas including schizophrenia, affective disorders, drug and alcohol abuse, child abuse, and behavior disorders. Current issues in diagnosis and measurement are also discussed. Finally, the future of family therapy research is discussed.

Sprenkle, D., & Moon, S. (Eds.). (1996). *Research methods in family therapy.* New York: Guilford Press.

This book is a collection of different research methods for family therapy. The first section focuses on qualitative methods, including ethnographies, grounded theory, phenomenology, critical theory, and focus groups. The next section focuses on quantitative methods and issues, including design, scale development, single-case experiments, meta-analyses, correlation and regression, and cost-effectiveness designs. The final section focuses on mixed methods. Included in this section are case study research, survey research, Delphi methods, program evaluation, and application of research to therapy practice.

Stanton, M., Todd, T., Steier, F., Van Deusen, J., Marder, L., Rosoff, R., Seaman, S., & Skibinski, E. (1980). *Family characteristics and family therapy of heroin addicts: Final report 1974–1978* (National Institute on Drug Abuse Grant No. R01-DA-01119). Philadelphia: Philadelphia Child Guidance Clinic.

This excellent report is the most comprehensive resource on the Philadelphia Child Guidance Clinic's research on the family therapy of heroin addicts. This report presents the recruitment of subjects, the complete research design, the differences in interactional patterns between addict and normal families, the breakdown of the different treatment modalities, and the study results. The study showed that paid family therapy and unpaid family therapy were superior to a paid family movie treatment and individual therapy in regard to days free from drug usage. Paid family therapy was also found to be superior to unpaid family therapy in terms of days free of drug usage.

Todd, T., & Stanton, M. (1983). Research on marital and family therapy: Answers, issues and recommendations for the future. In B. Wolman & G. Stricker (Eds.), *Handbook of family and marital therapy.* New York: Plenum Press.

This chapter provides an outcome research review with a focus on identifying future needs for specific research based on clinically relevant questions. An excellent summary of the conclusions that can safely be drawn from existing research is presented. A number of critical methodological issues that are currently facing the field are highlighted, and recommendations are given.

Tomm, K. (1983). The old hat doesn't fit. *Family Therapy Networker, 7*(4), 39–41.

The author contends that the methods of traditional science, based on assumptions of unbiased observation and linear cause-and-effect relationships, are poor tools for dealing with the phenomena of family therapy, which involve the observer as an active participant in systems of circular interaction. He suggests several possible directions that a new science should take, including more emphasis on process research and increased respect for subjective data. This is a provocative article that, in good systems fashion, gives the reader no final answers or comfortable closure.

Whisman, M., Jacobson, N., Fruzzetti, A., & Waltz, J. (1989). Methodological issues in marital therapy. *Advances in Behavior Research and Therapy, 11*, 175–189.

This article discusses both the strengths and challenges facing marital therapy researchers. Strengths include the use of assessment instruments having good reliability and validity, simultaneous use of self-report and observational measures, increased use of clinical significance measures, and the use of detailed treatment manuals. Challenges offered include assessing the individual in addition to the marital dyad, evaluating nonstandardized treatments, and describing inclusionary and exclusionary criteria in research. Suggestions are also made for the improvement and standardization of current research methodology.

Wynne, L. (1988). *The state of the art in family therapy research: Controversies and recommendations.* New York: Family Process Press.

This book is split into six sections. The first section addresses the conceptual framework of family therapy research. The second section addresses the selection of variables appropriate for family therapy research. The third section gives suggestions on designing an outcome study. The fourth section gives suggestions for approaching process research. The fifth section discusses data analysis as it pertains to family therapy research. The book concludes with an overview of the "state-of-the-art" research being done in family therapy at the time. Criteria for good research are also given.

REFERENCES

Alexander, J., Barton, C., Schiavo, R., & Parsons, B. (1976). Behavioral intervention with families of delinquents: Therapist characteristics and outcomes. *Journal of Consulting and Clinical Psychology, 44*, 656–664.

Alexander, J., Holtzworth-Munroe, A., & Jameson, P. (1994). The process and outcome of marital and family therapy: Research review and evaluation. In A. Bergin & S. Garfield (Eds.), *Handbook of psychotherapy and behavior change* (4th ed.). New York: Wiley.

Allred, G., & Kersey, F. (1977). The AIAC, a design for systematically analyzing marriage and family counseling: Progress report. *Journal of Marriage and Family Counseling, 3*, 17–26.

Atkinson, B., Heath, A., & Chenail, R. (1991). Qualitative research and the legitimization of knowledge. *Journal of Marital and Family Therapy, 17*, 175–180.

Beck, D., & Jones, M. (1973). *Progress on family problems: A nationwide study of clients and counselors' views on family agency services.* New York: Family Service Association of America.

Boss, P., Dahl, C., & Kaplan, L. (1996). Phenomenological methodology in family therapy research. In D. H. Sprenkle & S. M. Moon (Eds.), *Research methods in family therapy.* New York: Guilford Press.

Bray, J., Williamson, D., & Malone, P. (1984). Personal authority in the family system: Development of a questionnaire to measure personal authority in intergenerational family process. *Journal of Marital and Family Therapy, 10,* 167–178.

Cavell, T., & Snyder, D. (1991). Iconoclasm versus innovation: Building a science of family therapy—comments on Moon, Dillon, and Sprenkle. *Journal of Marital and Family Therapy, 17,* 167–171.

Colapinto, J. (1979). The relative value of empirical evidence. *Family Process, 18,* 427–441.

Dickey, M. (1996). Methods for single-case experiments in family therapy. In D. H. Sprenkle & S. M. Moon (Eds.), *Research methods in family therapy.* New York: Guilford Press.

Doherty, W. J. (1995). *Soul searching: Why psychotherapy must promote moral responsibility.* New York: Basic Books.

Eysenck, H. (1952). The effects of psychotherapy: An evaluation. *Journal of Consulting Psychology, 16,* 319–324.

Fischer, J., & Corcoran, K. (1994). *Measures for clinical practice: A sourcebook. Volume 1: Couples, families and children.* New York: Free Press.

Fisher, L. (1982). Transactional theories but individual assessment: A frequent discrepancy in family research. *Family Process, 21,* 313–320.

Fredman, N., & Sherman, R. (1987). *Handbook of family measurements for marriage and family therapy.* New York: Brunner/Mazel.

Garfield, S., & Bergin, A. (1994). Introduction and historical overview. In A. Bergin & S. Garfield (Eds.), *Handbook of Psychotherapy and behavior change* (4th ed.). New York: Wiley.

Gurman, A. (1983a). Family therapy research and the new "epistemology." *Journal of Marital and Family Therapy, 9,* 227–234.

Gurman, A. (1983b). The old hatters and new wavers. *Family Therapy Networker, 7*(4), 37.

Gurman, A., & Kniskern, D. (1978). Research on marital and family therapy: Progress, perspective and prospect. In S. Garfield & A. Bergin (Eds.), *Handbook of psychotherapy and behavior change* (2nd ed.). New York: Wiley.

Gurman, A., & Kniskern, D. (1981). Family therapy outcome research: Knowns and unknowns. In A. Gurman & D. Kniskern (Eds.), *Handbook of family therapy.* New York: Brunner/Mazel.

Gurman, A., Kniskern, D., & Pinsof, W. (1986). Research on the process and outcome of marital and family therapy. In S. Garfield & A. Bergin (Eds.), *Handbook of psychotherapy and behavior change* (3rd ed.). New York: Wiley.

Jacobson, N. (1978). A review of the research on the effectiveness of marital therapy. In T. Paolino & B. McCrady (Eds.), *Marriage and marital therapy: Psychoanalytic, behavioral and systems theory perspective.* New York: Brunner/Mazel.

Joanning, H., Thomas, F., Quinn, W., & Mullen, R. (1992). Treating adolescent drug abuse: A comparison of family systems therapy, group therapy, and family drug education. *Journal of Marital and Family Therapy, 18,* 345–356.

Kazdin, A. (1992). Drawing valid inferences from case studies. In A. Kazdin (Ed.),

Methodological issues and strategies in clinical research. Washington, DC: American Psychological Association.

Kazdin, A. (1994). Methodology, design, and evaluation in psychotherapy research. In A. Bergin & S. Garfield (Eds.), *Handbook of psychotherapy and behavior change* (4th ed.). New York: Wiley.

Keeney, B. (1983). *Aesthetics of change.* New York: Guilford Press.

Kerlinger, F. (1986). *Foundations of behavioral research* (3rd ed.). New York: Holt, Rinehart & Winston.

Kniskern, D. (1983). The new wave is all wet. *Family Therapy Networker,* 7(4), 38, 60–62.

Kniskern, D. (1985). Climbing out of the pit: Further guidelines for family therapy research. *Journal of Marital and Family Therapy, 11,* 159–162.

L'Abate, L., & Bagorozzi, D. (1993). *Sourcebook of marriage and family therapy evaluation.* New York: Brunner/Mazel.

Lambert, M., & Hill, C. (1994). Assessing psychotherapy outcomes and processes. In A. Bergin & S. Garfield (Eds.), *Handbook of psychotherapy and behavior change* (4th ed.). New York: Wiley.

Lyness, K., & Sprenkle, D. H. (1996). Experimental methodology in marital and family therapy research. In D. H. Sprenkle & S. M. Moon (Eds.), *Research methods in family therapy.* New York: Guilford Press.

Mills, S., & Sprenkle, D. (1995). Family therapy in the post-modern era. *Family Relations, 44*(4), 368–376.

Moon, S., Dillon, D., & Sprenkle, D. (1990). Family therapy and qualitative research. *Journal of Marital and Family Therapy, 16,* 357–373.

Newfield, N., Sells, S., & Smith, T. (1996). Ethnographic research methods: Creating a clinical science of the humanities. In D. H. Sprenkle & S. M. Moon (Eds.), *Research methods in family therapy.* New York: Guilford Press.

Olson, D. (1976). Bridging research, theory, and application: The triple threat in science. In D. Olson (Ed.), *Treating relationships.* Lake Mills, IA: Graphic.

Olson, D. (1981). Family research and family therapy: Bridging two different worlds. In E. Filsinger & R. Lewis (Eds.), *Assessing marriage: New behavioral approaches.* Beverly Hills, CA: Sage.

Parloff, M. (1980). *The efficacy and cost-effectiveness of psychotherapy* (Office of Technical Assessment, Document 052-003-00783-5). Washington, DC: U.S. Government Printing Office.

Paul, G. (1967). Strategy of outcome research in psychotherapy. *Journal of Consulting Psychology, 31,* 109–118.

Piercy, F., Laird, R., & Mohammed, Z. (1983). A family therapist rating scale. *Journal of Marital and Family Therapy, 9,* 49–59.

Piercy, F., & Nickerson, V. (1996). Focus groups in family therapy research. In D. H. Sprenkle & S. M. Moon (Eds.), *Research methods in family therapy.* New York: Guilford Press.

Piercy, F., & Sprenkle, D. (1990). Marriage and family therapy: A decade review. *Journal of Marriage and the Family, 52,* 1116–1126.

Pike, C., MacKinnon, D., & Piercy, F. (1996). Cost effectiveness research in family therapy. In D. H. Sprenkle & S. M. Moon (Eds.), *Research methods in family therapy*. New York: Guilford Press.

Pinsof, W. (1981). Family therapy process research. In A. Gurman & D. Kniskern (Eds.), *Handbook of family therapy*. New York: Brunner/Mazel.

Pinsof, W., & Wynne, L. (1995). The efficacy of marital and family therapy: An empirical overview, conclusions, and recommendations. *Journal of Marital and Family Therapy, 21,* 585–613.

Rafuls, S., & Moon, S. (1996). Grounded theory methodology in family therapy research. In D. H. Sprenkle & S. M. Moon (Eds.), *Research methods in family therapy*. New York: Guilford Press.

Rahilly, D. (1993). A phenomenological analysis of authentic experience. *Journal of Humanistic Psychology, 33,* 49–71.

Rediger, S. (1996). Critical theory: The emancipatory interest in family therapy. In D. H. Sprenkle & S. M. Moon (Eds.), *Research methods in family therapy*. New York: Guilford Press.

Russell, C., Olson, D., Sprenkle, D., & Atilano, R. (1983). From family symptom to family system: Review of family therapy research. *American Journal of Family Therapy, 11,* 3–14.

Schwartz, R., & Breunlin, D. (1983). Why clinicians should bother with research. *Family Therapy Networker, 7*(4), 22–27.

Shadish, W. (1992). Do family and marital psychotherapies change what people do? A meta-analysis of behavioral outcomes. In T. D. Cook, H. M. Cooper, D. S. Cordray, H. Hartmann, L. V. Hedges, R. J. Light, T. A. Louis, & R. Mosteller (Eds.), *Meta-analysis for explanation: A casebook*. New York: Russell Sage Foundation.

Shadish, W., Ragsdale, K., Glaser, R., & Montgomery, L. (1995). The efficacy and effectiveness of marital and family therapy: A perspective from meta-analysis. *Journal of Marital and Family Therapy, 21,* 345–360.

Shields, C. (1986). Critiquing the new epistemologies: Toward minimum requirement for a scientific theory of family therapy. *Journal of Marital and Family Therapy, 12,* 359–372.

Sprenkle, D. (1976). The need for integration among theory, research and practice in the family field. *Family Coordinator, 24,* 261–263.

Sprenkle, D., & Bischoff, R. (1995). Research in family therapy: Trends, issues, and recommendations. In M. Nichols & R. Schwartz (Eds.), *Family therapy: Concepts and methods* (3rd ed.). Needham Heights, MA: Allyn & Bacon.

Sprenkle, D., & Moon, S. (1996). *Research methods in family therapy*. New York: Guilford Press.

Todd, T., & Stanton, M. (1983). Research on marital and family therapy: Answers, issues and recommendations for the future. In B. Wolman & G. Stricker (Eds.), *Handbook of family and marital therapy*. New York: Plenum Press.

Tomm, K. (1983). The old hat doesn't fit. *Family Therapy Networker, 7*(4), 39–41.

Tomm, K. (1986). On incorporating the therapist in a scientific theory of family therapy. *Journal of Marital and Family Therapy, 12,* 373–378.

Touliatos, J., Perlmutter, B., & Straus, M. (1990). *Handbook of family measurement techniques.* London: Sage.

Wampler, K. (1982). Bringing the review of the literature into the age of quantification: Meta-analysis as a strategy for integrating research findings in family studies. *Journal of Marriage and the Family, 44,* 1009–1023.

Wells, R., & Dezen, A. (1978a). The results of family therapy revisited: The nonbehavioral methods. *Family Process, 17* 251–274.

Wells, R., & Dezen, A. (1978b). Ideologies, idols (and graven images?): Rejoinder to Gurman and Kniskern. *Family Process, 17,* 283–286.

Wynne, L. (1983). Family research and family therapy: A reunion? *Journal of Marital and Family Therapy, 9,* 113–117.

15

~

Ethical, Legal, and Professional Issues

LORNA L. HECKER
FRED P. PIERCY

As the family therapy field has developed, training procedures have become more explicit, replicable, and assessable; however, there are fewer detailed reports on the content and process of important nontherapy areas of interest, such as ethical, legal, and professional issues, intended to supplement the development of well-rounded family therapists.

A Delphi survey of experienced family therapy educators and program directors conducted by Winkle, Piercy, and Hovestadt (1981) resulted in the identification of specific areas of ethics and professional development within a model family therapy curriculum. Similarly, the American Association for Marriage and Family Therapy (AAMFT) specifies studies that include ethical, legal, and professional issues as requirements within its own model curriculum (AAMFT, 1994).

This chapter first defines some key terms and concepts, and then identifies several specific ethical, legal, and professional issues in family therapy. We also suggest learning activities for each component. As in other chapters, we also identify research issues, followed by an annotated bibliography of key books, chapters, and articles.

KEY TERMS AND CONCEPTS

American Association for Marriage and Family Therapy (AAMFT). AAMFT is the largest professional association specifically for marriage and family therapists. Founded in 1942, AAMFT represents the interests of family therapy on a variety of issues. For example, AAMFT has an important credentialing function; the designations of "Clinical Member" and "Approved Supervisor" are sought-after symbols of professional stature. AAMFT's Commission on Accreditation for Marriage and Family Therapy Education is officially recognized by the U.S. government as the accrediting body for graduate education in the field. More information about AAMFT may be secured from its national office at 1133 15th Street, N.W., Washington, DC 20036-4601. The phone number for AAMFT is 202-452-0109; fax number is 202-223-2329. The history of AAMFT is discussed by Mudd (1967).

American Family Therapy Academy (AFTA). AFTA serves an important networking function for senior clinicians and researchers in the field of family therapy. More information about AFTA may be secured from its national office at 2020 Pennsylvania Avenue, N.W., #273, Washington, DC 20006. The AFTA phone number is 202-994-2776.

Confidentiality. Confidentiality is based on the belief that persons have the right to privacy. When they enter a professional relationship with a family therapist, it is generally expected that the family therapist will hold as private personal information about the clients, as well as access to this information. Confidentiality is referred to in the *AAMFT Code of Ethics* (AAMFT, 1991).

Criminal versus tort law. Crimes are prosecuted by the state. For example, some states have now made having sexual relations with one's clients a felony. A therapist who violated this law would be prosecuted under criminal law. Tort law is wrongful conduct toward another person, for which one may be held financially liable. This wrongful conduct may be intentional or nonintentional (through carelessness). In some states, having sex with one's clients may be both a crime and a tort. The most common type of tort known to therapists is *malpractice.*

Disclosure statement. A written statement that a therapist gives to a client(s) generally lists the following: the therapist's qualifications, office policies regarding money and session time, and the therapist's view on the process of therapy. The goal of a disclosure statement is to help clients have informed consent regarding marital and family therapy. For specific examples of disclosure statements see Huber (1994), and Schlossberger and Hecker (1996).

Duty to warn. Therapists generally have a duty to warn only when (1) there is a likelihood that clients will cause harm to themselves or others; (2) a special relationship exists between the client and therapist; and (3) there is a foreseeable victim (Lamb, Clark, Brumheller, Frizzell, & Surrey, 1990). See *Tarasoff* for more background information on duty to warn.

Expert testimony. Subject to the rules of evidence, which vary by jurisdiction, almost anyone who "has knowledge or experience in matters not generally familiar to the public" can serve as an expert witness (Schwitzgebel & Schwitzgebel, 1980, p. 238). Generally, expert witnesses may offer opinions or inferences, whereas lay witnesses may not (Woody & Associates, 1984). (See the discussion of courtroom testimony in "Key Issues and Teaching Tools and Techniques" for key citations.)

Informed consent. The procedure in which clients or subjects choose whether to participate in therapy or research after being informed of certain facts usually includes (1) the fact that their involvement must be voluntary; (2) the nature of the therapy/research; (3) the costs and benefits of participation; and (4) the fact that they may withdraw from participation at any time. For a discussion of legal and ethical issues in informed consent to therapy, see Bray, Shepherd, and Hays (1985). Some states are now requiring therapists to give clients a type of informed consent called a disclosure statement.

Libel. Written defamation of character constitutes libel. Possible defenses for this tort, according to Schultz (1982), include (1) that the revelation was true; (2) that an informed consent form was signed; (3) that the doctrine of "qualified privilege" was invoked; or (4) that there was an overarching social duty to release the information.

Malpractice. Legal liability for improper treatment through civil law constitutes malpractice. The four key elements that constitute malpractice include (1) a therapist–patient relationship existed; (2) the therapist's conduct fell below the acceptable standard of care; (3) the conduct was the proximate cause of injury; and (4) an injury actually occurred (Schultz, 1982).

Managed care. A system in which an insurer manages the delivery of physical and mental health care costs in a variety of possible ways constitutes managed care. For example, the insurer may identify preferred providers who may agree to limit fees, limit the number of reimbursable sessions, or stipulate what services are reimbursable.

National Council on Family Relations (NCFR). The NCFR is a national organization concerned with theory, research, practice, and public policy as they relate to the family. The national office of NCFR is located at 3989 Central Avenue, N.E., Suite 550, Minneapolis, MN 55421. The phone number for NCFR is 612-781-9331; fax number is 612-781-9348.

Privileged communication. Those statements made by persons within a protected relationship (e.g., therapist–client) that the law protects from forced disclosure on the witness stand (Black, 1979) are called privileged communication. *Privilege is a legal right to privacy owned by the client.* Often there is gross misunderstanding regarding the extent of privileged communication for clients of family therapists, because states vary greatly in their statutes related to privileged communication. These statutes are generally found in the certification and licensure laws for marriage and family therapists within each state. See Arthur and Swanson (1993), Watkins (1989), Herlihy and Sheeley (1987), and Gumper and Sprenkle (1981) for more detailed information on confidentiality and privilege.

Slander. Oral defamation of character constitutes slander. Slanderous statements must be proved (1) to have been made public, and (2) to have been injurious to the reputation of the plaintiff. (See Libel for defenses against claims of defamation of character.)

Tarasoff v. Regents of the University of California. Tarasoff (1976) was an important legal case that pitted the patient's right to privacy against the therapist's duty to protect members of society. In essence, the California court questioned the limitations of privileged communication between a therapist and his or her client. The court noted that a psychotherapist treating a dangerous client has the duty to give threatened persons such warnings as are essential to avert foreseeable danger. For more information on this case and its implications, see Monahan (1993), Stein (1990), Ciccone (1985), and Schultz (1982). The *Tarasoff* case gave rise to what is commonly called therapists' "duty to warn."

KEY ISSUES AND TEACHING TOOLS AND TECHNIQUES

Ethical Issues

Family Therapy Theory and Interventions:
Ethical Decision Making in Marriage and Family Therapy

Comments on the Issue. The field of family therapy saw the beginning of specialized debates in the 1980s (e.g., Dell, 1986a, 1986b; Imber-Black, 1986) concerning ethics of systems theory and particular interventions used by family therapists. For example, in relation to ecosystemic epistemology, Dell (1980; 1982) asserted that constructs such as power and personal responsibility are epistemologically flawed. Taggart (1982) suggested that individual responsibility is an "epistemological error." A debate, led largely by feminists (e.g., Bograd, 1984; Goldner, 1985a, 1985b; Goodrich, Rampage, Ellman, & Halstead, 1988; Hare-Mustin, 1980) then centered around issues of responsibility: if the buck is passed from the individual to the system, who is personally responsible for symptomatic behavior?

In addition, paradoxical interventions have been considered by some to be dishonest, manipulative, and dangerous. Others find paradox to be a viable, ethical therapeutic intervention. For more information on paradox, its uses, and ethical debates on the issue, see Solovey and Duncan (1992),

Fisch (1990), Brown and Slee (1986), Fisher, Anderson, and Jones (1981), Haley (1976), O'Shea and Jessee (1982), Raskin and Klein (1976), and Rohrbaugh, Tennen, Press, and White (1981).

The debates regarding ecosystemic epistemology, the feminist critique of family therapy, and paradox highlight the need for the field of family therapy to focus on how MFTs accomplish their goals. The feminist debate, for example, brought into question how much families' sociological and political context should be included therapy.

One important issue to be addressed involves how therapists' morals influence goals, interventions, and outcome. Also, marriage and family therapists lack a good model for ethical decision making in the complex arena of family therapy. The field is making some progress in this area (e.g., Zygmond & Boorhem, 1989; Woody, 1990), but more work needs to be done in integrating philosophy of ethics (Fine & Ulrich, 1988) within marriage and family therapy. This work should include training in which family therapists learn how their moral beliefs and values influence their work.

Learning Activity. Present the class with the following scenario: "You have just been given a watch by one of your clients. Do you accept or reject the watch?" Ask students to give their reasons for accepting or rejecting the watch. This will lead to an interesting discussion of the ethical factors involved in the weighing of the decision to accept or reject gifts. The diversity of answers provides a good segue into discussing the complexities of ethical decision making in therapy. Note how student values and beliefs relate to how they respond to their client giving them the gift.

Ethical Codes

Comments on the Issue. The function of ethical codes is threefold. Broadly, codes (1) define the role of the profession, (2) help guide the conduct of the profession, and (3) serve as a basis for sanctions (Schlossberger & Hecker, 1995). Family therapy trainees should be familiar with the *AAMFT Code of Ethics* (AAMFT, 1991), *Procedures for Handling Ethical Matters* (AAMFT, 1992b), and *Decision Tree: AAMFT Ethics Cases* (AAMFT, 1992a). It may also be helpful to read the evolution of AAMFT ethical codes (Preister, Vesper, & Humphrey, 1994). In addition, family therapist trainees can benefit by reviewing cases illustrated in the *AAMFT: Ethics Casebook* edited by Brock (1994).

Learning Activity 1. The instructor assigns students to read AAMFT's *Procedures for Handling Ethical Matters* (AAMFT, 1992b), prior to class for background information on ethical complaints. The *Decision Tree: AAMFT Ethics Cases* (AAMFT, 1992a) is also distributed to students. The instructor can then illustrate all the possible official actions that might take place in the life of the following fictitious ethical complaint:

> At your suggestion, a female client of yours wrote the AAMFT Executive Director a notarized letter stating that Dr. X, a former therapist whom she saw for divorce therapy and sex-related issues, had had sex with her "as part of therapy" on repeated occasions. This woman felt guilty and taken advantage of, and asked the Executive Director to take appropriate disciplinary action. The Executive Director referred his letter to the AAMFT Ethics Committee.

Through discussing all the possible steps in AAMFT's procedures, family therapy trainees can become sensitized to the safeguards, appeals, and possible consequences built into AAMFT's system for handling ethical violations.

Learning Activity 2. Educators can use cases illustrated in *AAMFT: Ethics Casebook* (Brock, 1994) to bring ethical issues to life. After reading case vignettes to the class, have students analyze which ethical principle(s) were violated. Then break the class into groups of six. Each group "becomes" a national ethics committee and discusses and acts upon the ethical violations reported in the *Ethics Casebook*. The "committee's" decisions are then presented to the entire class and discussed. Finally, the instructor reads the results illustrating the ethical violations from *AAMFT: Ethics Casebook*.

Learning Activity 3. Students may be assigned to watch one or more movies containing questionable ethics related to therapy. Possible movies include *Prince of Tides, House of Games, Basic Instinct, Final Analysis, What About Bob?,* and *Suddenly Last Summer,* to name a few. Students then write short papers related to violations within the *AAMFT Code of Ethics* (AAMFT, 1991) that they note in the movie, as well as to questionable ethics not covered by the code.

Legal Issues

Family Law

Comments on the Issue. It is essential that family therapists have a working knowledge of family law. Because family law statutes vary from state to state, we recommend developing a relationship with a competent local attorney to serve as a consultant regarding changes in statutes and precedents. Because individual judges are typically given considerable latitude to interpret laws, knowledge about the inclinations and decisions of particular judges is frequently as important as knowledge of the laws themselves. Areas of special concern include trends in a particular state regarding custody decisions and the criteria utilized, precedents regarding awarding joint custody, policies and trends regarding child support, and mechanisms for changing decrees after a divorce.

In addition, family therapists should have current knowledge of state codes regarding privileged communication, mental health records, and patient access to records.

Learning Activity 1. The experience of actually observing divorce court proceedings can provide a student with an excellent "feel" for divorce and custody issues. In addition, local attorneys are often willing to speak to family therapy trainees about issues related to family law. Ask the attorney if he or she has a training tape for witnesses that illustrates lawyer tactics to lead witnesses. This education help students prepare for courtroom testimony.

Learning Activity 2. Collect legal questions throughout the course of your class that you have not been able to answer. Invite a local attorney to speak on family law and state statute. Send the attorney the unanswered questions prior to his or her lecture so that he or she may address them during the presentation.

Malpractice and Legal Liability

Comments on the Issue. Background readings regarding a therapist's legal liability include Huber (1994), Smith (1994), Stromberg (1988), Stromberg and Dellinger (1993), Conte and Karasu (1990), and Vesper and Brock (1991). Important topics related to the legal liability of the practicing family therapist include malpractice, contract law, torts, constitutional law, and criminal law. Family therapists should also be aware of how to responsibly use forms related to informed consent, disclosure statements, therapeutic contracts, confidentiality, and releases. To prepare lectures on "defensive" and legally informed family therapy, review Robert Woody's works (1982, 1988a, 1988b, 1991).

The following list comprises common types of malpractice claims in therapy, summarized by Stromberg and Dellinger (1993, p. 3):

- Misdiagnosis.
- Practicing outside of one's area of competence.
- Negligent or improper treatment.
- Physical contact or sexual relations with patients.
- Failure to prevent patients from harming themselves or others.
- Improper release of hospitalized patients.
- Failure to consult another practitioner or refer a patient.
- Failure to supervise students or assistants.
- Abandonment of patients.

Basic precautions to decrease liability in practice are (Stromberg & Dellinger, 1993, p. 4):

- Define realistically your areas of expertise and practice.
- Maintain competence in your practice.
- Choose and handle patients carefully.
- Support patients, consult, and refer when appropriate.
- Follow up when an unusual incident occurs in treatment.
- Terminate treatment carefully and with proper reasons.
- Keep complete records.

Because of increased litigation and increased regulation of the helping professions, family therapists increasingly need to pay special attention to keeping good client records. For information on record-keeping issues and tactics, see Engelberg (1994); Eberlein (1990); Gelman (1992); Remley (1989); Snider (1987); and Soisson, Vandecreek, and Knapp (1987). The general trend is toward clear, concise records that support one's diagnosis, course of therapy, management of client's/clients' condition(s), termination summary, and aftercare plans.

Ethical and responsible management of dangerous and suicidal family members is also an important area of legal liability. Some therapists have used "antisuicide," "no-harm," or "nonviolence" contracts when dealing with these potentially life-threatening client problems. Generally these contracts are written promises clients sign stating that they will comply with a series of therapeutic or interventive steps if they feel suicidal or homicidal. There are several limitations to "no-harm" and similar contracts. First, the therapist must trust that the client will follow through on the contract in the midst of suicidal, homicidal, or violent ideation. Second, the contracts are not legally binding. Third, the contracts may falsely lower a therapist's vigilance about a particular client. Finally, it seems that the contracts may serve the need of decreasing therapist anxiety more than decreasing client anxiety. Nevertheless, they may be a good tool to strengthen a therapeutic alliance around these issues. For more specific information on issues regarding suicidal clients, see Bonger (1991) and Richman (1986). For more specific information on violence in marital therapy, see Costa and Holliday (1993), Gutsche and Murray (1991), and Weidman (1986). An example of a no-harm contract for therapeutic use follows:

NO-HARM CONTRACT

I, _____ agree that I will not do anything that would cause harm to myself or to anyone else, for the following length of time: _____. I realize that I am responsible for my own actions, and if I find things in my life becoming too difficult, I will contact a therapist at the "Center for Families." If I cannot reach a therapist at the "Center for Families," I will contact one of the sources on a list my therapist has given to me, including going to a hospital emergency room.

Client signature	Date

Witness signature	Date

Learning Activity. Therapeutic situations with legal ramifications (e.g., a difficult client who does not want to be terminated or referred) may be role-played and discussed. However, due to the important and delicate legal issues involved, it is also desirable for a lawyer with expertise in these areas to be invited into class as a guest speaker/discussant. Here are some useful questions to pose to an attorney:

- If a therapist learns a child is on drugs, is the therapist legally bound to inform the parents?
- Can therapists keep separate "private notes" on a client that would not be considered part of a client's record?
- If a murder was committed by a client X years ago, and he or she divulges the information in therapy, is the therapist bound to divulge this information to the authorities?
- What is the best way to learn/stay apprised of state statutes?
- If I learn that another therapist previously sexually abused my client, and my client refuses to report the therapist, am I bound to inform the therapist's professional agency? What if therapists having sex with client is illegal in my state? Do I contact authorities?
- How does privilege or confidentiality change when there is more than one person in the therapy room?

Courtroom Testimony

Comments on the Issue. Several fine articles have been written to help the family therapist prepare to testify in court (e.g., Bernstein, 1979; Brodsky, 1977; Brodsky & Robey, 1973; Gardner, 1982; Meyerstein & Todd, 1980; Nichols, 1982). Use these to prepare a lecture on courtroom testimony. Family therapists should be able to establish credibility by (1) having background information ready on themselves, (2) recanting their professional experience, (3) discussing their professional standing (license, organizations, specialties, etc.), and (4) testifying regarding the basis of their opinions of the client(s). In addition, the family therapist must be able to answer fundamental questions about the field of marriage and family therapy.

Learning Activity 1. Because establishing professional credibility is essential, the therapist needs to give his or her lawyer questions about information he or she wants to come out in court. To practice this, students should be asked to bring to class a list of 5–10 questions that an attorney might ask them about their professional qualifications (they are asked to project their qualifications 5 years from now). The instructor then plays the role of the attorney.

Learning Activity 2. A second simulation activity involves the instructor as prosecuting attorney putting selected students "on the witness stand" and asking them questions in an attempt to discredit them as witnesses. If a student has trouble responding, other students may try. These role plays are brief, generally nonthreatening, and have generated a great deal of discussion. Students are prepared for the very real world of the adversarial court system by learning to grapple with how to handle such questions (adapted from Brodsky, 1977) as the following:

Is it possible that you may have some biases in this case?
Are you testifying in a custody case and have no children yourself?
Are you divorced? Who has custody of your children?
How much are you being paid to say this today?
Have you conducted follow-up studies on the consistency of your own
  judgments?
Is it not true that family therapists disagree among themselves as to
  what brings about change?

Certification, Licensure, and Freedom of Choice Laws

Marriage and family therapy is an evolving profession, as evidenced by 36 states having some form of certification or licensure to protect the practice of marriage and family therapy. As mental health dollars shrink, we will see more competition between helping profession disciplines. Continued certification or licensure laws, coupled with freedom of choice laws will be important to the continued development of the field. Licensing laws prohibit the actual *practice* of marriage and family therapy without a license; certification legislation prohibits the use of the professional *title* without a certificate. Under certification laws, some states will protect the title "Certified Marriage and Family Therapist," whereas others protect the more generic term "Marriage and Family Therapist" (AAMFT, 1993). State governing bodies establish educational and training criteria for MFTs, often influenced by the standards of the AAMFT. AAMFT has a model act to aid in the licensure/certification process entitled *The Model Marriage and Family Therapy Licensure Act* (AAMFT, 1992c).

Freedom of choice laws (sometimes called vendorship laws) allow consumers to choose among the various mental health disciplines and disallow third party payors from discriminating against any one mental health discipline (AAMFT, 1993). Freedom of choice laws, coupled with MFT certification or licensure, will continue to make marriage and family therapy a competitive treatment provider.

Learning Activity. The move toward licensure in marriage and family therapy has both pros and cons. Have students generate a debate on the pros and cons of certification or licensure. Possible pros and cons include the following:

Pros	Cons
Protects the public.	Does not guarantee that the public will be protected.
Licensure protects both the MFTs and the public.	Ethical codes already protect MFTs and the public.
Licensure will establish confidence in the MFT profession.	Clients will suffer due to competition between disciplines.
Licensure will make MFTs more salable.	Because licensure increases the specialty designation of MFTs, practices will be more limited.
Licensure provides more employment options.	Licensure plays into the world of third-party payers, who will set more restrictions on practice.
Licensure clearly defines the limits of MFT practice.	Some practitioners have a larger scope of practice than others and will be hurt by legislation.
The profession will not survive without licensure.	The profession will be better off without licensure.

Lawyer and Therapist as an Interdisciplinary Team

Comments on the Issue. Bernstein (1977) has written about lawyer–therapist cooperation in such areas as child custody, the blended family (Bernstein, 1981), and child neglect (Harris & Bernstein, 1980). Bernstein asserts that the therapist must become familiar with the pragmatics of legal maneuvering. Equally important is the task of educating a lawyer about family therapy so that months of therapeutic interventions will not be undone in the courtroom. The family therapist should be aware of the advantages and practical application of such cooperation, as well as the problems in reconciling adversarial and therapeutic roles.

Learning Activity. Opportunities for lawyer–therapist cooperation (e.g., preparation for child neglect cases; see Harris and Bernstein, 1980) may be role-played and discussed. Again, a family lawyer as guest speaker/discussant also would be helpful.

Professional Issues

Family Therapy: Profession or Professional Specialty?

Comments on the Issue. Many people believe that family therapy, with its unique history, professional associations, journals, and code of ethics, is now to be considered a viable profession, as are psychology, psychiatry, and social work. Others believe that family therapy is a legitimate specialty of each of these professions, but is not itself a profession. The question of family therapy as a profession or a professional specialty has far-reaching ramifications for family therapists in such areas as training, licensure, third-party payments, job security, and professional identity.

Learning Activity. Students should read Shields, Wynne, McDaniel, and Gawinski's article (1994) regarding the marginalization of family therapy, as well as responses to it (Anderson, 1994; Hardy, 1994). Students are then divided into two teams. One team is assigned to defend the Shields et al. (1994) position supporting integration of family therapy within the traditional mental health establishment, while the other team attacks this position, using the positions of Hardy (1994) and Anderson (1994).

Professional Survival into the 21st Century: Health-Care Reform and Its Implications for Marriage and Family Therapists

Comments on the Issue. Increasing health-care costs have led to the restructuring of health-care benefits within the United States. The reverberations of this restructuring have led some practitioners to respond to the changes with a sense of foreboding, loss, or anger, whereas others have responded to the changes as an arena of opportunity. (See the March/April 1994 *Family Therapy Networker* for more reflection on this issue.)

Although it is unclear exactly what direction health-care reform will take into the 21st century, present reforms have led practitioners of family therapy well into the arena of managed care. Generally, managed care includes health maintenance organizations, preferred provider organizations, and more restrictive insurance reimbursement regulations. For a more detailed debate on health-care reform and family therapy, see Crane (1995a), Patterson and Sherger (1995), and a response by Crane (1995b). For more information on managed care and reimbursement issues, see Browning and

Browning (1994), Todd (1994), and Small (1991). General trends regarding health-care reform suggest the following predictions:

- MFTs will need to continue to gain recognition as independent providers by lobbying for state recognition (certification, licensure) and by educating those in charge or managing mental health-care services (Crane, 1995a).
- MFTs must know how to provide diagnosis of major emotional disorders and be able to communicate in this language in order to facilitate business with other mental health providers, provider groups, and managed care (Crane, 1995a). Family therapists will also need to navigate the ethical issues that can arise from a clash in systems theory and the medical model of DSM-IV (American Psychiatric Association, 1994; Denton, 1989).
- Marketing services to fulfill needs will be paramount to survival. This may mean offering extremely specialized services, or offering "vertically integrated" (Crane, 1995a, p. 123) services, which means a client can gain access to many types of services once they enter a mental health-care practice.
- Reimbursement for services will occur in two ways: There will be a fee-for-service system (which is more common presently), with movement toward a capitated system, whereby a therapist or therapy practice will be paid a set amount for assuming all the mental health needs of a client or client group (Patterson & Scherger, 1995), with movement toward the latter.
- Brief therapy models will thrive in an era of decreased economic resources.
- In addition, cost-effectiveness research as outlined by Pike and Piercy (1990), and cost–benefit analysis (Yates, 1994) will support the cost-effectiveness of family interventions. Although it intuitively makes sense that MFTs can treat more people more cost-efficiently, we need more research in this area.
- MFTs continually will need to understand and traverse insurance territory. Coverage questions MFTs should know when querying about insurance coverage of clients include the following:

1. Are services covered by MFTs? Master's or doctoral level? Certification or licensure required?
2. Is marital or family therapy covered? What nervous or mental disorders are covered? Is group therapy covered?
3. Are outpatient services covered? Inpatient?
4. Must the service provider be supervised by an M.D., or does a referral need to be made by an M.D.?
5. What is the total amount insurance will pay yearly mental health services?
6. Is there a deductible that must be satisfied? If so, how much must be satisfied, and how often must the deductible be met (yearly?)?

7. Is there a limit or "usual and customary" restriction on the provider's charge?
8. Does this patient have any preexisting conditions that might preclude coverage of any mental health services?
9. What percentage of mental health services are covered?
10. Is there a restriction on the number of visits covered?
11. How do I make a claim? Do I pay the provider directly? Are there any special forms needed? What specific information do I need in order to process a claim?
12. Are there specific restrictions if the client is covered by alternate insurance in addition to this policy?

Ethical Issues Regarding Reimbursement. Several ethical (and potential legal) issues arise as a result of family therapists traversing the waters of insurance and managed care reimbursement:

- Adhering to brief therapy models despite client circumstances to appease the reimburser.
- Abandoning theory other than what fits into the reimburser's schema.
- Diagnosing clients with a disorder. For further information regarding this ethical dilemma see Denton (1989), Strong (1993), and Kaslow (1993).
- Raising fees so the insurance company pays both payment and copayment is insurance fraud. Not collecting copayments is generally considered fraud. Fees must also be standard to all clients.
- Signing off on insurance claims must be done within reimburser guidelines.
- Giving diagnoses for someone in marital or family therapy to ensure reimbursement when *V* codes are not covered.
- Releasing client information to reimbursers without following confidentiality guidelines; a release must be obtained from client.
- Taking on clients who have severe problems when you know reimburser will only allow *X* sessions can be problematic. At the end of that time, what does the therapist do if the client needs more sessions and the reimburser refuses to pay?

Licensure and Legislative Awareness

Comments on the Issue. The pros and cons of professional licensure (Gross, 1978; Kosinski, 1982) and the current state of family therapy licensure and certification are important professional issues with which family therapy trainees should be familiar. The licensure issue should also be understood in a larger context—that of legislative awareness. Dorken

(1981), for example, provides excellent suggestions on how to affect a state legislature.

Learning Activity 1. One class simulation could involve the class "becoming" a state AAMFT board faced with the task of initiating a certification or licensure bill for the next legislative session. The class should deal with whether they want a certification or a licensure bill, how to generate funds to support it, how to build a legislative network, how to choose the bill's sponsor, and how to lobby with legislators. In effect, they learn experientially the pragmatic intricacies of undertaking this important yet formidable task.

Learning Activity 2. A second simulation could involve assigning each student to testify in front of a "legislative subcommittee" (the class) for 3 minutes on the merits of a family therapy certification bill they previously were assigned to read. In critiquing these legislative testimonies, important "do's" and "don'ts" should be identified and discussed.

Journals and Publishing

Comments on the Issue. Current English-language family therapy journals and newsletters, as well as their editors' names and addresses, are included here. For additional details on family related journals, see Hanks, Matocha, and Susman (1992).

- *American Journal of Family Therapy.* Dr. Richard Sauber, Editor. Suite 115, 1050 NW 15th Street, Boca Raton, FL 33432.
- *Australian and New Zealand Journal of Family Therapy.* Max Cornwell, Editor. P.O. Box 633, Lane Cove, New South Wales, Australia 2066.
- *Contemporary Family Therapy: An International Journal.* William C. Nichols, Ed.D., Editor, Box 3667, Tallahassee, FL 32315-3667.
- *Family Process.* Peter Steinglass, M.D., Editor, 149 East 78th Street, New York, NY 10021.
- *Family Relations.* Mark A. Fine, Ph.D., Editor, Department of Psychology, University of Dayton, Dayton, OH 45469-1430.
- *Family Systems Medicine.* Donald A. Bloch, M.D., Editor, 40 West 12th Street, New York, NY 10021.
- *Family Therapy.* Martin Blinder, M.D., Editor, 130 Melville Avenue, San Anselmo, CA 94960.
- *Family Therapy Case Studies.* Michael Durrant, Editor, Eastwood Family Therapy Centre, P.O. Box 630, Epping, New South Wales, Australia, 2121.
- *Family Therapy Networker.* Richard Simon, Editor, 7703 13th Street, N.W., Washington, DC 20012.

- *Journal of Couples Therapy.* Barbara Jo Brothers, Ph.D., Editor, 3500 St. Charles Street, New Orleans, LA 70115.
- *Journal of Divorce and Remarriage.* Craig A. Everett, Ph.D., Editor, 1050 East River Road, Tucson, AZ 85718.
- *Journal of Family Psychology.* Howard A. Little, Editor, Temple University, 249 Weiss Hall, Philadelphia, PA 19122.
- *Journal of Family Psychotherapy.* Terry S. Trepper, Ph.D., Editor, Family Studies Center, Purdue University Calumet, Hammond, IN 46323-2094.
- *Journal of Family Therapy.* c/o Academic Press Limited, 24-28 Oval Road London, NWI 7DX, England, UK.
- *Journal of Feminist Family Therapy.* Lois Braverman, ACSW, Editor, 3833 Woods Drive, Des Moines, IA 50312.
- *Journal of Marital and Family Therapy.* Douglas H. Sprenkle, Ph.D., Editor, Purdue University, Marriage and Family Therapy Program, Fowler Building, West Lafayette, IN 47907.
- *Journal of Sex and Marital Therapy.* Editors, 65 East 76th Street, Suite 1A, New York, NY 10021.
- *Journal of Systemic Therapies.* Don Efron, Sr., Coeditor, Box 2484, Station B, London, Ontario, Canada, N6A467.
- *Journal of Strategic and Systemic Therapies* Don Efron, Sr., Coeditor, Box 2484, Station B, London, Ontario, Canada, N6A467.

Family therapy trainees should be familiar with these journals, as well as the process of getting their own names in print.

Learning Activity 1. Students should be assigned readings that will sharpen their writing skills (Becker, 1986; Piercy, McDaniel, & Sprenkle, 1996; Zinsser, 1994) and demystify the publication process (Berardo, 1981; Sporakowski, 1982). In addition, students should read about how prolific family therapists manage journal article rejections (Piercy, Moon, & Bischof, 1994). In small groups, they should be asked to discuss the tasks involved in having their own theses or dissertations published. In the class discussion that follows, the instructor should fill in any steps not mentioned by the students.

Learning Activity 2. To increase students' professionalization, another assignment is the writing of a publishable 15-page paper on a relevant area of interest. This assignment may be introduced as follows:

Each of you will choose an ethical, legal, or professional issue in family therapy of interest to you, read widely on that issue, and then write a scholarly, referenced term paper of publishable quality. To be publishable, your paper should go beyond a simple review of the current research and theory related to your issue. You should tackle your issue in some creative and imaginative way that would contribute to, rather than rehash, the literature related to your chosen topic. The following titles are only examples, but should provide a flavor for the theoretical originality or unique application of existing information that would make for a publishable paper:

"Ethical Issues Inherent for Family Therapists in Managed Care Practice"

"The Role of the Therapist's Values in Family Preservation Programs"

"Being an Advocate for Family Therapy: Guidelines for Legislative Testimony"

"The Ethics of a Not-Knowing Stance to Therapy"

"Beginning Therapists: Traversing the Ethical Issue of Inexperience"

"Writing Systemic Case Notes within an Individual-Oriented Agency"

"Accepting Gifts in Family Therapy: Accepting Generosity at the Risk of a Dual Relationship?"

"Suggestions for Educating Potential Employers about Why They Need a Family Therapist on the Team"

Person of the Therapist

Comments on the Issue. Training programs emphasize the professional development of trainees. Yet, therapy is a "personal encounter within a professional frame" (Aponte, 1994, p. 3). Thus, it seems that the person of the therapist should be deemed an appropriate part of the "professional development" of the marriage and family therapist.

The interface of family therapists' work and family lives on the person-of- the therapist issue is worth exploring. How does their work affect their own lives and those of their families? How do their families of origin affect their choice of a profession and their day-to-day work? What happens to their work when they experience marital or family problems? Although some have speculated on such questions (e.g., Charny, 1982; Piercy & Wetchler, 1987; Polson & Piercy, 1993; Wetchler & Piercy, 1986), there are few clear-cut answers.

The spirituality or religious life of the therapist also impacts his or her work. For many, it is difficult to not face overlap between therapeutic and religious views. Some see religion and family therapy as naturally intertwined and the spiritual life of the clients an important area for all family therapists to explore (Stander, Piercy, MacKinnon, & Helmeke, 1994). Others have taken a position that "true" religious psychotherapy would require extended expertise and training in both religion and therapy (Brandsma, Pattison, & Muysken, 1986). Thus, it is unclear how, if, or when to integrate religion in family therapy.

Learning Activity 1. Students are asked to read Aponte (1994) and discuss the following questions:

- Is it important for therapists to assess their personal emotions and reactions in therapy? Why or why not?
- Should every therapist be required to go to personal therapy? Why or why not?
- What do you expect to get from doing family therapy?
- Aponte suggests that therapists should "develop the capacity for personal *intimacy, mutuality, and commitment* with clients inside professional boundaries" (1994, p. 4). What do you think he means by this statement?

Learning Activity 2. Students are asked to take the questionnaire developed by Wetchler and Piercy (1986) to identify work-related enhancers and stressors of the marital and family lives of family therapists. Then the instructor presents and discusses the findings of Wetchler and Piercy's survey of 110 Indiana family therapists (which employed the same questionnaire). Finally, the group brainstorms ways family therapists may reduce stressors to their own marital and family lives. The reader will find a variety of other useful procedures to help trainees explore work–family interfaces in Piercy and Wetchler (1987).

Learning Activity 3. Ask students to read Stander et al. (1994) and Youngren (1993) and discuss the following questions:

- Should religion be integrated into family therapy? How?
- How do you respond to the belief that if you are going to practice religion in family therapy, then you must be an expert on both religion *and* family therapy?
- How does one work with the triangle of God, the family, and the therapist?
- Do your religious beliefs, or lack thereof, influence your selection of a family therapy theory/model?

Establishing a Private Practice: Public Relations

Comments on the Issue. Family therapists considering going into private practice should be familiar with public relations procedures (Kilgore, 1979), office forms and procedures, financing, fee structures, collection procedures, and means of making contact with potential clients and referral sources (e.g., cards, brochures, speaking engagements, media, and personal contacts). An excellent source for such information is Keller and Ritt's (1994) *Innovations in Clinical Practice: A Source Book.*

Learning Activity 1. A successful family therapist should be asked to discuss his or her own experiences in setting up a practice and developing a caseload. If possible, the therapist should share copies of business forms and discuss the technical aspects of carrying on a private practice.

Learning Activity 2. The ethical and pragmatic considerations of one current public relations trend—the family therapist as expert on a radio or TV talk show—should be examined. Specifically, the difference between therapy and public education should be explored, in addition to appropriate answers to difficult interview questions. Mock talk show interviews could be held to illustrate ethical dilemmas and to practice appropriate responses (cf. Kilgore, 1979; Myers-Walls & Piercy, 1985).

Job Hunting

Comments on the Issue. For those students interested in academic or agency positions, three broad job-hunting skills are necessary. The first is "getting sellable." Since many jobs have sources of applicants, students should use their academic careers to seek out experiences and develop skills that will allow them to stand out in the job market. This process involves the more-than-is-expected activities of running community groups, publishing articles, making speeches, attending workshops, joining professional organizations, holding offices, and reading journals and books that are not assigned.

Second, a "sellable" applicant must get his or her "foot in the door." Getting the attention of a prospective employer involves the development of a well-organized and compelling curriculum vita. Third, the job interview—the final step in most selection processes—is a critical one (see Darley & Zanna, 1981).

Learning Activity. Students are asked to specify in small groups their rights within a job interview, the skills they want to emphasize, and the questions they want to ask during the interview (McGovern, 1976). Finally, mock job interviews are held in groups of three. Upon completion of each interview, the interviewee should be given feedback regarding his or her answers and style of presentation.

RESEARCH ISSUES

Several studies have examined ethical issues in the field of marriage and family therapy. For example, researchers have conducted surveys about the ethical dilemmas faced by family therapists (Brock & Coufal, 1994; Green & Hansen, 1986, 1989). Nickell, Hecker, Ray, and Bercik (1995) explore marriage and family therapists' sexual attraction to clients and provide guidelines for training programs in addressing this issue. Clearly, ethical, legal, and professional issues are operationalizable and researchable. Examples of possible research questions include the following:

- What are the effects of a giving professional disclosure statements on the process and outcome in family therapy?
- What is the relationship between knowledge of ethical codes and the ethical behavior of family therapists?
- What factors correlate with credibility in the courtroom testimony of family therapists?
- What are the ethics of operating within the managed care network?
- What are therapists' policies regarding seeing clients who are seeing other therapists and are dissatisfied with the therapists or the therapy?
- What are therapists' policies regarding other ethical and legal issues?
- To what extent do family therapists (who may also be licensed as psychologists or psychiatrists) manipulate DSM-IV codes to gain third-party payments?
- What do family therapists perceive as ethical restraints related to advertising?

Questions such as these reflect important areas of inquiry for the family therapy researcher. In the years ahead, we expect to see much more research on such ethical, legal, and professional questions.

KEY BOOKS, CHAPTERS, AND ARTICLES

Becker, H. S. (1986). *Writing for social scientists.* Chicago: University of Chicago Press.

In this clear, readable book, Becker shares his own experiences with writing and provides a variety of useful insights. He humorously hits the mark in discussing the foibles of beginning writers and seems to have pinpointed the elusive work habits that contribute to good writing. Although most of Becker's examples are drawn from the sociological literature, this is an excellent source for family therapists struggling with the writing process.

Bernstein, B. E. (1979). Lawyer and therapist as an interdisciplinary team: Trial preparation. *Journal of Marital and Family Therapy, 5*(4), 93–100.

This article reviews trial preparation and illustrates examination and cross-examination, opinion testimony, and hypothetical questions. Bernstein's illustrations underline potential hazards of an adversarial court system, and his practical suggestions provide a means of averting these hazards.

Brock, G. W. (Ed.). (1994). *American Association for Marriage and Family Therapy: Ethics casebook.* Washington, DC: AAMFT.

This is an excellent source for learning about the ethical codes of AAMFT. The book covers the evolution of AAMFT's ethical codes, research on ethical practices of MFTs, and the ethical principles, with case examples. This is must-reading for any MFT.

Brodsky, S. L. (1977). The mental health professional on the witness stand: A survival guide. In B. D. Sales (Ed.), *Psychology in the legal process.* New York: Spectrum.

Brodsky provides useful suggestions for coping with cross-examination. He examines the "gambits" that lawyers use to discredit witnesses and provides the reader with excellent "responses that degambitize."

Brodsky, S. L., & Robey, A. (1973). On becoming an expert witness: Issues of orientation and effectiveness. *Professional Psychology, 3,* 173–176.

This article is frequently cited in the literature and, although dated, is still quite helpful in preparing the therapist for the witness stand.

Denton, W. (1989). A family systems analysis of the DSM-III-R. *Journal of Marital and Family Therapy, 16*(2), 113–125.

This article discusses the difference in scientific paradigms between DSM-III-R and family systems theory. Denton nicely articulates ethical dilemmas for family therapists arising from the use of the DSM. He also suggests the need for a family diagnostic classification system.

Doherty, W. J. (1995). *Soul searching: Why psychotherapy must promote moral responsibility.* New York: Basic Books.

Doherty concisely outlines his view of morality in the practice of psychotherapy. He proposes seven principles that therapists of any discipline may use as a framework for making moral decisions. Throughout the book, Doherty shares examples from his own clinical work that illustrate his grappling with moral issues. The book is both an invitation and a challenge for therapists to be forthright about their values and to regard morality as an irreducible element in clinical practice.

Doherty, W. J., & Boss, P. G. (1991). Values and ethics in family therapy. In A. S. Gurman & D. P. Kniskern (Eds.), *Handbook of family therapy* (Vol. 2). New York: Brunner/Mazel.

This is a comprehensive and thoughtful chapter on family therapy ethics. It presents a nice history of the development of ethics in the field of MFT and points out major issues relevant to ethics within the practice, theory, and research of family therapy.

Dorken, H. (1981). Coming of age legislatively in 21 steps. *American Psychologist, 2,* 167–173.

Family therapists reading this article will learn a lot about legislative activism from Dorken, a psychologist.

Framo, J. (1968). My families, my family. *Voices, 4*(33), 18–27.

Framo provides a telling commentary of how events in his own life have spilled over into his professional work. This should be required reading for all beginning family therapists.

Framo, J. (1975). Personal reflections of a family therapist. *Journal of Marriage and Family Counseling, 1,* 15–27.

This is a moving article in which Framo traces his development as a family therapist. In a very personal style, Framo deals with issues regarding professional identity and the interface between values and therapy.

Gardner, R. (1989). *Family evaluation in child custody mediation, arbitration, and litigation.* Cresskill, NJ: Creative Intelligence.

An excellent guide by a therapist with considerable experience in child custody litigation. This book provides detailed, useful information on many aspects of child custody issues.

Hanks, R. S., Matocha, L., Susman, M. B. (Eds.). (1992). *Publishing in journals on the family: A survey guide for scholars, practitioners, and students.* Binghamton, NY: Haworth.

This handbook is a must for anyone who wishes to publish as a family scholar. This book outlines the major journals relating to the family, as well as providing editor's names, addresses, types of articles accepted, review period time, acceptance rates, and circulation information.

Huber, C. H. (1994). *Ethical, legal and professional issues in the practice of marriage and family therapy* (2nd ed.). New York: Macmillan College Publishing.

This is a good resource for beginning family therapists. It introduces excellent foundational information.

Karpel, M. A. (1980). Family secrets: I. Conceptual and ethical issues in the relational context. II. Ethical and practical considerations in therapeutic management. *Family Process, 19,* 295–306.

Ethical issues regarding family secrets and confidentiality in family therapy are discussed. Means of dealing with secrets in family therapy are also presented.

Kilgore, J. (1979). The marriage and family therapist's use of media for public education. *Journal of Marital and Family Therapy, 5*(4), 87–92.

Kilgore presents some helpful suggestions for the family therapist who wishes to impart information to the public through radio, TV, and the printed word. His application of Anon's P-LI-SS-IT approach (see Chap. 5, "Key Clinical Terms" section) is particularly useful in determining what information to provide.

Lefferts, R. (1992). *Getting a grant in the 1990s: How to write successful grant proposals.*

This book helps to demystify the process of writing grant proposals. All steps of grant writing are detailed clearly identified in this useful guide.

Lemmon, J. A. (Ed.). (1984). Ethics, standards, and professional challenges [Special issue]. *Mediation Quarterly, 4.*

Five excellent articles discuss ethical issues in mediation. The article on neutrality in mediation is especially useful in its examination of a neutral versus proponent role for the mediator.

Margolin, G. (1982). Ethical and legal considerations in marital and family therapy. *American Psychologist, 37,* 788–802.

Margolin identifies and cogently discusses such important ethical and legal issues as (1) therapist responsibility, (2) confidentiality, (3) privileged communication, (4) informed consent, (5) therapist values, and (6) training and supervision.

Meyerstein, I., & Todd, J. C. (1980). On the witness stand: The family therapist and expert testimony. *American Journal of Family Therapy, 8*(4), 43–51.

The authors discuss the application of certain family therapy skills to courtroom testimony. This article is well written and useful.

Peterson, M. R. (1992). *At personal risk: Boundary violations in professional–client relationships.* New York: Norton.

This book is the first of its kind to explore boundary violations in depth. It is excellent reading and exposes the vulnerabilities within the professional–client relationship in an illuminating and educational manner.

Piercy, F., & Wetchler, J. (1987). Family-work interfaces of psychotherapists: I. A summary of the literature. II. A didactic–experiential workshop. *Journal of Psychotherapy and the Family, 3*(2), 17–32.

This article reviews the literature on the interfaces of therapists' work and family lives. Part II outlines a useful workshop that can easily be adapted to family therapists. The workshop helps therapists examine the effects of their present family lives and family of origin on their work, as well as the potential effects of their work on them personally and on their spouses and/or children.

Ryder, R., & Hepworth, J. (1990). AAMFT Ethical Code: Dual relationships. *Journal of Marital and Family Therapy, 16*(2), 127–132.

This article explores limitations that the AAMFT Code of Ethical Principles placed on dual relationships. The authors argue that, rather than restricting dual relationships, family therapists should have training to understand the complexity of relationships and issues of complexity and power, both within the therapy relationship and within training. Ryder and Hepworth provide an interesting analysis of dual relationship issues.

Schlossberger, E., & Hecker, L. (1996). HIV and family therapists' duty to warn: A legal and ethical analysis. *Journal of Marital and Family Therapy, 22,* 27–40.

This is the first article in the field to address the thorny issues related to duty to warn when a family therapist is working with an HIV-seropositive client. Of particular interest is the authors' delineation between duty to warn when clients are engaging in *legally permissible dangers* versus *illegal dangers.* The authors conclude that the therapist has no legal duty to intervene when clients pose dangers that laws grant them the right to pose. The authors also discuss ethical ramifications of such situations.

Schneider, J. G. (1994, August). Legal issues involving "repressed memory" of childhood sexual abuse. *The Psychologist's Legal Update, 5,* pp. 3–13.

This is must-reading for any practicing clinician. This issue discusses repressed memory lawsuits and gives guidelines for performing therapy with abuse victims that protects the therapist from performing leading therapy techniques, which may lead to false memory problems.

Vesper, J. H., & Brock, G. W. (1991). *Ethics, legalities, and professional practice issues in marriage and family therapy.* Needham Heights, MA: Allyn & Bacon.

This text has a particularly good emphasis on legal issues in MFT and less so on ethical decision making. Overall, it is an excellent reference.

Wetchler, J. L., & Piercy, F. P. (1986). The marital/family life of the family therapist: Stressors and enhancers. *American Journal of Family Therapy, 14*(2), 99–109.

This interesting study examines the number and relative strength of stressors and enhancers of marital and family life for 110 family therapists in Indiana. More enhancers were reported than stressors. The results also were examined in terms of respondents' (1) gender, (2) work setting, (3) theoretical orientation, (4) number of hours worked, (5) income, and (6) age.

REFERENCES

American Association for Marriage and Family Therapy (AAMFT). (1991). *AAMFT code of ethics.* Washington, DC: Author.

American Association for Marriage and Family Therapy (AAMFT). (1992a). *Decision tree: AAMFT ethics cases.* Washington, DC: Author.

American Association for Marriage and Family Therapy (AAMFT). (1992b). *Procedures for handling ethical matters.* Washington, DC: Author.

American Association for Marriage and Family Therapy (AAMFT). (1992c). *The Model Marriage and Family Therapy Licensure Act.* Washington, DC: Author.

American Association for Marriage and Family Therapy (AAMFT). (1993). *Marriage and family therapy: Regulating the profession* [Brochure]. Washington, DC: Author.

American Association for Marriage and Family Therapy (AAMFT). (1994). *Commission on Accreditation for Marriage and Family Therapy Education: Manual on accreditation* (Version 8.1). Washington, DC: Author.

American Psychiatric Association. (1994). *Diagnostic and statistical manual of mental disorders* (4th ed.). Washington, DC: Author.

Anderson, H. (1994). Rethinking family therapy: A delicate balance. *Journal of Marital and Family Therapy, 20*(2), 145–149.

Aponte, H. J. (1994). How personal can training get? *Journal of Marital and Family Therapy, 20*(1), 3–15.

Arthur, G. L., & Swanson, C. D. (1993). *Confidentiality and privileged communication.* Alexandria, VA: American Counseling Association.

Becker, H. S. (1986). *Writing for social scientists.* Chicago: University of Chicago Press.

Berardo, F. M. (1981). The publication process: An editor's perspective. *Journal of Marriage and the Family, 43,* 771–779.

Bernstein, B. E. (1977). Lawyer and counselor as an interdisciplinary team: Preparing the father for custody. *Journal of Marriage and Family Counseling, 3*(3), 29–40.

Bernstein, B. E. (1979). Lawyer and counselor as an interdisciplinary team. *Journal of Marital and Family Therapy, 5*(4), 93–100.

Bernstein, B. E. (1981). Malpractice: Future shock of the 1980s. *Social Casework: The Journal of Contemporary Social Work, 62,* 175–181.

Black, H. C. (1979). *Black's law dictionary* (5th ed.). St. Paul, MN: West.

Bograd, M. (1984). Family systems approaches to wife battering: A feminist critique. *American Journal of Orthopsychiatry, 54,* 558–568.

Bonger, B. (1991). *The suicidal patient: Clinical and legal standards of care.* Washington, DC: American Psychological Association.

Brandsma, J. M., Pattison, E. M., & Muyskens, J. L. (1986). Roles, contracts, and covenants: An analysis of religious components in psychotherapy. In D. K. Kentsmith, S. A. Salladay, & P. A. Miya (Eds.), *Ethics in mental health practice.* Orlando: Grune & Stratton.

Bray, J., Shepherd, J., & Hays, J. (1985). Legal and ethical issues in informed consent to psychotherapy. *American Journal of Family Therapy, 13*(2), 50–60.1

Brock, G. W. (Ed.). (1994). *American Association for Marriage and Family Therapy: Ethics casebook.* Washington, DC: AAMFT.

Brock, G. W., & Coufal, J. D. (1994). A national survey of the ethical practices and attitudes of marriage and family therapists. In G. W. Brock (Ed.), *American Association for Marriage and Family Therapy: Ethics casebook.* Washington, DC: AAMFT.

Brodsky, S. L. (1977). The mental health professional on the witness stand: A survival guide. In B. D. Sales (Ed.), *Psychology in the legal process.* New York: Spectrum.

Brown, J. E., & Slee, P. T. (1986). Paradoxical strategies: The ethics of intervention. *Professional Psychology: Research and Practice, 17,* 487–491.

Browning, C., & Browning, B. (1994). *How to partner with managed care.* Los Alamitos, CA: Duncliff's International.

Charny, I. (1982). The personal and family mental health of family thought. In F. Kaslow (Ed.), *International book of family therapy.* New York: Brunner/Mazel.

Ciccone, J. R. (1985). Privilege and confidentiality: Psychiatric and legal considerations. *Psychiatric Medicine, 2*(3), 272–285.

Conte, H. R., & Karasu, T. B. (1990). Malpractice in psychotherapy: An overview. *American Journal of Psychotherapy, 44*(1), 232–246.

Costa, L., & Holliday, D. (1993). Considerations for treatment of marital violence. *Journal of Mental Health Counseling, 15*(1), 26–36.

Crane, D. R. (1995a). Health care reform in the United States: Implications for training and practice of marriage and family therapy. *Journal of Marital and Family Therapy, 21*(2), 115–125.

Crane, D. R. (1995b). Marriage and family therapy in health care reform: A response to Patterson and Scherger. *Journal of Marital and Family Therapy, 21*(2), 137–140.

Darley, J. M., & Zanna, M. (1981). An introduction to the hiring process in academic psychology. *Canadian Psychology, 22,* 228–238.

Dell, P. (1980). Researching the family theories of schizophrenia: An exercise in epistemological confusion. *Family Process, 19,* 321–335.

Dell, P. (1982). Beyond homeostasis: Toward a concept of coherence. *Family Process, 21,* 21–41.

Dell, P. (1986a). In defense of lineal causality. *Family Process, 25*(4), 513–524.

Dell, P. (1986b). Toward a foundation for addressing violence. *Family Process, 25*(4), 527–529.

Denton, W. H. (1989). DSM-III-R and the family therapist: Ethical considerations. *Journal of Marital and Family Therapy, 15,* 367–377.

Dorken, H. (1981). Coming of age legislatively in 21 steps. *American Psychologist, 2,* 167–173.

Eberlein, L. (1990). Client records: Ethical and legal considerations. *Canadian Psychology, 31*(2), 155–166.

Engleberg, S. (1994). Client confidentiality for marriage and family therapists. In G. Brock (Ed.), *American Association for Marriage and Family Therapy: Ethics casebook.* Washington, DC: AAMFT.

Fine, M. A., & Ulrich, L. P. (1988). Integrating psychology and philosophy in teaching a graduate course in ethics. *Professional Psychology: Research and Practice, 19*(5), 542–546.

Fisch, R. (1990). "To thine own self be true . . . " Ethical issues in strategic therapy. In J. K. Zeig & S. G. Gilligan (Eds.), *Brief therapy: Myths, methods, and metaphors.* New York: Brunner/Mazel.

Fisher, L., Anderson, A., & Jones, J. E. (1981). Types of paradoxical interventions and indications/contraindications for use in clinical practice. *Family Process, 20,* 25–35.

Gardner, R. (1982). *Family evaluation in child custody litigation.* Cresskill, NJ: Creative Therapeutics.

Gelman, S. R. (1992). Risk management through client access to case records. *Social Work, 37*(1), 73–79.

Goldner, V. (1985a). Feminism and family therapy. *Family Process, 24,* 31–47.

Goldner, V. (1985b). Warning: Family therapy may be dangerous to your health. *Family Therapy Networker, 9,* 19–23.

Goodrich, T. J., Rampage, C., Ellman, B., & Hallstead, K. (1988). *Feminist family therapy: A casebook.* New York: Norton.

Green, S. L., & Hansen, J. C. (1986). Ethical dilemmas in family therapy. *Journal of Marital and Family Therapy, 12,* 225–230.

Green, S. L., & Hansen, J. C. (1989). Ethical dilemmas faced by family therapists. *Journal of Marital and Family Therapy, 15,* 149–158.

Gross, S. (1978). The myth of professional licensing. *American Psychologist, 33,* 1009–1016.

Gumper, L. L., & Sprenkle, D. H. (1981). Privileged communication in therapy: Special problems for the family and couples therapist. *Family Process, 20,* 11–23.

Gutsche, S., & Murray, M. (1991). The feminist meets the cybernetician: An integrated approach to spousal violence. *Journal of Strategic and Systemic Therapies, 10*(3–4), 76–91.

Haley, J. (1976). *Problem-solving therapy.* San Francisco: Jossey-Bass.

Hanks, R. S., Matocha, L., & Susman, M. B. (Eds.). (1992). *Publishing in journals on the family: A survey guide for scholars, practitioners, and students.* New York: Haworth.

Hardy, K. V. (1994). Marginalization or development? A response to Shields, Wynne, McDaniel, and Gawinski. *Journal of Marital and Family Therapy, 20*(1), 139–143.

Hare-Mustin, R. T. (1980). Family therapy may be dangerous to your health. *Professional Psychology, 11,* 935–938.

Harris, J. C., & Bernstein, B. E. (1980). Lawyer and social worker as a team: Preparing for trial in neglect cases. *Child Welfare, 59,* 469–477.

Herlihy, B., & Sheeley, V. L. (1987). Privileged communication in selected helping professionals: A comparison among statutes. *Journal of Counseling and Development, 65*(9), 479–483.

Huber, C. H. (1994). *Ethical, legal and professional issues in the practice of marriage and family therapy* (2nd ed.). New York: Macmillan College Publishing.

Imber-Black, E. (1986). Maybe "lineal causality" needs another defense lawyer: A feminist response to Dell. *Family Process, 25*(4), 523–525.

Karpel, M. A. (1980). Family secrets: I. Conceptual and ethical issues in the relational context. II. Ethical and practical considerations in therapeutic management. *Family Process, 19,* 295–306.

Kaslow, F. (1993). Relational diagnosis: An idea whose time has come? *Family Process, 32*(2), 255–259.

Keller, P. A., & Ritt, L. G. (Eds.). (1994). *Innovations in clinical practice: A source book.* Sarasota, FL: Professional Resource Exchange.

Kilgore, J. (1979). The marriage and family therapist's use of media for public education. *Journal of Marital and Family Therapy, 5*(4), 87–92.

Kosinski, F. A. (1982). Standards, accreditation, and licensure in marital and family therapy. *Personnel and Guidance Journal, 60,* 350–352.

Lamb, D. H., Clark, C., Drumheller, P., Frizzell, K., & Surrey, L. (1990). Applying "Tarasoff" to AIDS-related psychotherapy issues. *Professional Psychology: Research and Practice, 20*(1), 37–43.

Margolin, G. (1982). Ethical and legal considerations in marital and family therapy. *American Psychologist, 37,* 788–802.

McGovern, T. V. (1976). Assertion training for job interviewing and management/staff development. In A. J. Lange & P. Jakubowski (Eds.), *Responsible assertive behavior.* Champaign, IL: Research Press.

Meyerstein, I., & Todd, J. C. (1980). On the witness stand: The family therapist and expert testimony. *American Journal of Family Therapy, 8*(4), 43–51.

Monahan, J. (1993). Limiting therapist exposure to *Tarasoff* liability: Guidelines for risk containment. *American Psychologist, 48*(3), 242–250.

Mudd, E. (1967). *The American Association of Marriage Counselors: The first 25 years.* Dallas, TX: American Association of Marriage Counselors.

Myers-Walls, J., & Piercy, F. (1985). Mass media and prevention: Guidelines for family life professionals. *Primary Prevention, 5*(2), 124–133.

Nichols, J. (1982). The mental health professional as expert witness. In P. A. Keller & R. G. Ritt (Eds.), *Innovations in clinical practice: A source book.* Sarasota, FL: Professional Resource Exchange.

Nickell, N., Hecker, L., Ray, R., & Bercik, J. (1995). Marriage and family therapists' sexual attraction to clients: An exploratory study. *American Journal of Family Therapy, 23,* 315–327.

O'Shea, M., & Jessee, E. (1982). Ethical, value, and professional conflicts in systems therapy. In L. L'Abate (Ed.), *Values, ethics, legalities and the family therapist.* Rockville, MD: Aspen Systems.

Patterson, J., & Scherger, J. E. (1995). A critique of health care reform in the United States: Implications for the training and practice of marriage and family therapy. *Journal of Marital and Family Therapy, 21*(2), 127–135.

Piercy, F., McDaniel, S., & Sprenkle, D. H. (1996). Teaching professional writing in family therapy: Three approaches. *Journal of Marital and Family Therapy, 22*(2), 163–179.

Piercy, F., Moon, S., & Bischoff, R. (1994). Difficult journal article rejections among prolific family therapists: A qualitative critical incident study. *Journal of Marital and Family Therapy, 20*(3), 231–245.

Piercy, F., & Wetchler, J. (1987). Family-work interfaces of psychotherapy: I. A summary of the literature. II. A didactic-experiential workshop. *Journal of Psychotherapy and the Family, 3*(2), 17–32.

Pike, C. L., & Piercy, F. P. (1990). Cost effectiveness research in family therapy. *Journal of Marital and Family Therapy, 16*(4), 375–388.

Polson, M., & Piercy, F. (1993). The impact of training stress on married family therapy trainees and their families: A focus group study. *Journal of Family Psychotherapy, 4*(1), 69–92.

Preister, S., Vesper, J. H., & Humphrey, F. G. (1994). The evolution of a professional code of ethics. In G. Brock (Ed.), *American Association for Marriage and Family Therapy: Ethics casebook.* Washington, DC: AAMFT.

Raskin, D. E., & Klein, Z. E. (1976). Losing a symptom through keeping it: A review of paradoxical treatment techniques and rationale. *Archives of General Psychiatry, 33,* 548–555.

Remley, T. P., Jr. (1989). Counseling records: Legal and ethical issues. In B. Herliha & L. L. Golden (Eds.), *Ethical standards casebook* (4th ed.). Alexandria, VA: American Association for Counseling and Development.

Richman, J. (1986). *Family therapy for suicidal people.* New York: Springer.

Rohrbaugh, M., Tennen, H., Press, S., & White, L. (1981). Compliance, defiance, and therapeutic paradox: Guidelines for strategic use of paradoxical interventions. *American Journal of Orthopsychiatry, 51,* 454–467.

Schlossberger, E., & Hecker, L. (1996). *Purposes, content, and uses of professional codes: Enhancing the identity of the family sciences.* Unpublished manuscript, Purdue University Calumet, Hammond, IN.

Schlossberger, E., & Hecker, L. (1996). HIV and family therapists' duty to warn: A legal and ethical analysis. *Journal of Marital and Family Therapy, 22,* 27–40.

Schneider, J. G. (1994, August). Legal issues involving "repressed memory" of childhood sexual abuse. *Psychologist's Legal Update, 5,* pp. 3–13.

Schultz, B. M. (1982). *Legal liability in psychotherapy.* San Francisco: Jossey-Bass.

Schultz, J. (1982). *Writing from start to finish.* Upper Montclair, NJ: Boynton/Cook.

Schwitzgebel, R. L., & Schwitzgebel, R. K. (1980). *Law and psychological practice.* New York: Wiley.

Shalett, J. S., & Everett, C. A. (1981). Accreditation in family therapy education: Its history and role. *American Journal of Family Therapy, 9*(4), 82–84.

Shields, C. G., Wynne, L. C., McDaniel, S. H., & Gawinski, B. A. (1994). The marginalization of family therapy: A historical and continuing problem. *Journal of Marital and Family Therapy, 20*(1), 117–138.

Small, R. F. (1991). *Maximizing third-party reimbursement in your mental health practice.* Sarasota, FL: Professional Resource Exchange.

Smith, S. R. (1994). Liability and mental health services. *American Journal of Orthopsychiatry, 64*(2), 235–251.

Snider, P. D. (1987). Client records: Inexpensive liability protection for mental health counselors. *Journal of Mental Health Counseling, 9*(3), 134–141.

Soisson, E. L., Vandecreek, L., & Knapp, S. (1987). Thorough record keeping: A good defense in a litigious era. *Professional Psychology: Research and Practice, 18*(5), 498–502.

Solovey, A. D., & Duncan, B. L. (1992). Ethics and strategic therapy: A proposed ethical direction. *Journal of Marital and Family Therapy, 18*(1), 53–61.

Sporakowski, M. J. (1982). From the editor. *Family Relations, 31,* 315–316.

Stander, V., Piercy, F. P., MacKinnon, D., & Helmeke, K. (1994). Spirituality, religion and family therapy: Competing or complementary worlds? *American Journal of Family Therapy, 22*(1), 27–41.

Stein, R. H. (1990). *Ethical issues in counseling.* Buffalo, NY: Prometheus Press.

Stromberg, C. D. (1988). *The psychologist's legal handbook.* Washington, DC: Council for the National Register of Health Service Providers in Psychology.

Stromberg, C., & Dellinger, A. (1993). Malpractice and other professional liability. *Psychologist's Legal Update, 3,* 1–15.

Strong, T. (1993). DSM-IV and describing problems in family therapy. *Family Process, 32*(2), 249–253.

Taggart, M. (1982). Linear versus systemic values: Implications for family therapy. In L. L'Abate (Ed.), *Values, ethics, legalities and the family therapist.* Rockville, MD: Aspen Systems.

Tarasoff v. Regents of University of California, 17 Cal. 3 d 425, 551 P 2d. 334, 131 Cal. Rptr. 14 (1976).

Todd, T. (1994). *Surviving and prospering with managed mental health care.* Sarasota, FL: Professional Resource Press.

Vesper, J., & Brock, G. (1991). *Ethics, legalities, and professional issues in marriage and family therapy.* Needham Heights, MA: Allyn & Bacon.

Watkins, S. A. (1989). Confidentiality and privileged communication: Legal dilemma for family therapists. *Social Work, 34*(2), 133–136.

Weidman, A. (1986). Family therapy with violent couples. *Social Casework: The Journal of Contemporary Social Work, 67*(4), 211–218.

Wetchler, J. L., & Piercy, F. P. (1986). The marital/family life of the family therapist: Stressors and enhancers. *American Journal of Family Therapy, 14*(2), 99–109.

Winkle, C. W., Piercy, F. P., & Hovestadt, A. (1981). A curriculum for graduate level marriage and family therapy education. *Journal of Marital and Family Therapy, 7,* 201–210.

Woody, J. D. (1990). Resolving ethical concerns in clinical practice: Toward a pragmatic model. *Journal of Marital and Family Therapy, 16*(2), 133–150.

Woody, R. H. (1983). Avoiding malpractice in psychotherapy. In P. Keller & L. Ritt (Eds.), *Innovations in clinical practice: A source book* (Vol. 2). Sarasota, FL: Professional Resource Exchange.

Woody, R. H., & Associates. (1984). *The law and the practice of human services.* San Francisco: Jossey-Bass.

Woody, R. H. (1988a). *Protecting your mental health practice: How to minimize legal and financial risk.* San Francisco: Jossey-Bass.

Woody, R. H. (1988b). *Fifty ways to avoid malpractice.* Sarasota, FL: Professional Resource Exchange.

Woody, R. H. (1991). *Quality care in mental health: Assuring the best clinical services.* San Francisco: Jossey-Bass.

Yates, B. T. (1994). Toward the incorporation of costs, cost-effectiveness analysis, and cost-benefit analysis into clinical research. *Journal of Consulting and Clinical Psychology, 62*(4), 729–736.

Youngren, J. N. (1993). Ethical issues in religious psychotherapy. *Register Report: The Newsletter for Health Service Providers in Psychology, 19*(4), 6–8.

Zinsser, W. K. (1994). *On writing well: An informal guide to writing nonfiction.* New York: Harper Perennial.

Zygmond, M. J., & Boorhem, H. (1989). Ethical decision making in family therapy. *Family Process, 28*(3), 269–280.

Author Index

Subject Index

CPSIA information can be obtained at www.ICGtesting.com
Printed in the USA
LVOW12*2124270314

379294LV00004B/25/A